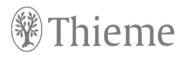

Neuroradiology

The Essentials with MR and CT

Second Edition

Val M. Runge, MD
Professor
Department of Diagnostic, Interventional, and Pediatric Radiology
University Hospital of Bern, Inselspital
University of Bern
Bern, Switzerland

1328 illustrations

Thieme
New York • Stuttgart • Delhi • Rio de Janeiro

Library of Congress Cataloging-in-Publication Data is available from the publisher.

Thieme Publishers New York
333 Seventh Avenue, New York, NY 10001 USA
+1 800 782 3488, customerservice@thieme.com

Georg Thieme Verlag KG
Rüdigerstrasse 14, 70469 Stuttgart, Germany
+49 [0]711 8931 421, customerservice@thieme.de

Thieme Publishers Delhi
A-12, Second Floor, Sector-2, Noida-201301
Uttar Pradesh, India
+91 120 45 566 00, customerservice@thieme.in

Thieme Publishers Rio de Janeiro,
Thieme Publicações Ltda.
Edifício Rodolpho de Paoli, 25º andar
Av. Nilo Peçanha, 50 – Sala 2508
Rio de Janeiro 20020-906 Brasil
+55 21 3172 2297

Cover design: Thieme Publishing Group
Typesetting by DiTech Process Solutions, India

Printed in USA by King Printing Company, Inc.   5 4 3 2 1

ISBN 978-1-68420-153-2

Also available as an e-book:
eISBN 978-1-68420-154-9

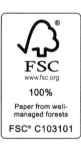

Contents

Foreword

From the first edition

Drs. Runge, Smoker, and Valavanis and their collaborators have done a superb job of distilling the essential aspects of Neuroradiology into a compact textbook. This book has a higher image to text ratio than most books I have read, making it the perfect companion for the neuroradiology PACS workstation. It should be required reading for residents prior to a neuroradiology rotation and for neuroradiology fellows before they begin their fellowship. However, it is so complete and image-rich that I plan to flip through the pages before the next time I sit for the Neuroradiology Certificate of Additional Qualification (CAQ) exam. It will also be of interest to neurology and neurosurgical trainees and attendings as an excellent review of the MRI and CT studies they encounter every day on their patients. *Neuroradiology: The Essentials with MR and CT* really covers the subspecialty from soup to nuts, from normal anatomy to disease, from the routine (e.g., stroke and multiple sclerosis) to cases that might only be seen once a year (e.g., glutaric acidemia type 1 and CADASIL). The image quality is excellent and the images are quite representative of what would normally be encountered in academic or community practice. The reader will note that there is a modicum of relevant MR physics interleaved in the discussion. This is reminiscent of Dr. Runge's previous MR physics textbooks. Since I believe this is Dr. Runge's sixteenth book, one expected clear, concise explanations of both MR physics and clinical neuroradiology and that's indeed the case. As noted above, this book should have a place next to the Neuroradiology PACS workstation for ready reference when one "just wants to be sure" or to flesh out the clinical aspects of the imaging findings for discussion with our clinical neuroradiology colleagues. However, I would be sure to bolt this book down because I suspect it will have a high tendency to "walk." I hope you enjoy reading it as much as I did.

William G. Bradley Jr., MD, PhD, FACR
Former Professor and Chairman, Department of Radiology
University of California San Diego
San Diego, California

Preface

Neuroradiology: The Essentials with MR and CT, Second Edition is written both to be read from cover to cover and to be used as a quick reference in the midst of a busy clinical day. The second edition adds many new figures, includes updates concerning 7T, and provides greater text detail particularly concerning brain aneurysms and AVMs. Designed as a practical educational resource for clinical neuroradiology, the text is divided into three sections: the brain, head and neck, and spine. Care has been taken for the text to be inclusive, yet focused on commonly encountered diseases, and to cover well the breadth of the field without gaps.

The diseases and their imaging presentations that one is likely to encounter in clinical practice, and which are essential to know, are included. The focus is on illustrating and describing the MR and CT appearances of these, discussing in depth the imaging findings. The text is written from a clinical radiology perspective, drawing on personal experience and covering common imaging findings often not well described in more traditional, academic textbooks.

The true basis of the text is that of clinical neuroradiology— that is, recognition of characteristic findings on both MR and CT of the disease processes we are likely to encounter in clinical practice, using as a basis excellent images and case materials from both modalities.

Val M. Runge, MD

Abbreviations

The following abbreviations are used with the figures, to enable rapid recognition of imaging technique and to permit the legends to be more concise.

ADC	Apparent diffusion coefficient	FLAIR	Fluid attenuated inversion recovery
ASL	Arterial spin labeling	GRE	Gradient recalled echo, specifically with
CBF	Cerebral blood flow		$T2^*$ weighting
CBV	Cerebral blood volume	MTT	Mean transit time
CE CT	Contrast-enhanced computed tomography	PD	Proton density weighted
CE MRA	Contrast-enhanced magnetic resonance	PET	Positron emission tomography
	angiography	STIR	Short tau inversion recovery
CE T1	Contrast-enhanced T1-weighted	T1	T1-weighted
CE T1 FS	Contrast-enhanced T1-weighted, with fat	T1 FS	T1-weighted, with fat suppression
	suppression	T2	T2-weighted
CT	Computed tomography	T2 FS	T2-weighted, with fat suppression
CTA	Computed tomography angiography	TOF	Time of flight magnetic resonance
DSA	Digital subtraction angiography		angiography
DWI	Diffusion weighted imaging	TTP	Time to peak

Acknowledgments

Some figures and text have been excerpted with permission from the following Thieme publications: *The Physics of Clinical MR Taught Through Images*, 4th edition; *Essentials of Clinical MR; Clinical 3T Magnetic Resonance*; and *Imaging of Cerebrovascular Disease*. A small number of figures, together with some source text, were also used from the following publication, for which Val M. Runge is the sole editor/author and who also owns the copyright: *Clinical Magnetic Resonance Imaging.*

1 Brain

1.1 Normal Anatomy and Common Variants

1.1.1 Normal Intracranial Anatomy

The frontal lobe is demarcated posteriorly from the parietal lobe by the central sulcus (▶ Fig. 1.1). On axial magnetic resonance (MR) images near the vertex, the central sulcus is readily identified. It is the major sulcus just behind the "L," the intersection of two sulci formed in part by the superior frontal sulcus. The precentral gyrus lies just anterior to the central sulcus and the postcentral gyrus just posteriorly. As a generalization,

the primary motor area (Brodmann area 4) is located in the precentral gyrus, and the primary somatesthetic (body's sensations) area (Brodmann areas 1, 2, and 3) in the postcentral gyrus. The parietal lobe is demarcated from the occipital lobe posteriorly by the parieto-occipital sulcus (fissure). The anatomy of the nuclei and white matter tracts is beyond the scope of this book, but see ▶ Fig. 1.2. The reader is referred to the many computer-based atlases, including *The Human Brain in 1969 Pieces* by Wieslaw Nowinski.

The pituitary gland is divided into anterior and posterior lobes. The anterior pituitary is referred to as the adenohypophysis and the posterior pituitary as the neurohypophysis. The normal

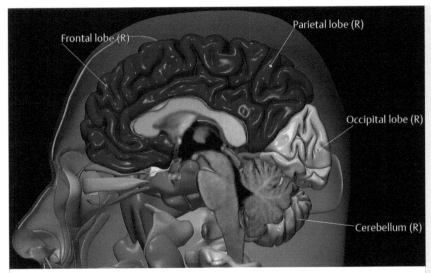

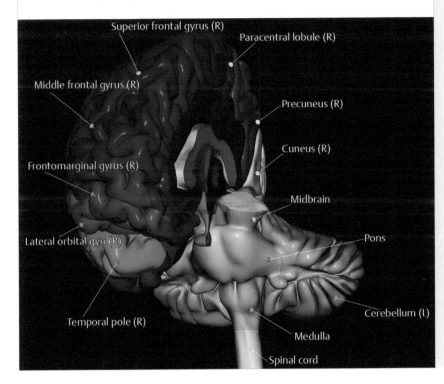

Fig. 1.1 Normal lobar and gyral anatomy. Important landmarks include the central sulcus, which separates the frontal lobe anteriorly from the parietal lobe posteriorly, and the sylvian fissure (the lateral sulcus), which divides the frontal and parietal lobes above from the temporal lobe below. The parietal and occipital lobes are separated by the parietooccipital sulcus. (Courtesy of Wieslaw Nowinski, DSc, PhD.)

(Continued)

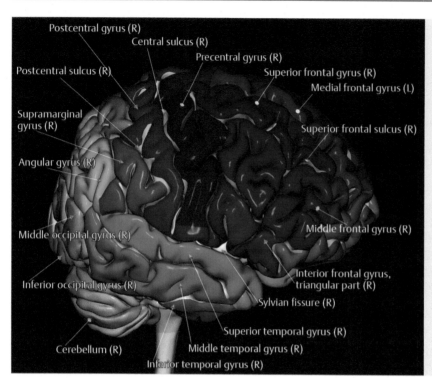

Postcentral gyrus (R)
Central sulcus (R)
Precentral gyrus (R)
Postcentral sulcus (R)
Superior frontal gyrus (R)
Medial frontal gyrus (L)
Supramarginal gyrus (R)
Superior frontal sulcus (R)
Angular gyrus (R)
Middle occipital gyrus (R)
Middle frontal gyrus (R)
Inferior occipital gyrus (R)
Interior frontal gyrus, triangular part (R)
Sylvian fissure (R)
Superior temporal gyrus (R)
Cerebellum (R)
Middle temporal gyrus (R)
Inferior temporal gyrus (R)

Fig. 1.1 (Continued)

pituitary is less than 10 mm in height, and demonstrates intense enhancement following intravenous contrast administration, due to the lack of a blood-brain barrier. A common variant in appearance of the pituitary is a slight upward convex superior margin, which can be seen in young women. On T1-weighted scans, the posterior pituitary is seen to be hyperintense in up to half of the normal patient population, a finding that is more common in younger patients (but not in the elderly).

The internal auditory canal (IAC) is a bony foramen within the petrous portion of the temporal bone. It contains the 7th (facial) and 8th (vestibulocochlear) nerve complexes. The 7th nerve lies in the anterior superior quadrant of the IAC, when viewed in cross-section, and runs laterally to the geniculate ganglion. The cochlear division of the 8th nerve lies in the anterior inferior quadrant. The superior and inferior vestibular nerves, also divisions of the 8th nerve, which supply information concerning equilibrium, lie in the superior and inferior posterior quadrants. As visualized in the axial plane, the cochlea is anterior and the vestibule posterior. There are three semicircular canals: the lateral (which has a horizontal orientation), superior, and posterior. The fluid (endolymph) within the cochlea, vestibule, and semicircular canals is normally isointense to cerebrospinal fluid (CSF) on MR.

1.1.2 Normal Arterial Anatomy

Three major arteries supply the cerebral hemispheres (▶ Fig. 1.3). The anterior cerebral artery (ACA) supplies the anterior two-thirds of the medial cerebral surface and 1 cm of superior medial brain over the convexity. The recurrent artery of Heubner, which originates from the A1 or A2 segment of the ACA, supplies the caudate head, anterior limb of the internal capsule, and part of the putamen. The posterior limb of the internal capsule, portions of the thalamus, the caudate, the

globus pallidus, and the cerebral peduncle are supplied by the anterior choroidal artery, which arises from the supraclinoid internal carotid artery. The middle cerebral artery (MCA) supplies the lateral portion of the cerebral hemispheres, the insula, and the anterior and lateral temporal lobes. The lenticulostriate arteries, which originate from the M1 segment of the MCA, supply the lentiform nucleus (globus pallidus and putamen) and the anterior limb of the internal capsule. The posterior cerebral artery (PCA) supplies the occipital lobe and the medial temporal lobe. The thalamoperforating and thalamogeniculate branches supply the medial portion of the thalami and the walls of the third ventricle. These small perforating branches arise from the P1 segment of the PCA with similar branches arising from the posterior communicating artery (▶ Fig. 1.4).

Three major but smaller vessels supply the cerebellum (▶ Fig. 1.5). The largest is the posterior inferior cerebellar artery (PICA), which supplies the tonsil, the inferior vermis, and the inferior cerebellum (with the exception of its most anterior extent). The anterior inferior cerebellar artery (AICA) supplies the anterior inferior portion of the cerebellum and is the smallest of the three vessels. It is commonly stated that the distribution of AICA is in continuum with PICA, with at times the distribution slightly larger or smaller. The superior cerebellar artery supplies the superior half of the cerebellum.

The circle of Willis is complete in only one quarter of the population. Variants include the following. A fetal origin of the posterior cerebral artery, with its origin from the internal carotid artery instead of the basilar artery, is seen in about one in five patients. The P1 segment of the posterior cerebral artery, which is the portion from the tip of the basilar artery to the junction with the posterior communicating artery (PCOM), is usually also hypoplastic in this circumstance. The PCOM is hypoplastic in one-third of patients. The anterior communicating artery (ACOM), which connects the two anterior cerebral arteries, is hypoplastic

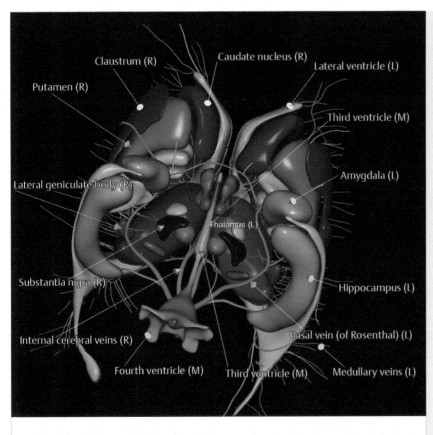

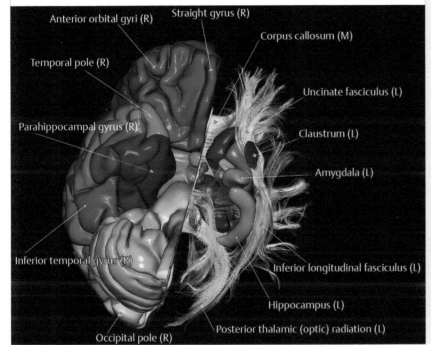

Fig. 1.2 Brain nuclei and white matter tracts, normal anatomy. Most relevant to MR interpretation are the locations of the caudate nucleus, putamen, globus pallidus (*light green,* immediately medial to the putamen and not labeled), hippocampus, and thalamus. Note also the location of the optic radiations. (Courtesy of Wieslaw Nowinski, DSc, PhD.)

in 15%. The A1 segment of the anterior cerebral artery, which begins at the carotid terminus and continues to the juncture with the ACOM, is hypoplastic in 10%.

The external carotid artery is the smaller of the two terminal branches of the common carotid artery. It arises anterior and medial to the internal carotid artery, then courses posterior laterally. There are many muscular branches, with the early branching of the external carotid artery allowing rapid recognition of this vessel in distinction to the internal carotid artery.

The internal carotid artery was traditionally divided into four major segments: the cervical, the petrous (horizontal), the cavernous (juxtasellar), and the intracranial (supraclinoid) portions. Today, there are seven recognized segments (C1 to C7): the cervical, petrous, lacerum, cavernous, clinoid, ophthalmic, and

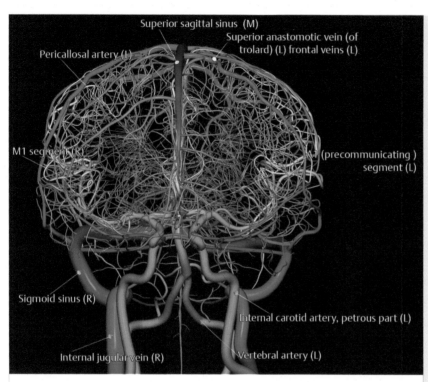

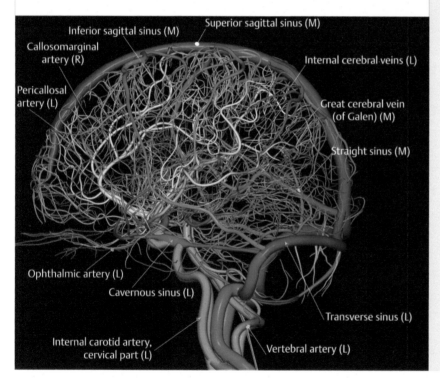

Fig. 1.3 Normal arterial and venous anatomy. Anteroposterior and lateral projections are illustrated. (Courtesy of Wieslaw Nowinski, DSc, PhD.)

communicating (terminal) segments. At its origin, the internal carotid artery is somewhat dilated, forming the carotid bulb. The petrous segment, C2, of the internal carotid artery has three sections: the ascending (vertical), the genu (bend), and the horizontal portions. The lacerum segment, C3, is still extradural. The cavernous segment, C4, is surrounded by the cavernous sinus. The meningohypophyseal artery arises from C4. The clinoid segment, C5, is very short, and begins after the artery exits from the cavernous sinus. C5 extends from the proximal dural ring to the distal dural ring. C6, the ophthalmic segment, extends from the distal dural ring (with this portion of the internal carotid artery thus considered intradural) to the origin of the PCOM. The ophthalmic artery arises from C6. C7 is that segment of the artery extending from the origin of the posterior communicating artery to the carotid terminus, where the vessel divides into the anterior and middle cerebral arteries. C6 and C7 together constitute the supraclinoid internal carotid artery.

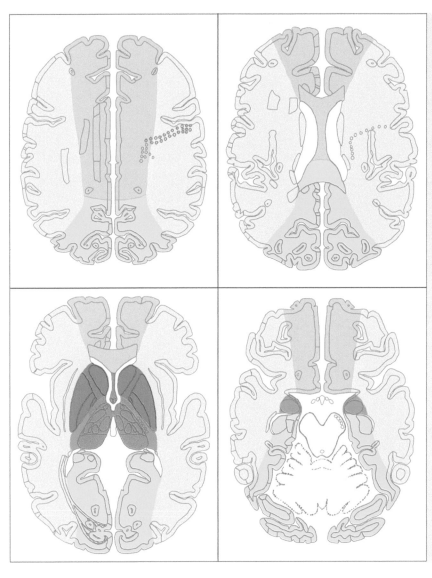

Fig. 1.4 Supratentorial arterial territories. Axial diagrams of the brain at four levels depict the major arterial territories of the supratentorial region, specifically the anterior cerebral artery (*blue*), middle cerebral artery (*pink*), and posterior cerebral artery (*yellow*) territories. In *red* is the vascular territory supplied by the penetrating branches of the middle cerebral artery (the lenticulostriate arteries). In *brown* is the territory supplied by the penetrating branches of the posterior cerebral arteries (the posterior thalamoperforators) and posterior communicating arteries (the anterior thalamoperforators). In *green* is the territory supplied by the anterior choroidal artery, which supplies amongst other structures the posterior limb of the internal capsule, the optic tract, and the hippocampus and amygdala. (Courtesy of Wieslaw Nowinski, DSc, PhD.)

There are many extracranial-intracranial vascular anastomoses. Two of these involve the ophthalmic artery. There are also multiple internal carotid-vertebral artery anastomoses, which represent persistent embryonic circulatory patterns. One of these is seen not uncommonly, as a normal variant, and is the persistent trigeminal artery (▶ Fig. 1.6). Pial-leptomeningeal anastomoses are also present, and are an important potential source of collateral blood flow in occlusive vascular disease.

1.1.3 Normal Venous Anatomy

Regarding the central venous anatomy of the brain, the paired internal cerebral veins and basal veins of Rosenthal join to form the vein of Galen. The latter is then joined by the inferior sagittal sinus, which lies along the free edge of the falx, to form the straight sinus, which drains to the confluence of the sinuses (torcular herophili). Superficial cerebral veins over the convexity join to form the superior sagittal sinus, which lies along the midline, which then drains to the confluence of the sinuses. Flow continues via the transverse sinuses, which are often asymmetric (with the right usually dominant), to the sigmoid

sinus, the jugular bulb, and then the internal jugular vein. There are three large named superficial veins. There is the superficial middle cerebral vein, which lies in the Sylvian fissure and drains into the cavernous or sphenoparietal sinus. The vein of Trolard joins the superior sagittal sinus and the superficial middle cerebral vein. The vein of Labbe joins the transverse sinus and the superficial middle cerebral vein. The venous system is currently best demonstrated (when considering computed tomography [CT] and MR) on two-dimensional (2D) time of flight (TOF) MR angiography.

1.1.4 Normal Myelination

Myelination begins in the brainstem, progresses to the cerebellum and cerebrum, with the order of myelination from central to peripheral, inferior to superior, and posterior to anterior. T1-weighted images are particularly useful to assess myelination in the first 9 months of life. With normal myelination, on T1-weighted images, white matter becomes higher in signal intensity. T2-weighted images are more useful to assess myelination after 6 months of age. However, it is important to note that longer repetition times (TRs) are required to evaluate the brain

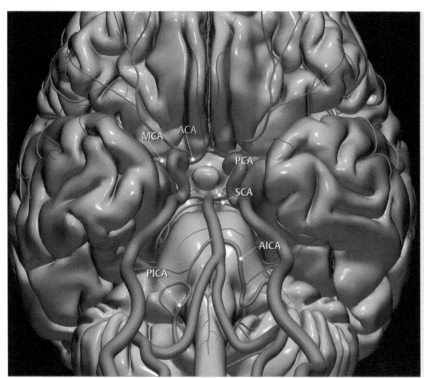

Fig. 1.5 Arterial supply of the posterior circulation, visualized on an anatomic drawing of the base of the brain. The posterior inferior cerebellar artery (PICA) originates from the vertebral artery. The two vertebral arteries join to form the basilar artery, with the major paired branches (in order from caudal to cranial) being the anterior inferior cerebellar artery (AICA), the superior cerebellar artery (SCA), and the posterior cerebral artery (PCA)—the latter marking the termination of the basilar artery. (Courtesy of Wieslaw Nowinski, DSc, PhD.)

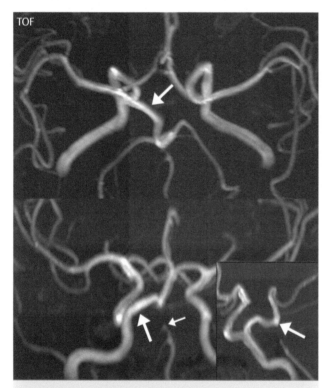

Fig. 1.6 Persistent trigeminal artery. Three projections from a 3D time-of-flight MRA of the circle of Willis are presented. The proximal basilar artery is small, and terminates in its mid-section (*small arrow*). The distal basilar artery is supplied from the right internal carotid artery, via a persistent embryonic connection (*large arrow*).

Myelination is quite specific for age from the newborn to 2 years of life; however, for simplification, the normal appearance is discussed at only four time frames. The dorsal pons, superior and inferior cerebellar peduncles, posterior limb of the internal capsule, and ventral lateral thalamus will demonstrate partial myelination, best seen on T1-weighted scans, in the newborn (▶ Fig. 1.7). The corpus callosum at this time is not myelinated, and will also appear thin.

At 6 months of age, on T1-weighted scans, the white matter of the cerebellum, the anterior limb and genu of the internal capsule, the white matter of the occipital lobe, and the posterior centrum semiovale will all appear normally myelinated with high signal intensity. The corpus callosum at this age will be partially myelinated, but will also still appear to be thin. At 6 months of age, on T2-weighted scans, only the posterior limb of the internal capsule will demonstrate low signal intensity, indicative of myelination.

At 12 months of age, on a T1-weighted scan, there will be a near adult pattern of myelination, specifically seen both in the deep and peripheral white matter. This pattern is reached by 9 months of age. On a T2-weighted scan, the deep white matter, specifically the internal capsule, corpus callosum, and corona radiata, will appear mature, with low signal intensity. Myelination is not yet complete at this age, as depicted on the T2-weighted scan, in the white matter of the frontal, temporal, parietal, and occipital lobes, together with the more peripheral subcortical white matter. These areas will still appear isointense to gray matter, not the low signal intensity (SI) on a T2-weighted scan indicative of mature myelination.

At 2 years of age, the deep and superficial white matter of the frontal, temporal, parietal, and occipital lobes will appear low SI on T2-weighted scans, similar to the adult pattern. The SI of these areas will however not be as low as the internal capsule, with that not occurring until 3 years of age. The deep white matter of the parietal lobes, surrounding the ventricular

under 2 years of age (with T2-weighted scans), when compared to the adult. On T2-weighted images, with normal myelination, white matter becomes lower in signal intensity. This is due to the lower water content as myelin matures.

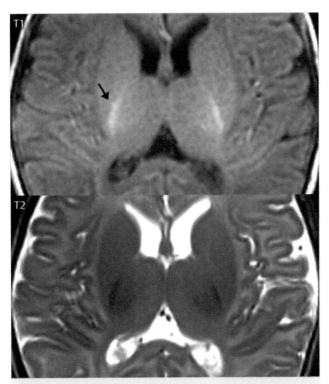

Fig. 1.7 Normal myelination in a newborn. At birth, the brain is principally not myelinated, with the appearance on MR strikingly different on both T1- and T2-weighted images when compared to the adult brain. Gray matter is predominantly of slightly higher signal intensity when compared to white matter on a T1-weighted scan in the newborn, with a principal indicator of early myelination being high signal intensity in the posterior limb of the internal capsule (*black arrow*).

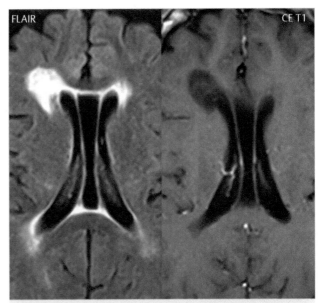

Fig. 1.8 Cavum septum pellucidi et vergae. In this patient with multiple sclerosis, and a prominent nonenhancing (chronic) right frontal plaque, the septum pellucidi are separated anteriorly, an extremely common normal variant. The division continues in this patient posteriorly, between the fornices, leading to a cavum septum pellucidi (anteriorly) and a cavum vergae (posteriorly).

trigones, is the last area to completely myelinate (the so-called zone of terminal myelination). Mild hyperintensity on T2-weighted scans in this region may persist up to 10 years of age.

1.1.5 Variants Involving the Septum Pellucidum

The septum pellucidum is a thin translucent plate, consisting of two laminae (leaves), that lies between the lateral ventricles. It extends from the corpus callosum superiorly to the fornix inferiorly. A cavum septum pellucidi is a common variant in which the two leaves are separated. This is a normal embryologic space, and is seen in all fetuses and premature infants. By 3 to 6 months of age only 15% of infants have a cavum septum pellucidi. The separation of leaves can persist into adulthood and as such is considered a normal variant.

A cavum septum vergae is also a normal embryologic space, like a cavum septum pellucidi but less common. It is essentially a posterior extension of a cavum septum pellucidi. It is seen as a midline cavity posterior to the columns of the fornix, which ends at the splenium of the corpus callosum. The internal cerebral veins lie inferiorly. When present in an adult, it is also considered to be a normal variant. The most common presentation is together with a cavum septum pellucidi, and in this instance the term cavum septum pellucidi et vergae (▶ Fig. 1.8) is used.

A cavum velum interpositum is a much less common variant, describing a cyst between the fornices superiorly and the roof of the third ventricle inferiorly. The internal cerebral veins lie within a cavum velum interpositum.

An absent septum pellucidum is rare, and almost always signifies major neurologic disease. It is associated with many congenital malformations, including septooptic dysplasia. An absent septum pellucidum can be an acquired abnormality, due to chronic hydrocephalus.

1.1.6 Physiological Calcification

The glomus portion of the choroid plexus, contained in the atria of the lateral ventricles, is the most frequent portion of the choroid plexus to calcify. Calcifications are usually globular and bilateral. Calcification and/or ossification is also commonly seen by CT in the falx (and less often in the pineal gland). These are all typically incidental findings. Because only dense, prominent calcification appears as low signal intensity on MR, calcification per se is less commonly visualized on MR. If the calcification is of sufficient size, it will however be seen on conventional MR. Ossification of the falx is well seen on MR due to visualization of the high signal intensity fat therein. Calcification and iron deposition are both dystrophic processes, and can occur together. Thus, sometimes what is seen as calcification on CT can be visualized as an abnormality on MR, but actually represents iron (hemosiderin) deposition.

1.1.7 Incidental Cystic Lesions

A pineal cyst is a common normal variant, and almost always asymptomatic. It is best visualized on thin section sagittal MR images. These are ovoid in shape, smoothly marginated, with a very thin wall, and rarely greater than 15 mm in diameter. The fluid therein will be homogeneous, with near CSF SI. On FLAIR,

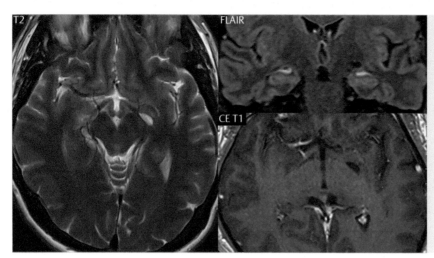

Fig. 1.9 Choroidal fissure cyst. These are considered a normal variant, and occur in the medial temporal lobe. They have CSF signal intensity on all MR pulse sequences, and expand slightly the choroidal fissure of the temporal lobe.

the cyst fluid will have slight high signal intensity. A thin uniform rim of contrast enhancement is common. Some large, but still asymptomatic, pineal cysts appear to have slight mass effect upon the adjacent colliculi.

Choroidal fissure cysts occur in the medial temporal lobe near the choroidal fissure (▶ Fig. 1.9). Their extra-axial location is easily confirmed on coronal images. Choroidal fissure cysts have a characteristic spindle shape when viewed in the sagittal plane.

1.1.8 Dilated Perivascular Spaces

The terms Virchow-Robin space and perivascular space are used interchangeably. This is a normal CSF space surrounding the perforating arteries entering the brain, and represents an invagination of the subarachnoid space. In the elderly, perivascular spaces may be more prominent. There are three common locations in which dilated perivascular spaces are seen. The first location is within the inferior third of the lentiform nucleus. In this instance the dilated spaces lie adjacent to the anterior commissure, following the course of the lenticulostriate arteries. Although usually less than 5 mm in diameter, larger dilated perivascular spaces can be seen in this location. These should be isodense on CT and isointense on MR to CSF. Differentiation can be difficult at times from chronic lacunar infarcts, with the latter the more common finding superiorly in the lentiform nucleus. The second common location for dilated perivascular spaces is within the white matter of the centrum semiovale. These follow the course of nutrient arteries, which lie along the white matter radiations. Thus, depending upon orientation relative to the slice, they may be seen either in cross-section or in plane, the latter as small radial structures. The third site, which is less common than the other two, is in the cerebral peduncle (near the substantia nigra). Although bilateral lesions may be seen here, typically the dilated perivascular space on one side is much larger than the other.

1.1.9 Other Incidental Lesions

Arachnoid granulations are small focal areas of arachnoid that protrude through the dura into the venous sinuses of the brain. CSF exits from the subarachnoid space via arachnoid granulations and enters the bloodstream, in part due to the normal higher pressure of CSF. These granulations also function as one-way valves. As MR has improved in terms of image quality and spatial resolution, visualization of arachnoid granulations within the transverse sinuses is not unusual. These should not be confused for venous thrombi.

A Tornwaldt cyst (▶ Fig. 1.10) is a common finding on MR of the brain, and is considered to be an incidental (benign) lesion. These vary in size, but are typically small. Tornwaldt cysts are thought to arise from the notochordal remnant, and occur in the posterior superior nasopharynx along the midline. They can be high signal intensity on T1-weighted scans, reflecting protein content.

Epidermoid cysts and small lipomas of the scalp are commonly encountered, incidentally. These entities have characteristic imaging appearances, on both CT and MR, and should be kept in mind when encountering a focal scalp lesion, due to their high incidence. The common small, painless lump under the skin seen incidentally on head CT is actually an epidermoid cyst, although often (incorrectly) termed "sebaceous cysts" by radiologists. The latter are much less common than epidermoid cysts, and affect the sebaceous glands, the oil glands in the skin.

1.2 Congenital Malformations

MR is the modality of choice for evaluation of all congenital malformations of the brain, with the exception of the craniosynostoses. In individual instances, some findings may be apparent on CT, with it thus being important to keep in mind the congenital malformations of the brain when interpreting CT.

1.2.1 Posterior Fossa Malformations

In a Chiari I malformation, there is displacement of the cerebellar tonsils > 5 mm below the level of the foramen magnum. This abnormality is not uncommon, and usually asymptomatic. On sagittal images the cerebellar tonsils are pointed or wedge-shaped (▶ Fig. 1.11). The fourth ventricle will be in normal position. Symptoms occur when there is obstruction of CSF flow through the foramen magnum. If there is crowding at the level of the foramen magnum, CSF flow studies can be obtained on MR to determine if the flow is abnormal and thus likely to contribute to symptoms (most frequently headache) (▶ Fig. 1.12). In symptomatic cases, there can be dilatation of the central canal of the

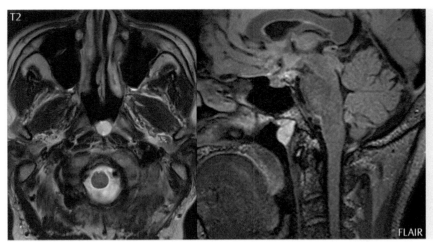

Fig. 1.10 Tornwaldt cyst. Axial T2-weighted and sagittal FLAIR scans reveal a well-circumscribed, round cyst along the midline in the upper posterior nasopharynx. This finding is considered incidental, of no clinical consequence.

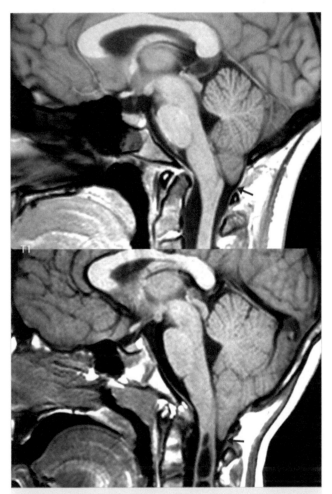

Fig. 1.11 Chiari I. In a Chiari I malformation, the cerebellar tonsils are pointed (*arrows*), and extend more inferiorly than normal, >5 mm below the level of the foramen magnum. Symptoms occur when normal CSF flow is prevented due to obstruction at the foramen magnum. Both patients in this instance have a paucity of CSF surrounding the cord at this level, and thus potentially could be symptomatic. The second patient however also demonstrates hydromyelia (dilatation of the central canal), consistent with altered CSF flow, with clinical symptomatology likely.

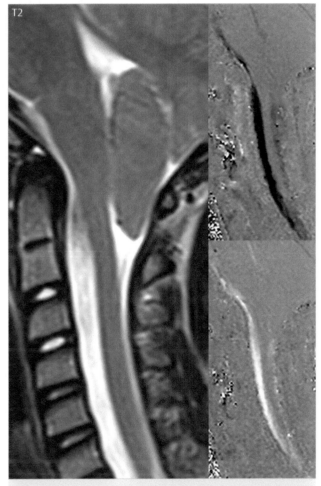

Fig. 1.12 Chiari I, with evaluation of CSF flow. The cerebellar tonsils are pointed, and extend below the C1 level. Note the normal configuration of the fourth ventricle. Phase contrast images at peak flow velocity in both the cranial and caudal directions are also illustrated. Flow is depicted as white or black, depending on direction, and is seen both anterior to the pons and anterior to the cord, establishing patency at the foramen magnum. An additional concordant finding is visualization of CSF anterior to the brainstem on the sagittal T2-weighted scan at that level.

spinal cord, specifically hydromyelia (more generally termed syringohydromyelia). Treatment is surgical, by suboccipital decompression with resection of the posterior arch of C1.

A Chiari I malformation is to be distinguished from tonsillar ectopia, specifically mild inferior displacement of the cerebellar tonsils seen in asymptomatic normal individuals. In this entity, the tonsils retain their normal globular configuration. In most normal individuals, the tonsils lie above the level of the foramen magnum, but they may lie as far as 5 mm below and still be normal.

The Chiari II malformation is a complex congenital brain anomaly, which involves principally the hindbrain (the medulla, pons, and cerebellum). Additional features involve the forebrain (the cerebral hemispheres, basal ganglia, and thalamic structures). In patients, a Chiari II malformation is associated with a neural tube closure defect in almost 100% of cases, usually a lumbosacral myelomeningocele. Characteristic features of a Chiari II malformation are subsequently described, not all features need be or are commonly present (▶ Fig. 1.13).

By definition, there will be a small posterior fossa with low insertion of the tentorium. The tentorial incisura may be widened, allowing the cerebellum to extensive superiorly, a "towering cerebellum." In this instance the folia of the cerebellum will have a vertical orientation. In a small number of cases the cerebellar hemispheres extend more anteriorly than normal, forming on an axial image the appearance of three bumps, the middle being that of the pons. The fourth ventricle is typically elongated (slitlike) and inferiorly displaced. A ballooned fourth ventricle is seen in 10%. Another defining feature is inferior displacement and elongation of the brainstem, tonsils, and vermis. The degree of displacement is often substantial. Cervicomedullary kinking,

overlapping of the medulla and cervical cord, may occur. There may be an enlarged foramen magnum and upper cervical canal, accompanied by a smaller C1 ring, with resultant compression of displaced brainstem, tonsils, and vermis at this level. Cervical (and thoracic) syringohydromyelia is common. Obstructive hydrocephalus is usually present, with most patients shunted. Callosal dysgenesis (usually partial agenesis of the corpus callosum) is seen in 75%. Fusion of the colliculi, "tectal beaking," is seen in the majority. The frontal horns may have a characteristic inferior pointing seen on coronal images. The massa intermedia is typically large. There is often hypoplasia or fenestration of the falx, with interdigitation of cerebral gyri. Stenogyria (multiple small cerebral gyri) is common. A Chiari III malformation is rare, with features of the Chiari II malformation together with a low occipital or upper cervical encephalocele.

In a Dandy-Walker malformation, there are three primary features. The posterior fossa is large, with the confluence of the sinuses/torcula high in position. Additionally, there is a large posterior fossa cyst that communicates with the fourth ventricle anteriorly. The third defining feature is vermian and cerebellar hemisphere hypoplasia, which can be present to a varying degree (▶ Fig. 1.14). On sagittal images, the residual vermis may be rotated superiorly (counterclockwise). The occipital bone may be scalloped and thinned. Imaging in the sagittal plane is essential for definition of the structural abnormalities. There is a spectrum of severity of findings, and thus the additional use, in the past, of the terms Dandy-Walker continuum and Dandy-Walker variant. The term Dandy-Walker spectrum has also been suggested more recently, specifically including mega cisterna magna as the entity with the mildest findings.

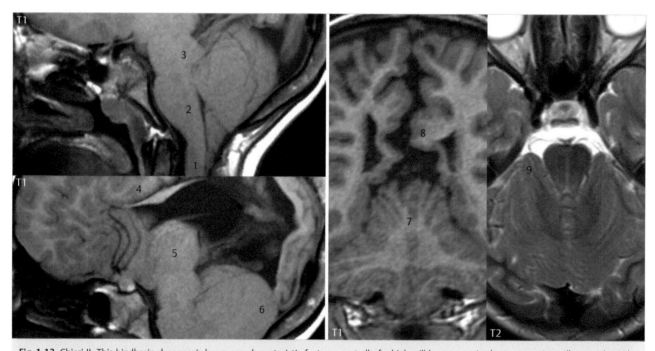

Fig. 1.13 Chiari II. This hindbrain dysgenesis has many characteristic features, not all of which will be present in the same patient. Illustrated are the peglike tonsillar herniation (1), a slitlike fourth ventricle (2), fusion of the colliculi with a beaklike appearance (3), partial agenesis of the corpus callosum (4), a large massa intermedia (5), low insertion of the tentorium (6), a towering appearance to the cerebellum with vertically oriented folia extending through a large tentorial incisura (7), partial agenesis of the falx with interdigitation of gyri (8), and anterior displacement of the cerebellar hemispheres relative to the pons (9).

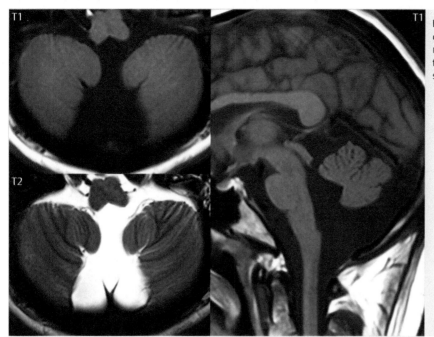

Fig. 1.14 Dandy-Walker malformation. There is dilatation of the fourth ventricle (which communicates with a posterior fossa cyst), hypoplasia of the inferior vermis, rotation of the vermis superiorly, and elevation of the torcula.

A mega cisterna magna is an enlarged CSF space posterior to the cerebellum, without mass effect, and with the cerebellar hemispheres, vermis and fourth ventricle specifically normal. These are common, and considered to be incidental findings. The primary differential diagnosis is a retrocerebellar (posterior fossa) arachnoid cyst. Although by definition there will be mild compression of the cerebellum, and scalloping of the calvarium may be present, most retrocerebellar arachnoid cysts are also asymptomatic. Like all arachnoid cysts, however, a discrete membrane separating the cyst from adjacent normal CSF is rarely seen on imaging. Retrocerebellar arachnoid cysts are most common along the midline. The size of the posterior fossa and position of the tentorium and straight sinus are usually normal, with the cerebellar vermis and hemispheres intact.

1.2.2 Cortical Malformations

Hemimegalencephaly is defined by hamartomatous overgrowth of a hemisphere. The lateral ventricle on the abnormal side is often large. Abnormalities of the brain on the side of involvement are common and include a thickened cortex and abnormal white matter signal intensity.

In heterotopic gray matter, there are displaced masses of gray matter, found anywhere from the embryologic site of development (periventricular) to the final destination after cell migration (cortical). The most common presentation is that of small focal regions of gray matter adjacent to the lateral ventricles (▶ Fig. 1.15). Important for diagnosis is that these small focal lesions are isointense to gray matter on all MR pulse sequences. The primary differential diagnostic consideration is tuberous sclerosis, specifically the subependymal nodules therein. The latter may demonstrate calcification, with the cortical involvement in tuberous sclerosis an additional differentiating feature. Less common forms of heterotopic gray matter include large nodular lesions and band heterotopia.

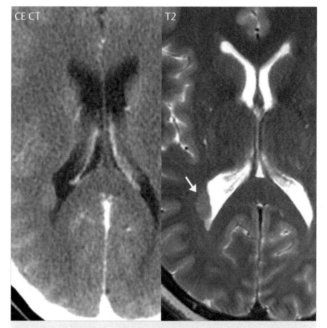

Fig. 1.15 Heterotopic gray matter. On CT, a small round lesion projects into the atrium of the lateral ventricle, with a suggestion that the attenuation is that of gray matter. On MR, this small heterotopic focus is isointense to and easily identified as gray matter. Isointensity to gray matter was confirmed on all pulse sequences (not shown).

The MR findings in focal cortical dysplasia (FCD) include blurring of the gray-white matter junction and an abnormal sulcal/gyral pattern (in a focal cortical distribution). In type 2, there is also focal cortical thickening (▶ Fig. 1.16). 10% of epilepsy patients have FCD. Of children less than 3 years of age, undergoing surgery for intractable epilepsy, 80% have FCD.

Lissencephaly type 1 or classic lissencephaly (previously known as the pachygyria-agyria complex) is a disorder of

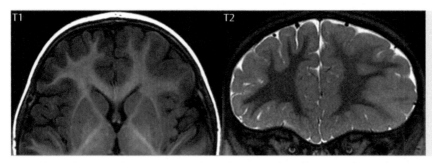

Fig. 1.16 Focal cortical dysplasia. There is focal cortical thickening and a relatively poorly defined transition between gray and white matter, seen in the left frontal lobe on axial and coronal scans, in this 18 month old with intractable seizures.

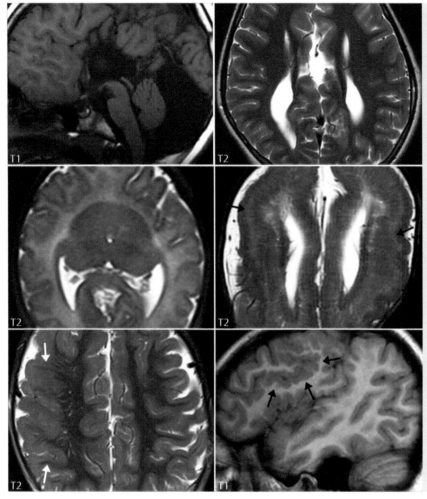

Fig. 1.17 Other congenital brain malformations. Six patients are illustrated. In the first there is near complete agenesis of the corpus callosum, with radially oriented gyri adjacent to the lateral ventricles. Many posterior fossa malformations are associated with callosal agenesis, and in this patient a large retrocerebellar cyst is also present. In the second patient, the lateral ventricles demonstrate a parallel orientation, a sign in the axial plane of callosal agenesis. Semilobar holoprosencephaly is illustrated in the third patient, with the interhemispheric fissure absent anteriorly and fused thalami. Rudimentary gyri and a smooth brain surface are seen in the fourth patient, with agyria, who also demonstrates the characteristic "cell-sparse" layer (*small black arrows*) underlying the cortex. The fifth patient demonstrates pachygyria, with a section (*white arrows*) of smooth thickened cortical gray matter with shallow sulci. The sixth patient has a focal area in the frontal lobe of polymicrogyria (*small black arrows*), with many very small gyri producing a cobblestoning appearance.

cortical formation, with arrested neuronal migration. On imaging, there is a thickened cortex, a smooth brain surface, a small number of shallow sulci, and decreased peripheral arborization of white matter (▸ Fig. 1.17). Histologically there is a four-layered cortex (as opposed to the normal six layers). On a T2-weighted scan, a hyperintense cell sparse zone may be recognizable, separating a thin gray matter cortical ribbon from a thicker underlying gray matter layer containing disorganized neurons. Incomplete lissencephaly (▸ Fig. 1.17), with focal areas of pachygyria (and otherwise normal brain), is much more common than complete lissencephaly.

Lissencephaly type 2, also known as cobblestone lissencephaly, is a distinct, separate entity from lissencephaly type 1. In type 2, there is a nodular or "pebbly" appearance to the brain surface, with broadened gyri and loss of sulci (thus the term lissencephaly). There are commonly associated ocular anomalies, with this entity usually occurring as part of a congenital muscular dystrophy. The brain is small and the cerebral white matter reduced in volume.

In polymicrogyria, an abnormality involving late neuronal migration, there are multiple small gyri along the brain surface (▸ Fig. 1.17). Due to their very small size, these may not be visualized on MR. The resultant imaging appearance is that of a focal region of brain with an irregular cortical surface, a thick layer of gray matter (cortex), and subtle irregularity at the gray-white matter interface. There will be a decreased number of

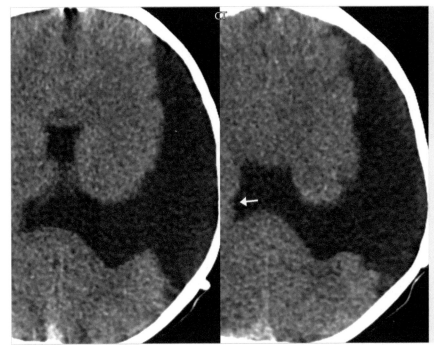

Fig. 1.18 Schizencephaly, "open lip." A large ventricular defect communicating with a large extra-axial CSF collection is seen on the left on CT in this 5-year-old child. The septum pellucidum is not present, a very common associated abnormality. Gray-white matter differentiation is not sufficient to identify on CT the gray matter lining the cleft. As well, there is only a hint of the defect on the right ("closed lip" schizencephaly), with a small ventricular dimple seen (*small white arrow*).

gyri, with the visible gyri being broad, thick, and relatively smooth. The involvement can be unilateral, bilateral, symmetric, or asymmetric. A perisylvian location is common. Anomalous venous drainage, often a large draining vein located in a deep sulcus, is common in regions of dysplastic cortex. On histology, in polymicrogyria, there is a derangement of the normal six-layered cortex.

Schizencephaly is characterized by the presence of a gray matter lined cleft, which extends from the cortex to the ventricular system. Schizencephaly can be either unilateral or bilateral. There is a spectrum of appearance, in terms of separation of the gray matter lined walls, from closed to open lip (▶ Fig. 1.18). A dimple in the wall of the ventricle can be an important clue for recognition of the closed lip form (▶ Fig. 1.19).

The septum pellucidum is commonly absent. MR is markedly superior to CT for detection of the gray matter lined cleft and associated abnormalities. Identification of the gray matter lining is important to differentiate schizencephaly from porencephaly. In the latter, there is an abnormal CSF space, due to destruction of brain, which can communicate with the ventricle but is not lined by gray matter. Porencephaly is caused by a vascular accident during the third trimester of fetal development, and as such often abuts the ventricle, with an intervening intact ependyma. The term porencephaly has also been used more generally to include any non-neoplastic cavity within the brain, not specifically in utero in etiology, including vascular insult, trauma, infection, and surgery.

1.2.3 Callosal Malformations

The corpus callosum (CC) is the largest interhemispheric commissure in the brain. The CC is divided into the genu (the "knee") anteriorly, the body, and the splenium posteriorly. There is an additional small named segment, the rostrum, which is a continuation of the genu, and projects posteriorly and inferiorly (coming from the Latin and meaning "beak," as

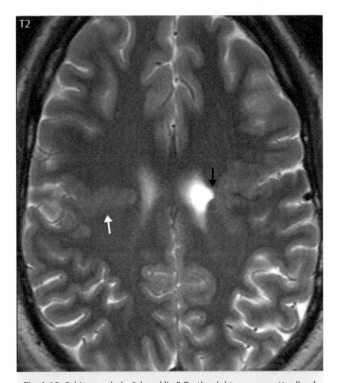

Fig. 1.19 Schizencephaly, "closed lip." On the right, a gray matter lined cleft (*white arrow*) is noted extending from the surface of the brain to the ventricle (continuity with the lateral ventricle was demonstrated on the adjacent section, not shown). On the left, a ventricular dimple (*black arrow*)—the ependymal margin of the contralateral cleft—is demonstrated, together with part of a gray matter lined cleft, in this patient with bilateral "closed lip" schizencephaly.

with a bird). Other links between the two cerebral hemispheres include the anterior and posterior commissures. The line connecting the two commissures, the AC-PC line, today defines the standard axial plane for MR imaging acquisitions.

The corpus callosum develops in the fetus between the 8th and 20th weeks, in an anterior to posterior fashion. The genu forms first, then the body, then the splenium, with the exception that the rostrum forms last. Total agenesis of the corpus callosum is due to an early insult, with partial agenesis due to a later insult during gestation. With total agenesis, axons that normally cross the midline instead run along the medial borders of the lateral ventricles, parallel to the interhemispheric fissure, forming the bundles of Probst (▶ Fig. 1.17). The lateral ventricles will be more widely separated than normal, and their orientation parallel. On a coronal image, there will be a crescent shape to the lateral ventricles, in particular the front horns, with the bundles of Probst lying medially. This appearance has been referred to as "devil's horns." There may be dilatation of the trigones of the lateral ventricles and the occipital horns, referred to as colpocephaly. Along the midline, as seen in the sagittal plane, there will be a radial orientation to the gyri adjacent to the body of the lateral ventricles.

The term callosal dysgenesis includes both partial and complete absence of the corpus callosum. In most instances, callosal dysgenesis is associated with another anomaly, with the most common being the Chiari II malformation. An excellent survey of the corpus callosum is obtained with sagittal imaging on MR imaging.

1.2.4 Holoprosencephaly and Related Disorders

Holoprosencephaly is a congenital malformation of the brain, characterized by failure of cleavage and differentiation involving the forebrain (prosencephalon). The prosencephalon separates early in development into the diencephalon (which includes the thalamus and hypothalamus) and the telencephalon (which includes the cerebral hemispheres and basal ganglia). Holoprosencephaly is somewhat artificially divided into three subcategories, which are subsequently discussed in order of decreasing severity. The septum pellucidum is absent in all. In alobar holoprosencephaly, the thalami are fused, the third ventricle is absent, the falx is absent (there is no interhemi-spheric fissure), and there is a single crescent-shaped ventricle connected to a large dorsal cyst. Alobar holoprosencephaly is rarely imaged. Infants are typically stillborn, or of short life span.

In semilobar holoprosencephaly, the interhemispheric fissure and falx are present posteriorly (▶ Fig. 1.17). There is partial separation of the thalami by a small third ventricle, with rudimentary temporal horns. The splenium of the corpus callosum is present. In lobar holoprosencephaly, the falx and interhemispheric fissure extend into the frontal region. The anterior falx is dysplastic. The frontal horns of the lateral ventricles have an abnormal configuration, and the frontal lobes may be hypoplastic. Inspection of both axial and coronal MR images is important, with the latter in particular useful to demonstrate frontal lobe abnormalities.

Septo-optic dysplasia is defined by the presence of an abnormality involving the septum pellucidum and hypoplasia of the optic nerves (▶ Fig. 1.20). There may be mild dysplasia to complete absence of the septum pellucidum. The optic chiasm and nerves will be small, together with a thin pituitary infundibulum. The degree of pituitary dysfunction is variable, with growth hormone deficiency most common.

1.2.5 Phakomatoses

In neurofibromatosis type 1 (NF1) focal areas of signal abnormality (FASI), with abnormal high signal intensity on T2-weighted scans, are seen in the brain in characteristic locations in the majority of preteen children. The most common location for this finding is the globus pallidus (▶ Fig. 1.21). Here the lesions are usually bilateral, but often asymmetric in size. The lesions of the globus pallidus may also be slightly hyperintense on T1-weighted scans. Similar lesions can also be seen, but are less common, in the thalamus, brainstem, and cerebellar white matter. With age, these abnormalities fade, and eventually may no longer be seen on MR. The other common abnormalities seen in NF1 include gliomas involving either the optic nerve or optic chiasm, and sphenoid wing dysplasia in association with a plexiform tumor. Optic chiasm lesions usually have bilateral contiguous optic tract involvement and may demonstrate optic nerve involvement. Cutaneous lesions in NF1 include cafe au lait spots, axillary freckles, hamartomas (Lisch nodules) of the iris, and multiple subcutaneous nodules (peripheral nerve tumors).

NF2 is a much less common disease, with the presence on MR of bilateral vestibular schwannomas being pathognomonic (▶ Fig. 1.22). Meningiomas, ependymomas, and other intracranial nerve tumors can also be seen.

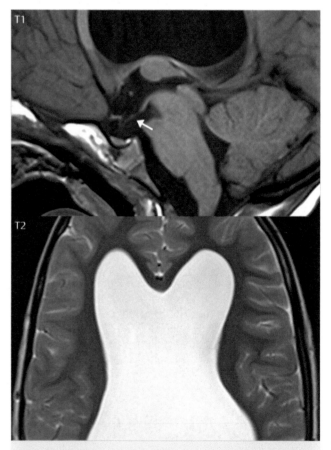

Fig. 1.20 Septo-optic dysplasia. This entity is characterized, in its most classic presentation, by absence of the septum pellucidum, which is well seen on axial scans, together with a small optic chiasm (*white arrow*), optic nerves, and pituitary—all well illustrated in the sagittal plane.

Tuberous sclerosis has a characteristic imaging presentation on MR, with both subependymal and parenchymal lesions. In a single patient, one or the other of these two abnormalities may dominate. Small subependymal nodules are common, with some projecting into the ventricular system. These are readily recognized on both T1- and T2-weighted scans, and may demonstrate calcification on CT Characteristically, there will also be multiple parenchymal lesions, which are best visualized on T2-weighted scans (specifically FLAIR) (▶ Fig. 1.23). These parenchymal hamartomas (tubers) involve both gray and white

matter, with their epicenter in the subcortical white matter. These are high signal intensity on T2-weighted scans. The term "gyral core" is used for an abnormality confined to the subcortical white matter core of an expanded gyrus. The term "sulcal island" is used to describe involvement of two adjacent gyri, with sparing of the normal intervening cortex lining the sulcus. Mild ventricular enlargement can be present.

CT may demonstrate peripheral calcifications and parenchymal hypodensity associated with parenchymal hamartomas. Brain tumors are seen in a small percent of cases. The most common of these is a subependymal giant cell astrocytoma (WHO grade I), characteristically occurring along the wall of the lateral ventricle with obstructive hydrocephalus due to blockage of the foramen of Monro (▶ Fig. 1.24). Cutaneous lesions seen in tuberous sclerosis include leaf-shaped hypopigmented spots (on the trunk and limbs), adenoma sebaceum (small red papules scattered over the face in a butterfly pattern), and

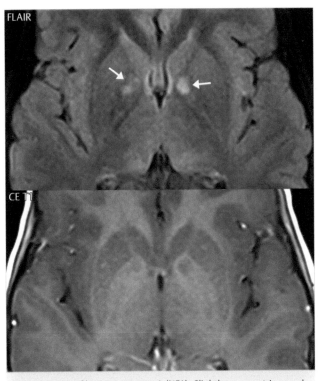

Fig. 1.21 Neurofibromatosis type 1 (NF1). Slightly asymmetric round foci of abnormal signal intensity (FASI) are seen on FLAIR in a very characteristic location, the anterior globus pallidus (*white arrows*). There is no abnormal contrast enhancement. Although FASIs may also occur in other locations, this appearance is pathognomonic for NF1.

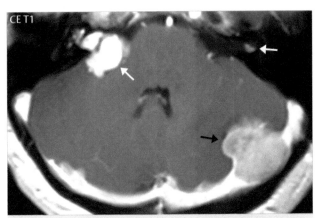

Fig. 1.22 Neurofibromatosis type 2 (NF2). Bilateral internal auditory canal enhancing lesions are noted (*white arrows*), each consistent with a vestibular schwannoma. The lesion on the patient's left is purely intracanalicular. The lesion on the right expands the internal auditory canal and has both intra- and extra-canalicular components. An additional, moderate in size, enhancing extra-axial lesion (*black arrow*) is noted, invading the left transverse sinus, consistent with a meningioma. Bilateral vestibular schwannomas are pathognomonic for NF2, with meningiomas often also seen, as in this patient.

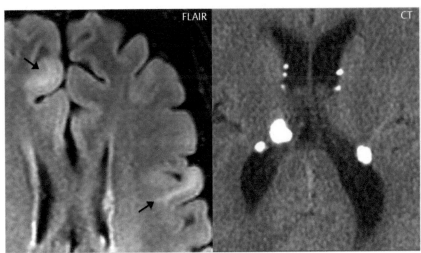

Fig. 1.23 Tuberous sclerosis. The two pathognomic findings in this disease entity are illustrated, with the respective modalities on which they are best visualized. On FLAIR, high signal intensity within the white matter of two gyri (*black arrows*) with overlying near normal gray matter is seen, consistent with cortical tubers. In a different patient, calcified subependymal nodules are well identified on CT.

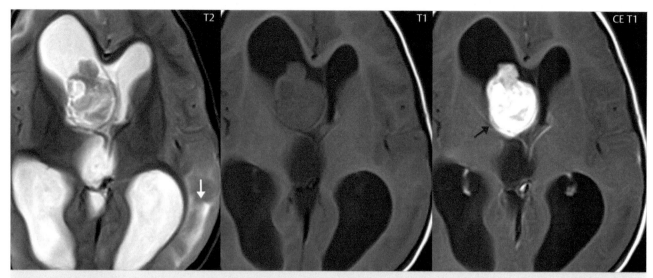

Fig. 1.24 Giant cell astrocytoma. A large, prominently enhancing (*black arrow*), intraventricular mass is noted, lying at the foramen of Monro. There is ventricular enlargement, but without interstitial edema, consistent with chronic compensated obstructive hydrocephalus. Abnormal high signal intensity (*white arrow*) on the T2-weighted scan within the white matter of an expanded gyrus is consistent with a cortical tuber, in this patient with tuberous sclerosis.

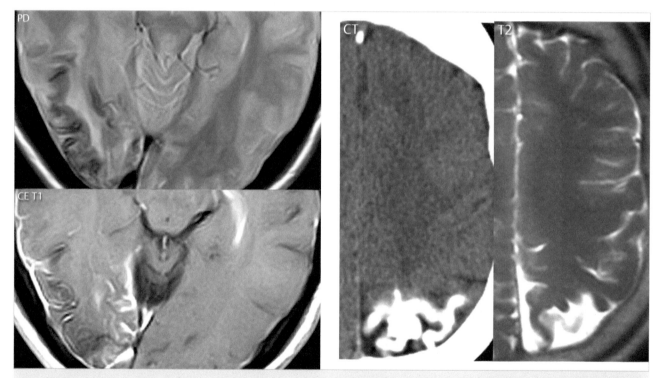

Fig. 1.25 Sturge-Weber syndrome. Subtle cortical/subcortical low signal intensity on both scans (**part 1**) reflects dense dystrophic calcification. There is mild associated gliosis, seen as subtle high signal intensity on the proton density-weighted image. Serpentine enhancement is seen post-contrast, reflecting the pial angioma, overlying the gyri and extending within the sulci in the right occipital lobe in this patient. Cortical calcification is seen on CT (**part 2**), with focal atrophy on MR, in a different patient, classic features for chronic disease in this phakomatosis.

rough thickened yellow skin over the lumbosacral region posteriorly (shagreen patch).

The Sturge-Weber syndrome is also known as encephalotrigeminal angiomatosis. On CT, focal cortical calcification is seen together with associated atrophy late in the disease process. MR demonstrates focal leptomeningeal enhancement, which markedly improves depiction of the disease and its extent of involvement (▶ Fig. 1.25). Late in the disease process gliosis is seen as abnormal high SI on T2-weighted scans in the adjacent white matter. The cutaneous lesion characteristic for Sturge-Weber is a "port wine stain"; however, this lesion need not be present.

Cerebellar hemangioblastomas can occur in adults in von Hippel-Lindau disease. Lesions characteristic of this autosomal dominant disease include CNS hemangioblastomas, clear cell

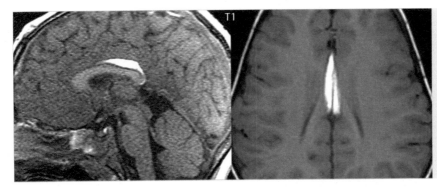

Fig. 1.26 Lipoma of the corpus callosum. Sagittal and axial T1-weighted images from two different patients are presented. A lipoma, with high signal intensity (isointense to subcutaneous fat), is noted along the midline, immediately superior to the corpus callosum. On the sagittal image the lesion extends posteriorly to wrap around the splenium.

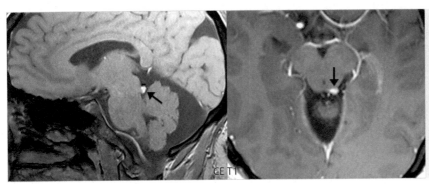

Fig. 1.27 Lipoma of the quadrigeminal plate. A common location for small incidental lipomas, such as that illustrated (*arrows*), is the quadrigeminal plate. In this instance, the lipoma is adjacent to the left inferior colliculus. Chemical shift artifact, seen as a small black line just superior to the lesion on the sagittal image, identifies the lesion as fat.

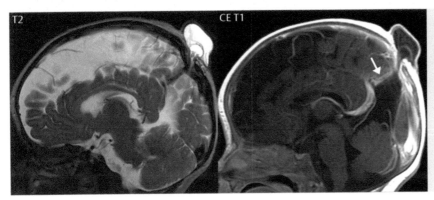

Fig. 1.28 Cephalocele, parietal. A small midline lesion, with a limited skull defect, is noted. In this instance, the lesion contains meninges and CSF without obvious brain tissue (a meningocele). Note the persistent falcine sinus (*arrow*), a common associated feature of atretic parietal cephaloceles.

renal carcinomas, pheochromocytomas, and cysts of the liver and pancreas.

1.2.6 Lipomas

Lipomas are rare congenital malformations with a very distinctive appearance and location, regardless of whether imaged by CT or MRI. Lipomas have low attenuation on CT (–50 to –100 HU), and there may be associated calcification. Small lipomas can go unrecognized on CT due to the relative poor detectability of dark objects (as opposed to bright objects) on a uniform background. On MR, lipomas will be isointense to fat on all pulse sequences. Their distinctive appearance, and high detectability, on MR is due to the high signal intensity on T1-weighted scans. Depending upon the bandwidth utilized for the pulse sequence, a chemical shift artifact may also be seen (in the readout [frequency encoding] direction). Scans with and without fat saturation can be used for definitive identification of fat. Lipomas are typically asymptomatic. More than half are associated with other brain malformations. The most common location (about half of all lipomas) is interhemispheric, lying

superiorly along the corpus callosum (▶ Fig. 1.26), and in this instance often associated with partial agenesis of the corpus callosum. Other characteristic but less common locations include the suprasellar cistern, the quadrigeminal plate cistern (▶ Fig. 1.27), and the cerebellopontine angle. Intracranial vessels and nerves may course through a lipoma.

1.2.7 Anomalies of the Skull

A cephalocele is a protrusion of cranial contents through a congenital defect. There are two main types, a meningocele (▶ Fig. 1.28), which contains meninges and CSF, and a meningoencephalocele (▶ Fig. 1.29), which also contains brain. These most commonly occur along the midline. More than 50% are occipital, the most common location, and 15% fronto-ethmoidal. A related entity to the latter, from an embryogenesis perspective, is a nasal dermal sinus. CT defines the bony defect, MR the associated soft tissues and specifically whether brain tissue is present.

Craniosynostosis is premature fusion of a skull suture. The cranial sutures normally begin to fuse at age 3 and are completely fused by age 6. Distortion of the shape of the calvarium

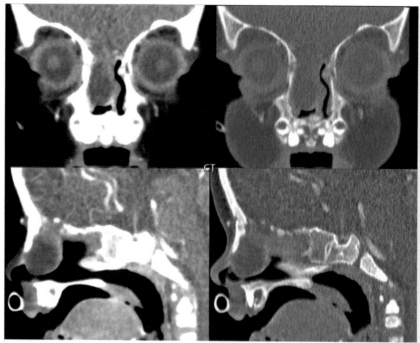

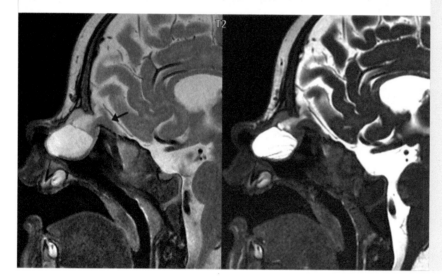

Fig. 1.29 Cephalocele, nasoethmoidal. In **part 1**, coronal and sagittal reformatted CT images are presented, reconstructed with soft tissue and bone algorithms. A well-delineated, somewhat heterogeneous, soft tissue mass—with a suggestion of two components (the more superiorportion being isodense to brain), extends through a bony defect into the nasal cavity (ethmoid region). The cribriform plate is deficient. In **part 2**, two different sagittal midline T2-weighted scans are presented: the first, a 2-mm FSE scan, and the second, a 1-mm CISS (FIESTA-C or bFFE) scan. Both display a linear structure (*arrow*), isointense to brain, that could be traced on adjacent images and is one of the two olfactory tracts. The tract enters the more superior of the two components of this cephalocele, with the more inferior containing only CSF. This anomaly is thus by definition a meningoencephalocele, containing meninges, CSF, and brain tissue.

is predictable based upon the suture(s) involved. Scaphocephaly (dolichocephaly) is due to synostosis of the sagittal suture, resulting in an increased AP dimension (▶ Fig. 1.30). Brachycephaly is used to describe an increase in transverse dimension of the skull, which can be due to synostosis of the coronal or lambdoid sutures bilaterally. Unilateral coronal or lambdoid synostosis is referred to by the term plagiocephaly, with the result being asymmetrical flattening of one side of the skull. Craniosynostosis is best evaluated by high-resolution, low radiation dose, CT with 3D reconstructions to assess the status of the sutures (▶ Fig. 1.31).

1.3 Inherited Metabolic Disorders

This section discusses a diverse group of disorders due to inborn errors of metabolism. Imaging is often suggestive of the general diagnosis, but rarely specific for the individual disease.

White matter is usually involved, although this may be secondarily. In the chronic phase for each, these diseases share a similar imaging appearance, with atrophy and usually generalized white matter abnormality. The specific genetic defect for each disease, and often its many variants, is usually today well known. These have not been discussed in detail below, as they contribute little to image interpretation.

1.3.1 Diseases Affecting White Matter

Metachromatic Leukodystrophy

The most common form of this disease presents in the second year of life. The imaging appearance is nonspecific, with symmetric abnormal high signal intensity in the cerebral white matter on T2-weighted scans. This progresses temporally, together with generalized cerebral atrophy.

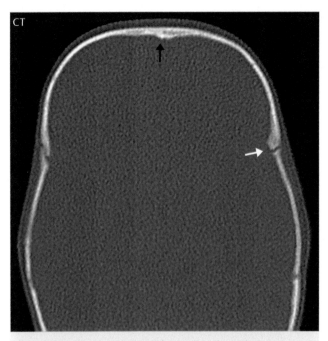

Fig. 1.30 Craniosynostosis (sagittal suture). In this pediatric patient, the sagittal suture is fused (*black arrow*), the most common suture to be involved, thereby producing scaphocephaly. The coronal suture is normal (*white arrow*). The result is a long, narrow head (increased AP, decreased LR, dimensions to the skull).

Krabbe Disease

Clinical symptoms begin between age 3 and 6 months. Early features on imaging can be helpful for diagnosis, with involvement of the thalamus, caudate nucleus, and dentate nucleus, in addition to the more nonspecific involvement of the white matter of the corona radiata. In the nuclei, high density is seen on CT, with this finding preceding the generalized low-density in white matter. The thalami may be high signal intensity on T1-weighted scans early in the disease process, another useful finding for diagnosis if present. This leukodystrophy is often associated with enlargement of optic and cranial nerves.

X-linked Adrenal Leukodystrophy

Of the many types of adrenoleukodystrophy, the childhood cerebral form is the most relevant and most common. This is a disease of young boys, with presentation between 5 and 12 years of age. Early clinical features include decreased visual acuity, gait disturbances, and mild intellectual impairment, with rapid disease progression. The most common imaging pattern is that of posterior white matter involvement, including specifically the periatrial (parieto-occipital) white matter, the fornix and the splenium of the corpus callosum. The pattern of spread is from posterior to anterior, as opposed to other leukodystrophies that extend from anterior to posterior (i.e., Alexander disease) (▶ Fig. 1.32).

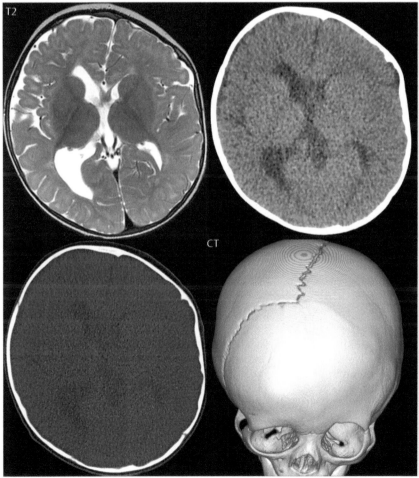

Fig. 1.31 Craniosynostosis (left coronal suture). CT reveals a normal right coronal suture, with bony bridging of the suture on the left. The result is an abnormal shape to the skull, which is asymmetrical, and termed plagiocephaly (which can involve either the coronal suture, as in this patient, or the lambdoid suture). No gross structural abnormalities are noted involving the brain. (Case provided courtesy of Ianina Scheer, MD, University Children's Hospital, Zürich.)

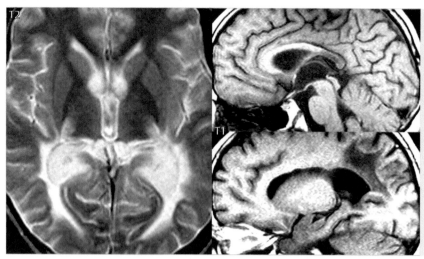

Fig. 1.32 Adrenoleukodystrophy. Images are presented from a young boy, with males almost exclusively involved in this X-linked disorder, the most common enzyme deficiency disease to present in childhood. The classic pattern of involvement is posterior-predominant, with involvement of the splenium of the corpus callosum, adjacent white matter, and fornix. These findings are reflected in the presented case with abnormal high signal intensity on T2- and low signal intensity on T1-weighted images.

As to be anticipated, these areas display low density on CT and increased signal intensity on T2-weighted MR scans. The anterior disease margin (the leading margin of demyelination) may display abnormal contrast enhancement, due to its inflammatory nature. In chronic disease, there is atrophy of the splenium. In 15% of patients, the pattern is predominantly frontal in location, with again abnormal contrast enhancement at the peripheral disease margin. In rare instances, the disease is predominantly unilateral.

Phenylketonuria

Imaging findings are nonspecific, with abnormal white matter hyperintensity on T2-weighted MR sequences due to delayed/defective myelination.

Maple Syrup Urine Disease

The classic form of this disease presents in the first few days of life. Profound edema is seen in regions of the brain that are normally myelinated at birth. There may be in addition generalized edema of the cerebral hemispheres.

Pelizaeus-Merzbacher Disease

The classic form of this disease, a hypomyelinating disorder, is X-linked recessive and presents within the first few months of life. In the most common form of the disease, myelination does not appear to progress further than that normally present at birth. The amount of myelination and white matter slowly decrease with time.

1.3.2 Disease Affecting Gray Matter: Huntington Disease

This autosomal dominant disease is characterized by degeneration and volume loss involving the corpus striatum (the caudate nucleus and putamen). The most common imaging finding is volume loss involving the head of the caudate nucleus, symmetrically, best demonstrated on thin section heavily T1- or T2-weighted (for good gray-white matter delineation) coronal

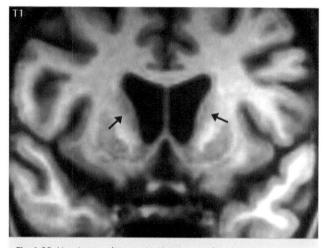

Fig. 1.33 Huntington disease. As Huntington disease progresses findings become apparent on MR and CT, the most notable being symmetric caudate head atrophy (*black arrows*). Diffuse cerebral volume loss also occurs with time.

images (▶ Fig. 1.33). In longstanding disease there is generalized cerebral atrophy. Huntington disease presents clinically in the fourth and later decades, with choreoathetosis and progressive dementia. MR findings are not seen early in the disease process.

1.3.3 Diseases Affecting Both White and Gray Matter

Canavan Disease

This autosomal recessive disease presents in the first few weeks of life due to marked hypotonia, with early development of macrocephaly and seizures. In infantile onset patients, imaging studies demonstrate a nonspecific, symmetric diffuse abnormality of the cerebral white matter. The subcortical white matter is involved early in the disease process, a possible differentiating finding. There is typically involvement of the globus pallidus, with the putamen spared. As with this general category of disease, end-stage findings include atrophy of both white matter and the cerebral cortex, and ventriculomegaly.

Alexander Disease

This disease was originally described as a disorder of infants, with macrocephaly. The infantile form has a rapid lethal course. Together with Canavan disease, it is one of the two leukodystrophies with macrocephaly. Subsequent to the discovery of the specific mutation involved, this disease was shown to have a large spectrum of phenotypes, with juvenile and adolescent forms, and survival into adulthood by some patients. In the infantile form, frontal white matter involvement predominates, with progressive posterior extension.

Mucopolysaccharidoses

In this category of disease, there is a deficiency of lysosomal enzymes necessary for the degradation of mucopolysaccharides. These diseases are thus multisystemic. Excretion in the urine of incompletely degraded mucopolysaccharides is characteristic. The imaging presentation is one of dilated perivascular spaces (an identifying feature), atrophy with varying degrees of hydrocephalus, together with white matter changes that are initially more focal in nature (▶ Fig. 1.34). These lesions progress with time to resemble a nonspecific metabolic disorder, but if treated early by bone marrow transplantation may regress. Stenosis at the craniovertebral junction is a known additional associated finding. The mucopolysaccharidoses include Hurler (most common), Hunter (next most common), Sanfilippo, and Morquio diseases.

Mitochondrial Encephalomyopathy with Lactic Acidosis and Stroke-like Episodes (MELAS)

This entity refers to a group of disorders that present with stroke-like symptoms. Presentation is most common in the second decade of life. Patients have in common deletions of mitochondrial DNA. The parietal and occipital cortex and subcortical white matter are most frequently involved, although any area of the brain may be affected. The imaging presentation is one of vasogenic edema, in involved regions, with subsequent resolution and development later of other regions of involvement. Lesions do not follow specific arterial distributions, a differentiating feature from thrombotic or embolic infarction.

Leigh Syndrome

This term is now known to refer to a symptom complex, with several different genetic causes. The unifying theme appears to be defective terminal oxidative metabolism. Clinical presentation is in the first year of life. The patterns of injury vary with the mutation.

Glutaric Acidemia Type 1

A prominent clinical feature of this autosomal recessive disease is presentation with an acute encephalopathy, typically by 18 months of age. Unlike the majority of the genetic metabolic disorders, imaging findings are more specific for this diagnosis, with identification and clinical follow-up critical for treatment. Open Sylvian fissures (due to hypoplasia of the frontal and temporal opercula) together with bilateral basal ganglia (most notably the putamen) involvement (T2 hyperintensity) and macrocephaly are characteristic (▶ Fig. 1.35). A suspicion on imaging of this diagnosis should prompt laboratory evaluation, with dietary intervention known to prevent the devastating neurologic consequences of this disease.

GM1 and GM2 Gangliosidoses

These are rare lysosomal storage diseases (▶ Fig. 1.36) caused by deficiency in activity of specific lysosomal enzymes, with GM2 gangliosidosis more widely known due to Tay-Sachs disease (one of the GM2 gangliosidoses, which also include Sandhoff disease). The thalami and white matter are involved early, with cerebral and cerebellar atrophy a late finding.

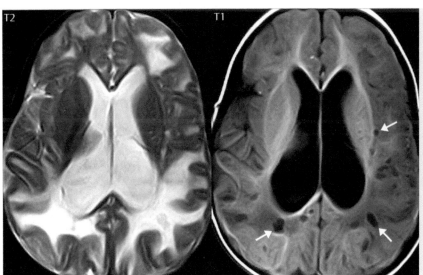

Fig. 1.34 Hunter syndrome. Late in the disease process, most of the leukodystrophies cannot be differentiated, and feature generalized cerebral atrophy (reflected by ventricular enlargement in this pediatric patient) together with patchy to diffuse abnormal high signal intensity white matter on T2-weighted scans. However, on the T1-weighted scan illustrated, there is a finding that is characteristic for the mucopolysaccharidoses, specifically Hunter and Hurler diseases, and that is the numerous strikingly enlarged dilated perivascular spaces (*arrows*).

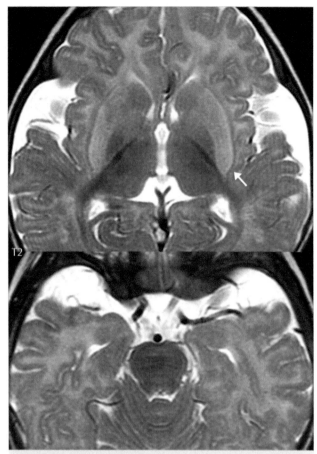

Fig. 1.35 Glutaric acidemia type 1. Widened CSF spaces, which include the sylvian fissures and the potential space anterior to the temporal lobes (with these two areas communicating) are characteristic for glutaric acidemia type 1, as shown. Additional typical findings, more difficult to recognize due to the age of this patient (6 months), include increased signal intensity on T2-weighted images in the periventricular white matter as well as the globus pallidus and putamen (*arrow*) bilaterally. Early recognition of this entity is important, as it is readily treated and otherwise leads to permanent sequelae.

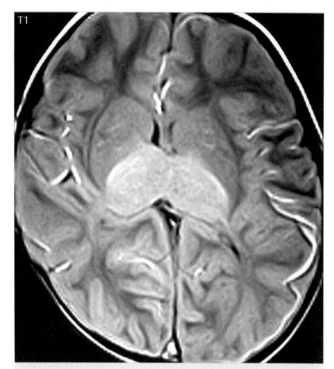

Fig. 1.36 GM1 gangliosidosis. Knowledge of the patient's age and presentation is critical for image evaluation in a patient suspected to have an inherited metabolic disorder. The image presented is from an 11-month-old patient with cessation of normal development at 3 months of age. Myelination would be appropriate in the axial image presented for a newborn, with high signal intensity in the posterior limb of the internal capsule, but is markedly delayed for a child near 1 year of age. At that time in development, myelination on T1-weighted images should appear near complete, with high signal intensity seen throughout the cerebral and cerebellar white matter.

1.4 Acquired Metabolic, Systemic, and Toxic Disorders

1.4.1 Acute Hypertensive Encephalopathy

This entity, also known by the term posterior reversible encephalopathy syndrome (PRES), is caused by acute severe hypertension. There is a predilection for involvement of the parietooccipital regions (the posterior circulation), with bilateral, symmetric abnormal high signal intensity (vasogenic edema) on fluid attenuated inversion recovery (FLAIR) involving the cortex and subcortical white matter in a nonvascular distribution (▶ Fig. 1.37). In prominent disease, the involvement of the cerebral hemispheres may be more extensive. Diffusion is usually not restricted. There may be accompanying involvement of the basal ganglia.

1.4.2 Wernicke Encephalopathy

This entity is caused by thiamine deficiency, and is seen in severe malnutrition, in particular with alcohol abuse. On FLAIR, in extensive disease, abnormal bilateral hyperintensity can be noted in the mamillary bodies, around the third ventricle, and in the medial thalami, tectal plate, and periaqueductal area (▶ Fig. 1.38). Involvement of the mamillary bodies is a distinctive feature. The mamillary bodies can also have abnormal contrast enhancement, as can occur in the other involved areas.

1.4.3 Hepatic Encephalopathy

This entity can occur with either acute or chronic liver disease, and is characterized on MR imaging by high signal intensity bilaterally within the globus pallidus on T1-weighted images (▶ Fig. 1.39). The signal intensity characteristics are thought to reflect manganese deposition. Similar findings can be seen with hyperalimentation.

1.4.4 Carbon Monoxide Poisoning

Inhalation of carbon monoxide (CO) results in impaired oxygen transport, with CO having 200 times the affinity for hemoglobin of oxygen. The hallmark of CO poisoning is symmetric injury to the globus pallidus. Initially vasogenic edema will be present, with mild enlargement of the nuclei. With time, this is replaced by gliosis and cystic encephalomalacia, with the chronic appearance being one of symmetric atrophy of the nuclei (▶ Fig. 1.40).

Pantothenate kinase-associated neurodegeneration (PKAN) can mimic the appearance of CO poisoning on CT and MR, with the term "eye of the tiger" used for the imaging presentation on T2-weighted scans and FLAIR. This progressive neurodegenerative disorder involves a mutation in the pantothenate kinase 2 gene, and today is classified within the category of neurodegeneration with brain iron accumulation (NBIA), of which PKAN is the most common type.

1.4.5 Osmotic Demyelination

This disease, previously referred to by the term central pontine myelinolysis, occurs due to too rapid correction of severe chronic hyponatremia (often in patients with alcoholism or malnutrition). In its classic presentation, there is abnormal symmetric involvement of the central pons, sparing the periphery, with high signal intensity on T2-weighted scans (▶ Fig. 1.41) (which may lag behind clinical symptoms by 1 to 2 weeks) and restricted diffusion (seen early in the disease

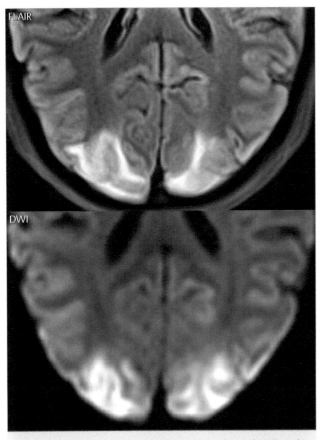

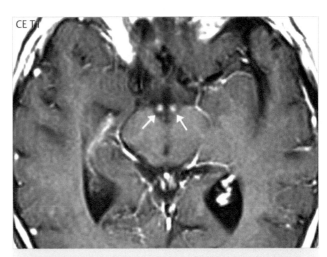

Fig. 1.37 Posterior reversible encephalopathy syndrome (PRES). In this entity, also known as acute hypertensive encephalopathy, symmetric abnormal high signal intensity is seen on FLAIR scans, consistent with vasogenic edema, posteriorly in the parietal-occipital regions involving cortical gray and subcortical white matter. On DWI, these areas are most commonly normal, but may be hyperintense (as illustrated), however, with the ADC map normal (no restricted diffusion).

Fig. 1.38 Wernicke encephalopathy. Involvement of the mamillary bodies, seen on FLAIR with abnormal hyperintensity (image not shown) and post-contrast with abnormal enhancement (illustrated, *arrows*), is the most characteristic finding in this disease from an imaging perspective.

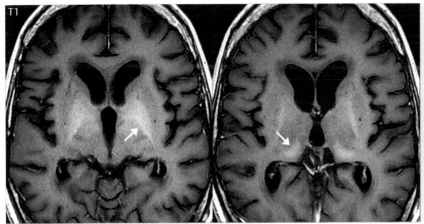

Fig. 1.39 Hepatic encephalopathy. Subtle abnormal high signal intensity (*arrow*, first image) is present bilaterally in the globus pallidus on a T1-weighted scan in this patient, consistent with manganese deposition. Presumably dependent on the amount of abnormal metal accumulation, the findings range in patients from somewhat subtle to striking hyperintensity. Also noted in this case is bilateral abnormal hyperintensity in the thalami (*arrow*, second image), which can also be seen in hepatic encephalopathy (involving any of the basal ganglia), but is less common.

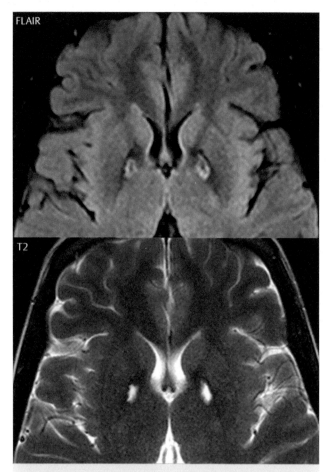

Fig. 1.40 Carbon monoxide poisoning (chronic). The globus pallidus is small (atrophic) bilaterally, with symmetric lesions therein demonstrating peripheral gliosis and central cavitation (fluid). On FLAIR, the gliosis is seen as abnormal high signal intensity, with central lower signal intensity due to fluid. On the heavily T2-weighted fast spin echo scan, the very high signal intensity fluid centrally within the lesions dominates the image appearance, with the gliosis less evident.

process). Extrapontine myelinolysis is most commonly seen in conjunction with central pontine myelinolysis (the term osmotic demyelination encompasses both entities), with symmetric involvement of the basal ganglia and cerebral white matter, and less commonly other areas.

1.4.6 Mesial Temporal Sclerosis

The etiology of mesial temporal sclerosis is unknown, with this entity likely the end result of several different possible insults. On pathology, there is atrophy of the hippocampus and adjacent structures, with disease bilateral in up to 20%. Mesial temporal sclerosis is a common cause of complex partial seizures. Thin section, high-resolution, coronal MR scans reveal atrophy of the hippocampus and ipsilateral fornix, with resultant mild enlargement of the adjacent temporal horn (▶ Fig. 1.42). Thin section coronal T2-weighted or FLAIR scans may also demonstrate hyperintensity of the involved hippocampus, with loss of the normal internal architecture common. 7 T offers improved anatomic depiction of the hippocampus, leading to higher confidence in the diagnosis of mesial temporal sclerosis and specifically the assignment of histologic subtype (▶ Fig. 1.43).

1.5 Hemorrhage

1.5.1 Parenchymal Hemorrhage

Hemorrhage has a specific but varied appearance on MR, dependent on time frame (▶ Fig. 1.44). The appearance is much more straightforward on CT. In normotensive young adults, vascular malformations are the most common cause of spontaneous hemorrhage. In adults, parenchymal hemorrhage is commonly due to hypertension (▶ Fig. 1.45), whereas subarachnoid hemorrhage is commonly due to rupture of an intracranial aneurysm. Typical locations for hypertensive hemorrhage include, in order of decreasing frequency, the basal ganglia (in particular the putamen), thalamus, pons (▶ Fig. 1.46), and cerebellar hemisphere (▶ Fig. 1.47). The descriptions of the appearance of hemorrhage in the literature are predominantly for parenchymal bleeds. To some extent, the appearance of subarachnoid hemorrhage is similar.

Hyperacute hemorrhage on CT is of moderate density, rapidly increasing further in density (attenuation) over the first few hours due to clot formation and retraction. After a few days, in the subacute time frame, a progressive loss in attenuation begins. By 1 to 4 weeks, a hematoma will be isodense to brain, and in the chronic phase may appear hypodense.

The subsequent description of hemorrhage on MR is for field strengths of 1.5 T and above, covering the vast majority of clinical systems today. Magnetic susceptibility effects, which cause decreased signal intensity depending on the time frame of the hemorrhage, are much less evident at lower field strengths. On MR, hemorrhage follows a regular well-defined temporal progression of changes in signal intensity (▶ Fig. 1.48).

Oxyhemoglobin (hyperacute) progresses to deoxyhemoglobin (acute), to intracellular methemoglobin (early subacute), then extracellular methemoglobin (late subacute), and eventually to hemosiderin (chronic). Oxyhemoglobin (hyperacute hemorrhage) has the signal intensity of fluid, high on T2- and low on T1-weighted scans. This imaging appearance is relatively nonspecific. Within hours, however, deoxyhemoglobin (acute hemorrhage) is evident with distinctive low signal intensity on T2-weighted scans. Deoxyhemoglobin does not have a unique appearance on T1-weighted scans, on which it appears isointense to mildly hypointense. Methemoglobin (subacute hemorrhage) has distinctive high signal intensity on T1-weighted scans, and bleeds can be further subdivided

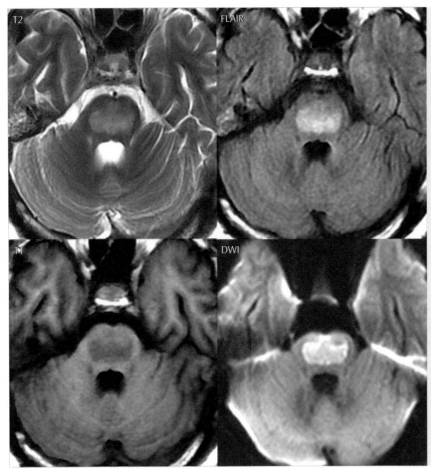

Fig. 1.41 Osmotic demyelination. There is abnormal high signal intensity centrally within the pons on the axial T2-weighted and FLAIR images presented, with corresponding abnormal low signal intensity on the T1-weighted scan. Note that the lateral and more posterior portions of the pons are spared, together with the more anterior (ventral) pons and the corticospinal tracts. There is also restricted diffusion (which can be seen acutely), with abnormal high signal intensity on DWI, in this comatose patient 1 week following rapid correction of hyponatremia.

temporally into intracellular and extracellular methemoglobin. Initially, in the intracellular phase, blood will be high signal intensity on a T1-weighted scan and low signal intensity on a T2-weighted scan (the latter due to a susceptibility effect). With red blood cell lysis, methemoglobin becomes extracellular in location, with distinctive high signal intensity on both T1- and T2-weighted scans (▶ Fig. 1.49).

With time, methemoglobin is converted into hemosiderin (and to a lesser degree ferritin), with chronic hemorrhage thus exhibiting pronounced low signal intensity on T2-weighted scans again due to susceptibility effects. The appearance of a chronic parenchymal hemorrhage on MR also depends on whether the central fluid collection is resorbed or not. If resorbed, a hemosiderin cleft will be left. If not resorbed, there will be a central fluid collection with high signal intensity on both T1- and T2-weighted scans, surrounded by a hemosiderin rim. With the passage of years, the fluid collection may change in appearance on T1-weighted scans from high to low signal intensity. It is important to note that the evolution of parenchymal hemorrhage on MR does not always follow the characteristic pattern described. Additional factors can be very

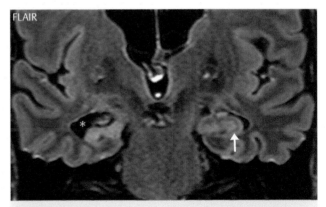

Fig. 1.42 Mesial temporal sclerosis. In **part 1**, on the coronal thin section (2.4 mm) FLAIR image, there is gross atrophy of the right hippocampus with enlargement of the adjacent temporal horn of the lateral ventricle (*asterisk*). Note the preservation of architecture and distinct layers of gray and white matter in the normal left hippocampus (*white arrow*). The diagnosis was confirmed in this instance by surgical pathology.

(Continued)

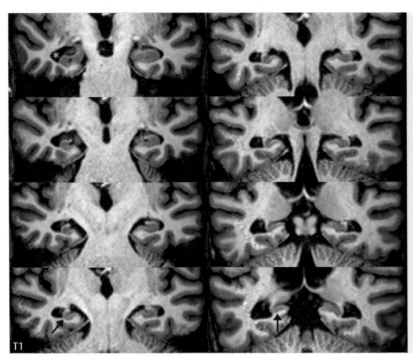

Fig. 1.42 (*Continued*) In **part 2**, thin section (1 mm) contiguous coronal T1-weighted scans confirm the atrophy of the right hippocampus and widening of the adjacent anterior temporal horn (*asterisk*). These sections also demonstrate that the right hippocampus is small, when compared to the left, throughout its extent from anterior to posterior (*black arrows*).

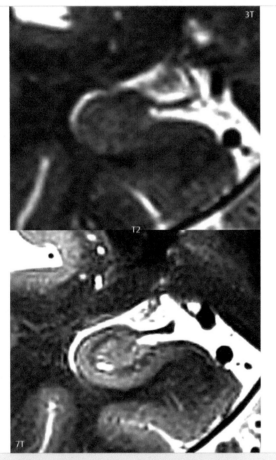

Fig. 1.43 Normal hippocampus, coronal thin section imaging comparing 3 T and 7 T. Note the markedly improved depiction of hippocampal structure (subfields) at 7 T, due to the higher achievable spatial resolution. Source: Springer E, Dymerska B, Cardoso PL, et al. Comparison of Routine Brain Imaging at 3 T and 7 T. *Invest Radiol.* 2016;51(8):469–482.

important, including dilution, clotting, and hematocrit. One key to the recognition of parenchymal hemorrhage, not discussed in detail, is the presence of edema surrounding the hematoma, which is seen in the hyperacute, acute, and early subacute stages.

1.5.2 Subarachnoid Hemorrhage

The appearance of acute subarachnoid hemorrhage on CT is generally well known, being well visualized with abnormal high attenuation. Depending on the amount of blood present, the sensitivity for detection of subarachnoid hemorrhage on CT can decrease rapidly with time following presentation. CT can be negative in patients with subarachnoid hemorrhage due either to a time delay (a few days) between the hemorrhage and imaging or the small quantity of blood present.

MR is actually more sensitive for subarachnoid hemorrhage than CT, although the imaging appearance is complex and recognition thus more difficult, particularly for radiologists with less experience. FLAIR is extremely sensitive to changes in the CSF, thus even very small amounts of subarachnoid hemorrhage will be seen as abnormal high signal intensity within the sulci. This appearance is however not specific for subarachnoid hemorrhage, and can be seen in any disease process that leads to a subtle change from normal in the composition of CSF. Meningitis produces this appearance, with administration of 100% O_2 in anesthetized ventilated patients another known cause. Regional versus global distribution of changes on FLAIR however aids in differentiation of these processes.

On T2* (susceptibility) weighted images, acute subarachnoid blood will be seen as low signal intensity, in distinction to normal high signal intensity CSF. In combination with the appearance on FLAIR, this finding is specific for acute subarachnoid hemorrhage (▶ Fig. 1.50). Depending on the time frame and the

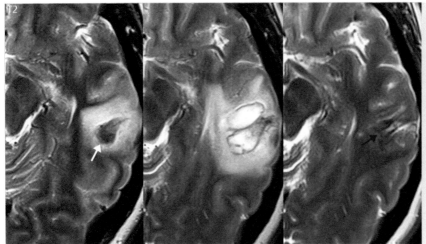

Fig. 1.44 Temporal evolution of parenchymal hemorrhage. On initial presentation, this posterior temporal hematoma (*white arrow*) demonstrates low signal intensity on the T2-weighted scan, indicative of deoxyhemoglobin. Also present is surrounding vasogenic edema, with abnormal high signal intensity. Two weeks later, temporal evolution has occurred to extracellular methemoglobin, with high signal intensity on the T2-weighted scan. Five months following presentation, there has been resorption of most of the fluid, together with resolution of the edema, leaving a low signal intensity hemosiderin cleft (*black arrow*).

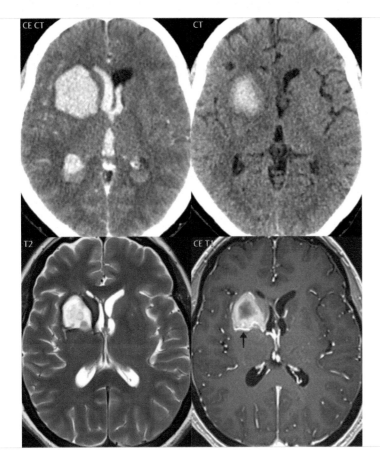

Fig. 1.45 Hypertensive hemorrhage. A large acute parenchymal hematoma is seen on the initial CT in this patient (left upper image), with its epicenter in the right putamen. There has also been extravasation of blood into the ventricular system, with hemorrhage seen in the frontal horns, third ventricle, and atria of the lateral ventricles. On the follow-up CT 3 weeks later, the hematoma is smaller and is in transition from hyperdense to isodense to brain. On the MR obtained after an additional 3 weeks, the hematoma is high signal intensity on both T2- and T1-weighted scans (consistent with methemoglobin), with a hemosiderin rim seen on the T2-weighted scan and a thin peripheral rim of enhancement (*black arrow*) post-contrast. Both are characteristic features on MR in a subacute hematoma, with the enhancement blending into the margin of the high signal intensity hemorrhage.

amount of hemorrhage, subarachnoid hemorrhage can also be seen as high signal intensity on T1-weighted scans, due to the presence of methemoglobin. By 3 days following presentation, high signal intensity is commonly seen on T1-weighted scans, a finding that typically persists for days to weeks. In comparison, the sensitivity of CT to subarachnoid hemorrhage decreases markedly following the first few days, with CT often normal thereafter.

Hemorrhage within the ventricular system is similarly well seen in the acute time frame by CT, and both acutely and later on following clinical presentation by MR. Blood clots are common within the ventricular system, with hyperdensity on CT

and a variable but characteristic appearance on MR depending on composition. Layering of a small amount of hemorrhage posteriorly in the atria of the lateral ventricles is commonly visualized on MR, a sign that can persist for days to weeks following hemorrhage.

1.5.3 Superficial Siderosis

In superficial siderosis, there is hemosiderin deposition in macrophages within the membranes lining the CSF spaces. The cause is recurrent subarachnoid hemorrhage, typically due to a hemorrhagic neoplasm, ruptured aneurysm, or vascular

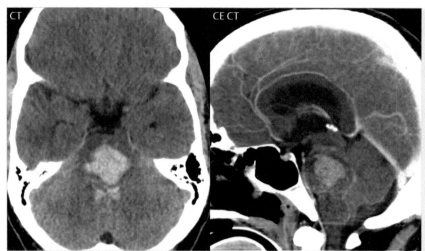

Fig. 1.46 Acute pontine hemorrhage. A large acute hemorrhage is seen centrally in the pons on axial unenhanced and sagittal enhanced CT. A small amount of hemorrhage is also seen in the fourth ventricle posteriorly, which is compressed due to mass effect. The pons and cerebellum, considered together, are the third most common site for hypertensive hemorrhage, after the putamen/external capsule (first) and the thalamus (second). This known hypertensive patient presented in hypertensive crisis.

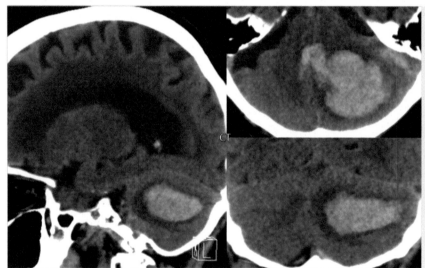

Fig. 1.47 Acute cerebellar hemorrhage, hypertensive. A large acute parenchymal hemorrhage is seen in the left cerebellar hemisphere, on sagittal, axial, and coronal reformatted images from a non-contrast CT exam. Note the vasogenic edema circumferential to this hematoma. Hemorrhage is also seen in the fourth ventricle on the axial image, with interstitial edema and ventricular enlargement noted on the sagittal image, due to extraventricular obstructive hydrocephalus (on the basis of the subarachnoid and ventricular hemorrhage).

malformation that has bled. The surface of the cerebellum is the most common site (▶ Fig. 1.51). Clinical symptoms occur rarely, and only when there is substantial deposition of hemosiderin. Possible symptoms include sensorineural hearing loss, pyramidal tract signs, and cerebellar dysfunction, together with cranial nerve dysfunction (most often cranial nerves II, V, VII, or VIII, with the severity of injury proportional to the cisternal length of the nerve). T2-weighted scans at 1.5 T and above demonstrate hypointensity of the involved leptomeninges or ependyma. Any sequence that improves the sensitivity to susceptibility (T2*), such as a gradient echo sequence or susceptibility weighted imaging, will also be more sensitive to the presence of superficial siderosis (as well as the use of 3 T as opposed to 1.5T).

1.6 Trauma

A few definitions are in order to introduce the topic of brain trauma. A cortical contusion is simply a bruise of the brain's surface. The inferofrontal and anteroinferior temporal portions of these two lobes of the brain are particularly vulnerable (▶ Fig. 1.52). The term "coup" is used to reference an injury that

lies directly beneath the area of impact. The term "contrecoup" is used for an injury that occurs remote from the site of impact, along a direct line but opposite to this site, caused by acceleration effects. Imaging of acute head injury is the province of CT. Acute intracranial hemorrhage and bone fractures are well seen and evaluated (▶ Fig. 1.53).

1.6.1 Parenchymal Injury

Diffuse axonal injury (DAI) and cortical contusion are the two most common findings in the setting of trauma with a closed head injury. Subcortical gray matter injury also occurs, but much less frequently. DAI occurs due to shearstrain forces with rapid deceleration. There are three common locations (given in order from the most to the least common, which also parallels the degree of severity of the injury from least to most): the gray-white matter junction, the corpus callosum (splenium), and the brainstem (▶ Fig. 1.54). CT is often normal in this setting.

Injuries at the gray-white matter junction will be seen as multiple small foci of abnormal high signal intensity on FLAIR

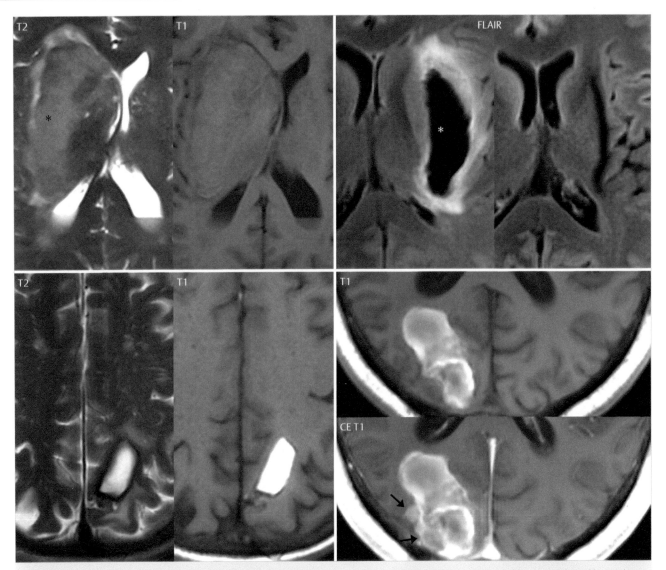

Fig. 1.48 Parenchymal hemorrhage on MR, the spectrum of signal intensity appearance. Initially, but for a very short time, a parenchymal hemorrhage contains oxygenated hemoglobin and is seen as a fluid collection, with slight hyperintensity on a T2-weighted scan. A large, basal ganglia, hyperacute hemorrhage (*black asterisk*) illustrates this appearance. There is a small amount of associated vasogenic edema and marked mass effect upon the right lateral ventricle. In the next patient, FLAIR scans are shown both on presentation and long term follow-up. This large, acute, left external capsule hematoma evolves from a fluid collection containing deoxyhemoglobin (*white asterisk*, with low signal intensity on T2-weighted scans), to a hemosiderin lined cleft (also low signal intensity). Note the associated vasogenic edema and mass effect in the acute stage. The third patient illustrates a subacute, extracellular methemoglobin hematoma, with high signal intensity on both T2- and T1-weighted scans, in the left parietal region. Note the peripheral hemosiderin rim, with low signal intensity, already present on the T2-weighted scan. The fourth patient illustrates on an unenhanced T1-weighted scan a methemoglobin hematoma in the right occipital lobe. This case emphasizes the importance of looking for the cause of a hemorrhage, as the post-contrast scan reveals the associated enhancing metastasis (*black arrows*).

scans. Most commonly these involve the frontal lobe. If the lesions are hemorrhagic, they will be well seen in the acute time frame on T2*-weighted gradient echo scans, due to the presence of deoxyhemoglobin. Susceptibility weighted imaging offers a further improvement in sensitivity to T2* effects, and in cases with hemorrhage will demonstrate more extensive injury. The second most common injury seen in DAI is a shear injury of the corpus callosum, with the majority involving the splenium. This injury and the subsequently described injury of the brainstem are usually not seen in isolation but with extensive shear injury at the gray-white matter junction. In the brainstem,

lesions are seen most often in the pons and the dorsolateral midbrain. Lesions in the brainstem carry a very poor prognosis, often with a fatal outcome.

In patients evaluated months to years following severe head trauma, the residual from DAI involving injury at the gray-white matter junction can be visualized, with high signal intensity on FLAIR due to gliosis and low signal intensity on T2*-weighted images due to the presence of hemosiderin. Encephalomalacia, with both gliosis and cystic changes, will be seen in areas of prior contusion. In severe injury, there may be resultant generalized cerebral atrophy.

1.6.2 Epidural Hematoma

The dura is the periosteum of the inner table and is strongly adherent to the skull. An epidural hematoma accumulates between the inner table of the skull and the dura, and is typically due to a skull fracture with laceration of a blood vessel. The most common location is temporal/parietal, due to laceration of the middle meningeal artery. Less common are posterior fossa lesions, due to an occipital skull fracture with secondary laceration of the transverse sinus. In 50% of cases there will be an intervening lucid interval after the initial trauma, with subsequent rapid progressive deterioration. The imaging appearance is that of a biconvex, elliptical fluid collection, which can cross the midline (falx) and the tentorium, with the venous sinuses displaced away from the skull (▶ Fig. 1.55).

In adults, epidural hematomas do not cross suture lines, although in children (and with venous lesions) this is not true.

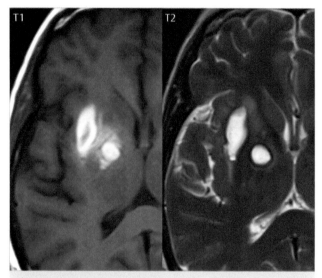

Fig. 1.49 Parenchymal hemorrhage, involving the globus pallidus and putamen (the lentiform nucleus). High signal intensity on both T1- and T2-weighted scans is consistent with extracellular methemoglobin, in this late subacute hypertensive hemorrhage. An additional characteristic finding is the faint hemosiderin rim, with low signal intensity on the T2-weighted scan.

CT is the exam of choice due to its ready availability and speed, particularly with accompanying life support systems. MR is more sensitive to coexisting parenchymal brain injuries, as well as subacute hemorrhage. On CT, an acute epidural hematoma will be hyperdense, with a hypodense component due to active bleeding in one-third of cases. On MR, the displaced dura may be identifiable, with the acute epidural hematoma itself having the signal intensity characteristics of oxy- or deoxyhemoglobin.

1.6.3 Subdural Hematoma

Subdural hematomas demonstrate a convex inward border (▶ Fig. 1.56). On MR, the general age of a lesion will be evident, due to the signal intensity of blood products therein, with blood in subdural hematomas following the described temporal progression of deoxyhemoglobin to intracellular methemoglobin to extracellular methemoglobin. There is no blood-brain barrier of course, thus macrophages freely enter the fluid collection and eventually remove the blood products therein. Chronic subdural hematomas on MR differ in their appearance from parenchymal hematomas. They are isointense to slightly hypointense with brain on T1-weighted images, with high signal intensity on T2-weighted scans (specifically hyperintense to CSF on FLAIR), and do not demonstrate hemosiderin deposition unless recurrent. A subdural hygroma, strictly defined, contains CSF and is the result of an arachnoid tear or insufficiency. With some chronic subdural hematomas there may be sufficient resorption of blood products to make differentiation from a hygroma, on the basis of signal intensity, difficult.

1.6.4 Nonaccidental Trauma (Child Abuse)

Nonaccidental trauma can be caused by direct impact injuries or shaking. Findings include skull fractures, subdural hematomas, and contusions. The skull fractures and accompanying scalp hematomas are well visualized by CT Otherwise, children in whom this entity is suspected are best evaluated by MR. Bilateral subdural hematomas of differing ages strongly suggest this diagnosis (▶ Fig. 1.57). Territorial infarcts and/or global hypoxic injury may also be present. FLAIR, T2* (gradient echo or

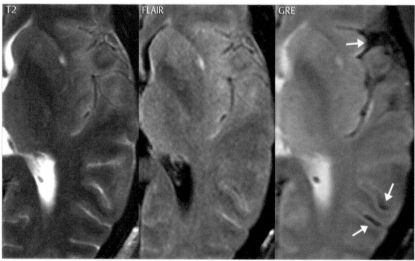

Fig. 1.50 Acute subarachnoid hemorrhage, MR. On initial inspection, the T2-weighted scan appears normal (other than a small external capsule chronic lacunar infarct). However, in retrospect (particularly in comparison with the GRE scan), the left sylvian fissure does not demonstrate the characteristic high signal intensity of CSF (it is isointense with brain), raising the suspicion of subarachnoid hemorrhage or other pathology. FLAIR confirms this finding, but also demonstrates abnormal high signal intensity in two sulci posteriorly, indicative of either blood or inflammatory changes. The GRE scan confirms that both findings represent subarachnoid hemorrhage (*arrows*), with abnormal low signal intensity due to T2* changes (seen with both deoxy- and intracellular methemoglobin).

susceptibility weighted imaging), and diffusion-weighted imaging (DWI) scans should all be obtained. The use of T2*-weighted scans is in part for the detection of chronic blood products, specifically the residual from prior hemorrhagic contusions.

1.6.5 Penetrating Injuries

Gunshot wounds to the brain cause a myriad of findings and are best and urgently so evaluated by CT (▶ Fig. 1.58). In addition to the defect at the entry site, there may be extensive skull fractures. The location of metal fragments from the bullet will be readily evident. Edema may be extensive. Parenchymal hemorrhage is almost always present and subdural hematomas common.

1.7 Herniation

Subfalcine herniation is the most common brain herniation, and is caused by a supratentorial mass on one side that shifts

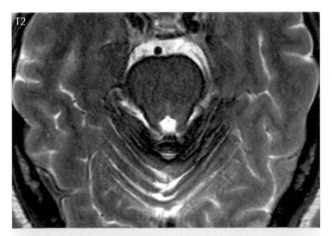

Fig. 1.51 Superficial siderosis. There is somewhat subtle abnormal hypointensity surrounding the pons, and outlining the superior cerebellar folia, due to superficial hemosiderin deposition from recurrent hemorrhage.

brain to the opposite side. Herniation of brain occurs across the midline under the inferior or "free" margin of the falx. The cingulate gyrus, anterior cerebral artery, and internal cerebral vein can be displaced to the contralateral side under the falx. The ipsilateral ventricle will be compressed and displaced toward the midline. The contralateral ventricle can enlarge (unilateral obstructive hydrocephalus), due to occlusion of the foramen of Monro. The herniated anterior cerebral artery can also be compressed against the free margin of the falx, and thus occluded with subsequent infarction of the cingulate gyrus.

Descending transtentorial herniation is the second most common cerebral herniation, and can caused by a large hemispheric mass, occurring subsequent to subfalcine herniation. The uncus of the temporal lobe will be displaced medially and encroach upon the suprasellar cistern. On imaging, both the ipsilateral ambient cistern (which lies lateral to the midbrain) and lateral portion of the prepontine cistern may be widened. With further mass effect, the uncus and hippocampus can both herniate through the tentorial incisura. Descending transtentorial herniation can be either unilateral or, in more severe cases, bilateral (▶ Fig. 1.59).

Tonsillar herniation is well visualized by MR, with the imaging findings including inferior displacement of the tonsils, pointing of the tonsils (in distinction to their normal rounded shape), and obliteration of CSF at the level of the foramen magnum (▶ Fig. 1.59).

1.8 Infarction

In young patients, the etiologies for cerebral infarction are many and varied, in distinction to adults. Leading causes include congenital and acquired heart disease, together with sickle cell disease. In the elderly, infarcts are most often due to atherosclerosis, with vessel occlusion due to either thrombosis or embolism (▶ Fig. 1.60).

Common areas of atherosclerotic involvement include the carotid bifurcation, distal internal carotid artery, and middle cerebral artery. Risk factors for infarction in an adult include high blood pressure, high cholesterol, smoking, diabetes,

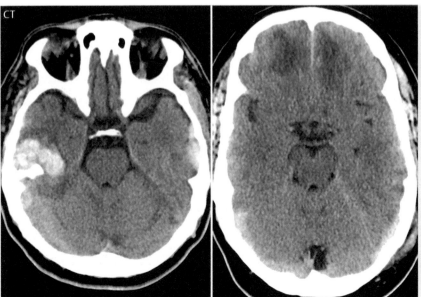

Fig. 1.52 Contusion, parenchymal. High velocity contusion injuries are illustrated in two different patients, showing characteristic areas of the brain involved. In the first, there is a large hemorrhagic contusion, with the area of hemorrhage surrounded by low density (edema), overlying the right petrous apex. Also noted is a small acute epidural hematoma on the left. In the second patient, low-density regions are noted in the low frontal lobes bilaterally, corresponding to nonhemorrhagic parenchymal contusions.

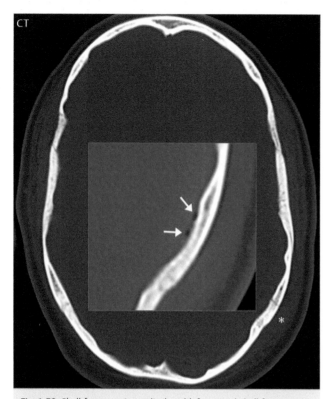

Fig. 1.53 Skull fracture. A nondisplaced left parietal skull fracture (*asterisk*) is seen on this axial CT image reconstructed with a bone algorithm. It is anterior to the lambdoid suture. The insert, a magnification of a portion of the image immediately superior to that displayed, reveals two small foci of pneumocephalus (*arrows*), an important clue to the radiologist to search for a nearby skull fracture in the setting of trauma. Note also the extracranial soft tissue swelling adjacent to the fracture.

obesity, cardiovascular disease, oral contraceptives, and cocaine. The clinical presentation is that of an acute neurologic deficit.

Infarction involving the precentral gyrus (primary motor cortex) leads to contralateral motor deficits (▸ Fig. 1.61). Infarction in the left inferior frontal gyrus (specifically in Broca's area, the part of the brain responsible for speech production) causes an expressive aphasia. Infarction in the left posterior superior temporal gyrus (specifically in Wernicke's area) causes receptive aphasia. The latter two statements apply to patients who are left-hemisphere dominant.

1.8.1 Arterial Territory Infarcts

Infarcts in the major arterial territories are easily recognized due to their arterial distribution and their involvement of both gray and white matter. MCA infarcts are most common, followed by PCA infarcts. Of the three major arterial territories, ACA infarcts are by far the least common. The MCA supplies the lateral cerebral hemispheres, with the lenticulostriate arteries (arising from the M1 segment) supplying the globus pallidus and putamen and the anterior limb of the internal capsule. The PCA can originate from the tip of the basilar artery (80%) or in the case of a fetal origin (20%) directly from the internal carotid artery. The PCA supplies the posteroinferior temporal lobe, medial parietal lobe, occipital lobe, and portions of the brainstem, thalamus, and internal capsule (▸ Fig. 1.62). The ACA supplies the anterior putamen, caudate nucleus, hypothalamus, corpus callosum, and medial surface of the cerebral hemisphere (▸ Fig. 1.63).

The posterior inferior cerebellar artery (PICA) arises from distal vertebral artery and supplies the retro-olivary (lateral) medulla, inferior vermis, tonsil, and posterior inferior portion of the cerebellar hemisphere (▸ Fig. 1.64). The most frequent cause of a PICA infarct is thrombosis of the vertebral artery. The anterior

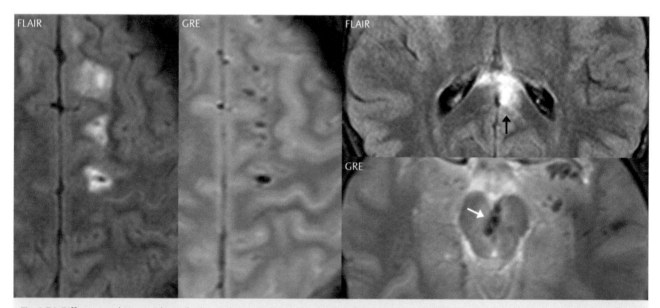

Fig. 1.54 Diffuse axonal injury. Edema (high signal intensity) and petechial hemorrhage (low signal intensity) are seen on T2-weighted scans at the gray-white matter junction of the frontal lobe in this patient who was involved in a high velocity auto accident. The GRE scan better visualizes the T2* effect due to this hemorrhage (deoxyhemoglobin). The FLAIR scan at the level of the splenium of the corpus callosum reveals edema therein (*black arrow*), a less frequent and more clinically significant injury. The GRE scan of the brainstem reveals hemorrhage (*white arrow*) within the cerebral peduncles, the least common area of involvement of the three illustrated, and the most severe clinically.

inferior cerebellar artery (AICA) supplies a small portion of the cerebellum, anteriorly and inferiorly. Its territory is often referred to as being in equilibrium with PICA, specifically the larger the PICA territory, the smaller the AICA territory (and vice versa). The remaining arterial territory in the cerebellum is that of the superior cerebellar artery (SCA), which supplies the superior half of the cerebellum (and parts of the midbrain) (▶ Fig. 1.65) and arises from the basilar artery just proximal to the posterior cerebral artery. The largest two cerebellar, arterial territories are that of the SCA and PICA. Concerning territorial infarcts in the cerebellum, PICA is most common, followed by the SCA, with infarcts of AICA being uncommon. In the elderly, chronic small cerebellar infarcts are commonly detected on MR, and are seen in both major territories.

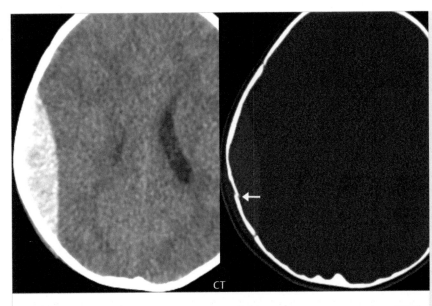

Fig. 1.55 Acute epidural hematoma. A large, extra-axial, high-density fluid collection (acute hemorrhage) is seen on the right, overlying the temporal and parietal lobes (**part 1**). Note the biconvex shape. On the image windowed for bone, an underlying, minimally displaced, skull fracture (*white arrow*) is noted. In a second patient (**part 2**), a smaller epidural hematoma is noted overlying the right frontal lobe (*black arrow*). The blood is noted to be predominantly methemoglobin (high signal intensity on a T1-weighted scan) on MR. CT demonstrated an adjacent skull fracture (not shown). However, not seen on CT was the petechial hemorrhage (deoxyhemoglobin) along the gray-white matter junction (*white arrows*), demonstrated on a coronal image, reflecting diffuse axonal injury in this patient with major trauma.

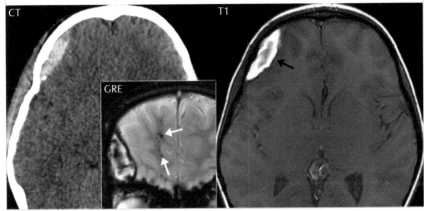

Fig. 1.56 Subdural hematoma. A small subdural hematoma is seen on the right, with a much larger subdural hematoma on the left. Note the obliteration of sulci on the left, best seen on the FLAIR scan, due to mass effect. Regardless, there is little midline shift. The large subdural hematoma exhibits many adhesions, best seen on the T2*-weighted gradient echo scan, important information to communicate to the neurosurgeon since drainage will likely require lysis of these adhesions.

1.8.2 Lacunar Infarcts

Lacunar infarcts are small, deep cerebral infarcts, most frequently seen with hypertension. They result from occlusion of small penetrating arteries arising from the major cerebral arteries, and most commonly involve the basal ganglia (▶ Fig. 1.66), internal capsule (▶ Fig. 1.67), thalamus (▶ Fig. 1.68), and brainstem (▶ Fig. 1.69). The blood supply to the pons is mainly from the basilar artery via small paramedian and circumferential penetrating branches. Infarcts in the pons are most frequently unilateral, paramedian, and sharply marginated at the midline. Bilateral pontine infarcts, which are less common, remain paramedian in

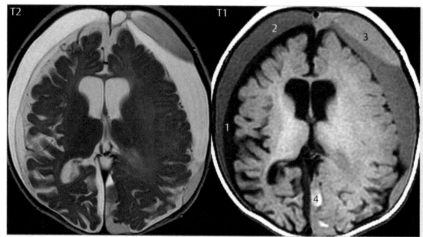

Fig. 1.57 Nonaccidental trauma. There are subdural hematomas of four different time frames (numbered 1 to 4, each with a characteristic signal intensity) in this infant, a pathognomic appearance for nonaccidental trauma. In addition, there is mild cerebral atrophy on the right, with the subdural hematomas causing mass effect on the left, reflected by obliteration of cerebral sulci together with the left atrium of the lateral ventricle

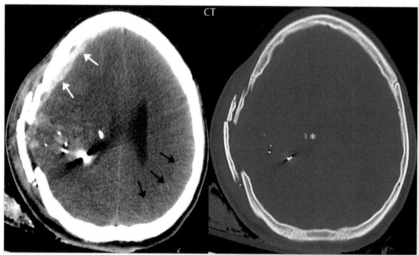

Fig. 1.58 Penetrating trauma, with extensive parenchymal injury. There are comminuted, displaced fractures involving the parietal and (more inferiorly) temporal bones, with accompanying scalp swelling. Hyperdense extra-axial fluid (an acute subdural hematoma, *white arrows*) overlies the right frontal lobe. There is leftward midline shift, with effacement of the right lateral ventricle. Scattered foci of intraparenchymal hemorrhage are seen surrounding metallic bullet fragments within the right frontal and parietal lobes. A small bone fragment (*asterisk*) is displaced medially adjacent to the right lateral ventricle. There is diffuse sulcal effacement. There is loss of gray-white matter differentiation in the right parietal region, indicative of more extensive injury (ischemia), best seen in comparison to the normal contralateral side (*small black arrows*).

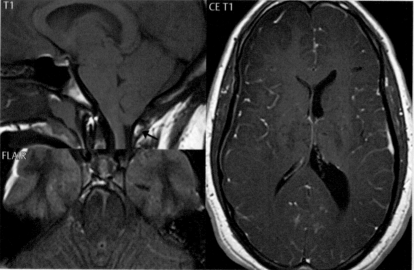

Fig. 1.59 Transtentorial and tonsillar herniation. On sagittal imaging the pons and cerebellum are compressed, with the latter caudally displaced, the fourth ventricle is small and the cisterna magna obliterated. The cerebral peduncles are compressed, with bilateral uncal herniation (demonstrated on the axial FLAIR image). The cerebellar tonsils extend to the level of C1 (*black arrow*, posterior arch). The cause in this instance is meningitis, with diffuse brain swelling. There is abnormal enhancement of the meninges postcontrast and obliteration of cerebral sulci, consistent with this diagnosis. A small subdural empyema is also noted on the right on both axial scans.

distribution. Lateral pontine infarcts are uncommon. The differential diagnosis for a unilateral pontine lesion includes multiple sclerosis (MS), whereas for bilateral central lesions the differential diagnosis includes central pontine myelinolysis and pontine glioma.

1.8.3 Medullary Infarcts

In the medulla, both lateral (▶ Fig. 1.69) and medial infarcts are seen. Lateral medullary infarcts, Wallenberg syndrome, present clinically with dysarthria, dysphagia, vertigo, nystagmus, ipsilateral Horner syndrome, and contralateral loss of pain and

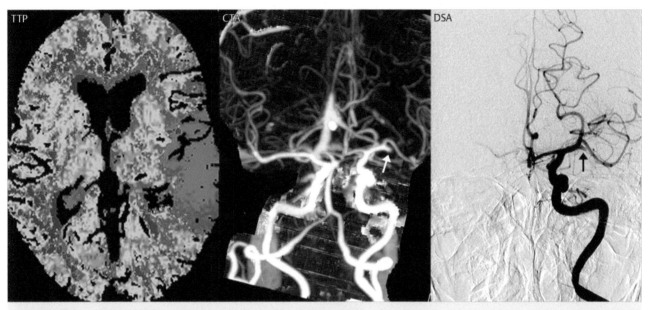

Fig. 1.60 Hyperacute distal MCA territory infarct, evaluation by CT. This 79-year-old woman presented 1.5 hours prior to the initial imaging evaluation with clinical signs of ischemia in the left MCA territory. The unenhanced CT (not shown) was grossly unremarkable. The time to peak (TTP) image reveals delayed perfusion in nearly the entire left MCA territory, with the exception of the lenticulostriate artery distribution. CBV was normal (not shown). CTA reveals thromboembolic occlusion (*white arrow*) of the distal left M1 segment of the MCA. The occlusion (*black arrow*) was confirmed on DSA. Following mechanical thrombectomy (3 hours following the CT), flow to the left MCA and its branches was fully restored (image not shown).

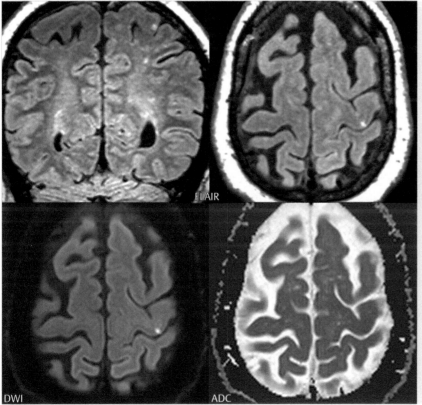

Fig. 1.61 Early subacute pinpoint cortical infarct, left precentral gyrus. The patient presented 6 days prior to the MR exam with right arm and facial paralysis. NIHSS = 3 (minor stroke), which improved to 0 (no stroke symptoms). CT at the time of symptom onset was negative. Multiple small focal areas of gliosis or edema (with high signal intensity) are seen on the coronal FLAIR, with a single focus within the precentral gyrus (seen on both the coronal and axial scans). The cortical location of the latter suggests possible clinical significance. The lesion is of high signal intensity on DWI, yet with little restricted diffusion, consistent with the clinical timing (cytotoxic edema, which is visualized as restricted diffusion, typically fades by 7 to 10 days following onset in ischemia).

temperature sense over the body. This is a known complication of chiropractic neck manipulation, due to dissection of the vertebral artery near the atlantoaxial joint. The arteries supplying the lateral medulla usually arise from the distal vertebral artery, but can originate from PICA. Thus, a lateral medullary infarct can on occasion be seen in a patient with a PICA infarct. Medial medullary infarction (▶ Fig. 1.70), Dejerine syndrome, presents with ipsilateral tongue weakness (with deviation of the tongue toward the infarct side), contralateral limb weakness, and contralateral loss of touch, proprioception, and vibration sense (due to involvement of the hypoglossal nerve, corticospinal tract, and medial lemniscus). The blood supply is from the anterior spinal artery.

1.8.4 Temporal Evolution

MR is markedly more sensitive than CT for detection of early brain infarcts, largely due to DWI. Within minutes, cytotoxic edema develops in an area of ischemia, which is visualized as high signal intensity on DWI with corresponding low ADC (restricted diffusion) on the calculated apparent diffusion coefficient map (▶ Fig. 1.71).

In cytotoxic edema, there is impaired function of the sodium potassium pump leading to a net flow of water into the cell. There is no change in overall water content of the tissue. Soon after development of a territorial infarct, there may be subtle loss of cortical sulci. A slight increase in thickness of cortical gray matter may also be visualized on T1-weighted scans. By 24 hours, vasogenic edema is present in 90% of brain infarcts, representing on overall increase in tissue water content. Vasogenic edema is seen with abnormal high signal intensity on T2-weighted scans and corresponding low signal intensity on T1-weighted scans, due to prolongation of both relaxation times. Vasogenic edema is seen as an area of low attenuation compared to normal adjacent brain on CT Vasogenic edema typically persists for weeks. During the second week, ADC values return to near baseline (and later rise above normal). However, an ischemic lesion may remain high signal intensity on DWI in the subacute time period due to "T2 shine through" (▶ Fig. 1.72)—with the high signal intensity due to the partial T2-weighting of the sequence (with the ADC map normal). MR is also markedly superior to CT for detection of lacunar

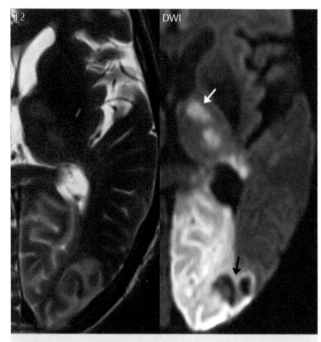

Fig. 1.62 Posterior cerebral artery (PCA) infarction, early subacute. There is both vasogenic edema and cytotoxic edema, as demonstrated by respectively high signal intensity on the T2- and the diffusion-weighted scans, in the entirety of the left PCA distribution. In this instance, infarcts of the same time frame are also seen in the left thalamus (*white arrow*), which is supplied by the posterior thalamo-perforators (which originate from the P1 segment of the PCA). There is also hemorrhage (*black arrow*) within the lesion, seen with low signal intensity due to a T2* effect.

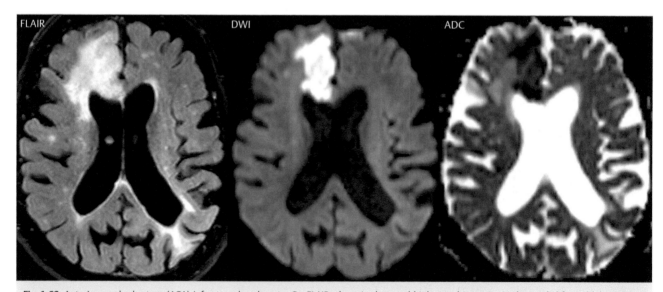

Fig. 1.63 Anterior cerebral artery (ACA) infarct, early subacute. On FLAIR, there is abnormal high signal intensity in the medial frontal lobe (ACA territory) on the right, involving both gray and white matter, with mild mass effect upon the frontal horn of the lateral ventricle. There is corresponding abnormal hyperintensity on DWI, reflecting cytotoxic edema (confirmed to be restricted diffusion on the ADC map). This anatomic distribution lies within, and forms part of, the ACA territory. Also present is loss of brain substance and mild gliosis in the left parietal region, consistent with a chronic watershed infarct.

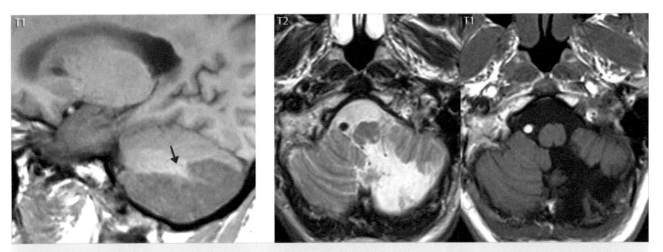

Fig. 1.64 Posterior inferior cerebellar artery (PICA) infarction. On a sagittal T1-weighted scan (**part 1**), abnormal low signal intensity (*arrow*) is seen involving the inferior half of the cerebellum, consistent with a subacute PICA territory infarct. This is the most common territorial infarct seen in the cerebellum. In a different patient (**part 2**), a chronic left PICA infarct is noted. There is absence of brain substance (cystic encephalomalacia) in the region of the posteroinferior cerebellum on the left. Note that the involved cerebellum includes the cerebellartonsil and a portion of the vermis. There is mild loss of substance involving the left medulla, with a tiny area of cystic encephalomalacia, with the lower medulla supplied by PICA in about half of cases. Note the spared anterior cerebellum at this level, in the AICA territory.

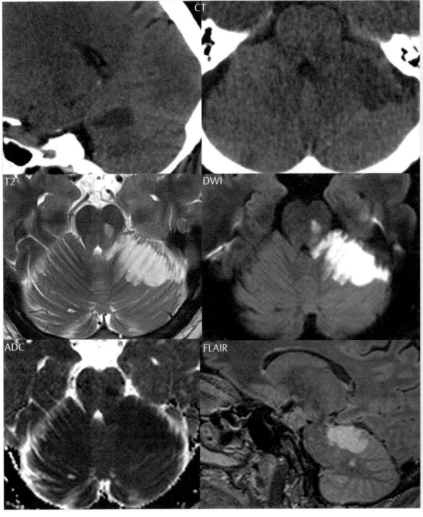

Fig. 1.65 Acute superior cerebellar artery (SCA) infarction, with an accompanying small unilateral pontine infarct. Hypodensity is seen on CT in a portion of the SCA territory, with hyperintensity on axial T2-weighted MR (and sagittal FLAIR), both due to vasogenic edema. Hyperintensity on DWI together with a low ADC confirms the presence of restricted diffusion. There is an additional small left sided pontine infarct, best seen on MR. The patient had a patent foramen ovale, likely the etiology for these infarcts. On imaging 1 hour after onset of symptoms (not shown), there was only restricted diffusion. The images shown are from follow exams acquired 1 day (CT) and 3 days (MR) following clinical presentation.

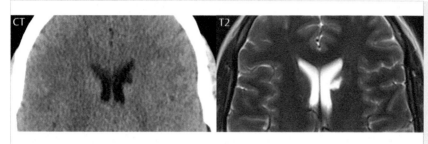

Fig. 1.66 Chronic lacunar infarct, caudate head. A focal very low attenuation lesion is seen within the caudate head on CT, with corresponding high signal intensity on the T2-weighted scan, consistent with a chronic cavitated infarct. A caveat however is that very low attenuation on rare occasion corresponds to edema in an early subacute infarct, with CT both less sensitive for detection of ischemia and also much less specific in regard to dating when compared to MR.

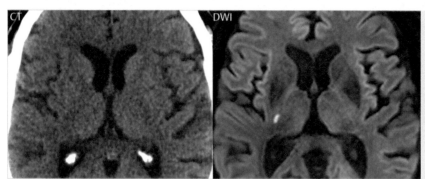

Fig. 1.67 Acute lacunar infarction, posterior limb of the internal capsule. The patient was hypertensive, and presented for CT (which was negative) with acute hypoesthesia involving the left side of the body. The MR was obtained 15 hours later, and reveals a small acute lacunar infarct in the internal capsule on the right. Due to the ability to detect cytotoxic edema, with diffusion weighted imaging, MR can detect even very small infarcts within 15 minutes of clinical symptomatology.

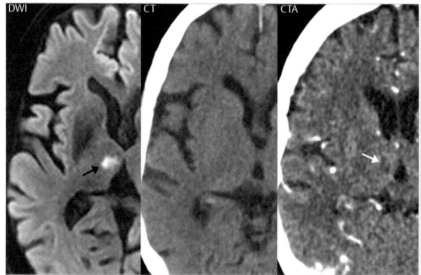

Fig. 1.68 Acute thalamic infarction. There is restricted diffusion, with abnormal high signal intensity on the diffusion-weighted image, in this small acute, right sided, lacunar infarct (*black arrow*). Unenhanced CT, obtained with a 4-mm slice thickness, does not visualize the lesion, which is common due to the lower sensitivity of this modality (and its insensitivity to cytotoxic edema). Note that on thinner section images (2 mm), obtained during bolus contrast administration (CTA), that the infarct (*white arrow*) can be recognized in retrospect due to slight lower attenuation in comparison with adjacent normal brain.

infarcts, and those involving the posterior fossa and brainstem. Time-of-flight (TOF) MR angiography (MRA) is often normal, even in large territorial infarcts. Vessel occlusion and/or stenoses can be seen, but are not common findings on MR studies, other than those obtained very early following presentation.

Cerebral infarcts are divided temporally into hyperacute (<6 hours) (▶ Fig. 1.71), acute (<24 hours), subacute, and chronic lesions. There is no consensus in the literature relative to these terms, with "acute infarction" often also used to refer to lesions 1 day to 1 week in age. Subacute is generally used to reference lesions in the first 1 to 2 months, and chronic lesions those >1 to 2 months in age. The term subacute is sometimes subdivided into early subacute (first week) (▶ Fig. 1.73) and late subacute (1 to 6 weeks in age) infarcts. This subdivision reflects in part that first week infarcts generally do not display blood-brain barrier disruption, whereas later subacute infarcts do—and thus

typically display abnormal contrast enhancement on MR. Mass effect, due to prominent vasogenic edema, is common in early subacute infarcts, and begins to fade by 2 weeks following onset.

1.8.5 Abnormal Contrast Enhancement

The patterns of abnormal contrast enhancement in brain infarcts on MR are well described in the literature. Intravascular enhancement reflects slow arterial flow, and is the earliest type of abnormal enhancement seen. Intravascular enhancement can be seen in the first day, and up to a week following presentation. A short segment of a single vessel, or of multiple enhancing vessels, may be seen. Meningeal enhancement, adjacent to the area of infarction, is the least common form of abnormal contrast enhancement, but can be seen from days 1 to 3. These two patterns of enhancement have been described for MCA and

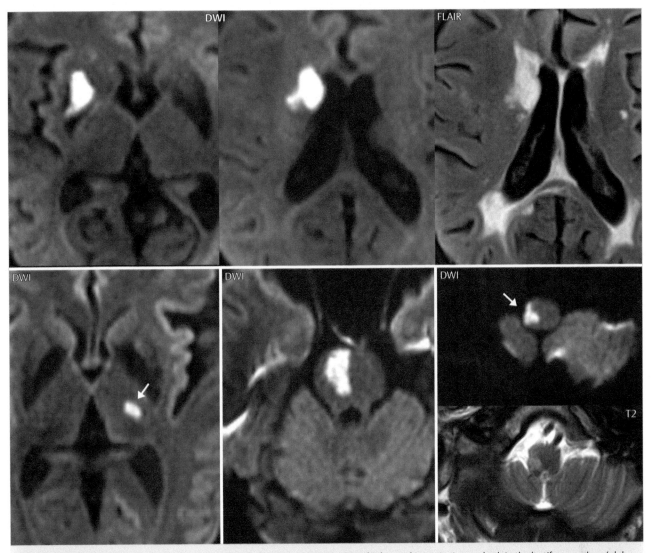

Fig. 1.69 The anatomic spectrum of lacunar infarction. In the first patient, on DWI, high signal intensity is seen both in the lentiform nucleus (globus pallidus and putamen) and the caudate head, a common imaging appearance. The caudate head lesion is also shown on FLAIR to be high signal intensity, dating this lesion as acute to subacute in time frame. The caudate infarct, however, cannot be differentiated on the basis of signal intensity on the FLAIR scan from the marked accompanying periventricular white matter gliosis. In the second and third patients, respectively, thalamic (*white arrow*) and pontine lacunar infarcts are seen with high signal intensity on DWI. Note the sharp demarcation, vertically along the median raphe, of the pontine infarct, a common imaging appearance. In the fourth patient, a lateral medullary infarct (*white arrow*) is seen with hyperintensity on both DWI and T2-weighted scans.

PCA infarcts. Parenchymal enhancement, which is gyriform in pattern for territorial infarcts (▶ Fig. 1.74), is common during the first month, but is not typically seen in the first week. There is considerable variation however in the timing of parenchymal enhancement. Parenchymal enhancement, due to blood-brain barrier disruption, may persist for up to 8 weeks on MR following presentation. Enhancement of territorial and lacunar infarcts in the subacute time frame is very common on MR. Abnormal enhancement on MR permits differentiation of subacute from chronic infarcts, together with the identification of subacute infarcts in the midst of chronic white matter ischemic changes. Parenchymal enhancement can also be seen on CT, but is often less evident, and is generally restricted to gyriform like enhancement in territorial infarcts.

1.8.6 CT in Infarction

Signs specific to CT, which help in detection of large early MCA distribution infarcts on that modality, include a hyperdense MCA (acute thrombosis), loss of the insular ribbon (loss of gray-white matter differentiation involving the insular cortex), and loss of definition of the basal ganglia (▶ Fig. 1.75). CT perfusion (with the addition of cerebral blood volume [CBV], cerebral blood flow [CBF], and mean transit time [MTT]) has added greatly to the detectability of larger, early infarcts by this modality (▶ Fig. 1.76). This scan is routinely performed in many centers to determine the mismatch between brain with markedly reduced CBF (< 12 cm^3/100 g/minute) in the irreversibly infarcted core, and potentially salvageable brain tissue in areas

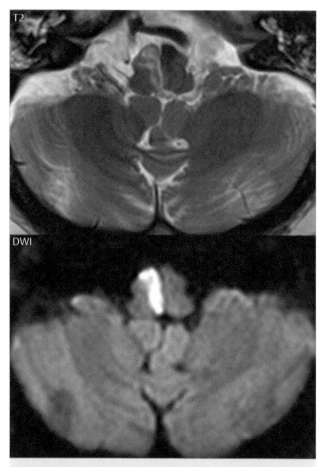

Fig. 1.70 Acute medial medullary infarct. Abnormal hyperintensity is noted in the right medial medulla on both T2- and diffusion-weighted scans, which corresponds to vasogenic and cytotoxic edema, respectively.

where CBF is reduced (12–22 cm³/100 g/minute, with normal being ≈ 50) or MTT prolonged, the ischemic penumbra (▶ Fig. 1.76). Treatment options in the acute time period include thrombolysis or thrombectomy, with the decision in part dictated by the presence and extent of an ischemic penumbra (tissue at risk) (▶ Fig. 1.76).

Without perfusion studies, early infarcts (< 24 to 48 hours) may be very difficult to detect on CT. Late subacute infarcts are usually isodense on CT, and thus also not apparent. In a very small number of cases on MR, a similar phenomenon is observed, with edema fading substantially on FLAIR. From personal experience, these infarcts are readily identifiable on postcontrast MR. Brain death is occasionally imaged on CT, with characteristic findings including global brain swelling and ischemia (with loss of gray-white matter differentiation), an important appearance to know and thus readily recognize prospectively (▶ Fig. 1.77).

1.8.7 Chronic Infarcts

With large chronic infarcts, findings include focal cerebral atrophy, with widened sulci and ex vacuo ventricular dilatation. Cystic encephalomalacia and gliosis are common (▶ Fig. 1.78). The former has CSF signal intensity on all pulse sequences, with the latter (gliosis) having high signal intensity on FLAIR and often noted surrounding the area of cystic change. Wallerian degeneration, also known as anterograde degeneration, describes the degeneration that occurs involving axons distal to the site of injury. This is reflected by loss of tissue volume, and in some instances by gliosis and thus abnormal high signal intensity on FLAIR. Wallerian degeneration is often seen in the corticospinal tract, in patients with a large chronic infarct involving the motor cortex. Gliosis can be seen in continuity in the posterior limb of the internal capsule, the cerebral

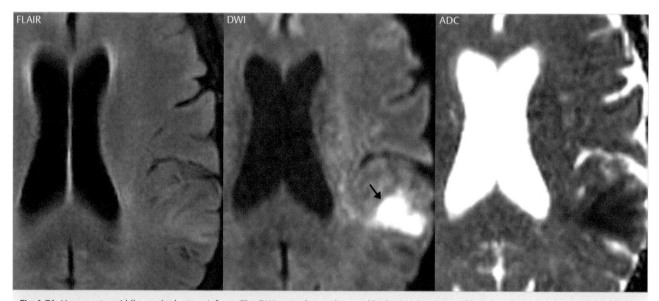

Fig. 1.71 Hyperacute middle cerebral artery infarct. The DWI scan shows abnormal high signal intensity (*black arrow*), confirmed to be restricted diffusion on the ADC map, consistent with cytotoxic edema in the posterior division of the left MCA. Given the early time frame of this hyperacute infarct (by definition < 6 hours), little vasogenic edema has developed, with only subtle hyperintensity on the FLAIR scan.

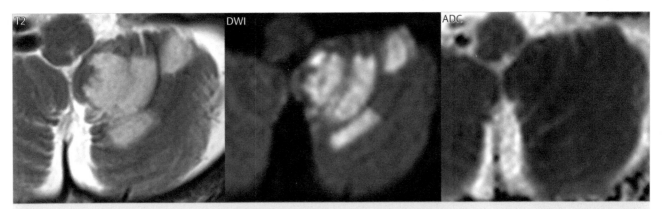

Fig. 1.72 Subacute PICA infarction. There is abnormal high signal intensity on T2- and diffusion-weighted axial scans in the left PICA territory. The ADC map however does not demonstrate restricted diffusion, thus identifying the findings on DWI to represent "T2 shine through". The absence of a true diffusion change dates the infarct to be more than 1 week old, thus late subacute in time frame.

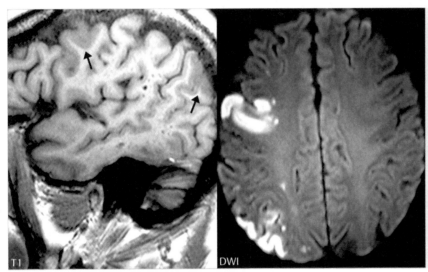

Fig. 1.73 MCA and watershed distribution early subacute infarcts. Vasogenic edema is noted on a sagittal T1-weighted scan, with abnormal low signal intensity, along several cortical gyri (*black arrows*). Cytotoxic edema is noted on the axial diffusion weighted scan, confirming the predominantly cortical distribution of ischemia. This infarct involves both the MCA territory in the frontal lobe and the watershed distribution in the parietal lobe (at the confluence of the arterial territories of the MCA, ACA, and PCA).

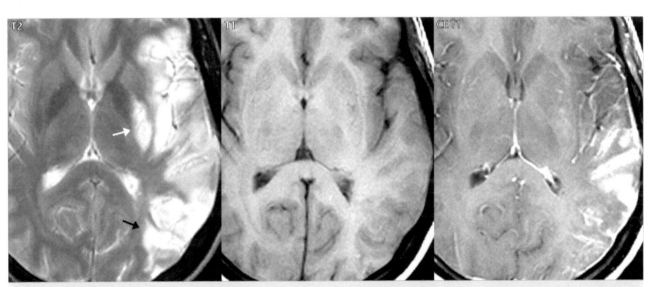

Fig. 1.74 Late subacute, enhancing, MCA infarct. A large infarct is identified on the T2-weighted scan, with extensive vasogenic edema reflected by abnormal high signal intensity, encompassing almost the entirety of the MCA territory at this level. Note the wedge shape of this territorial infarct, with involvement of both cortical gray and underlying white matter. Also included in this infarct is a portion of the lentiform nucleus more centrally (*white arrow*) and the watershed territory more posteriorly (*black arrow*). Post-contrast, a portion of the lesion demonstrates gyriform enhancement (due to blood-brain barrier disruption), characteristic for a late subacute infarct.

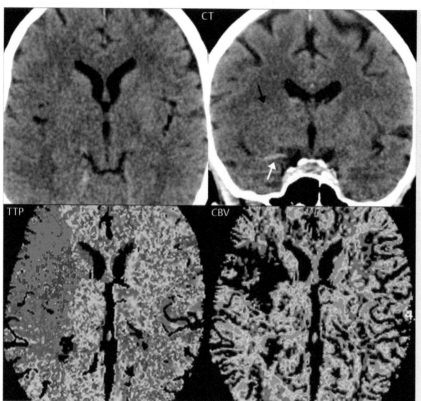

Fig. 1.75 Hyperacute middle cerebral artery infarct, with only subtle findings on conventional CT. There is mild hypodensity involving the right lentiform nucleus (seen both on the axial and coronal unenhanced CT, *black arrow*) together with a hyperdense right MCA sign (*white arrow*). A large hyperacute right MCA distribution infarct is confirmed on CBV and TTP maps, from the perfusion CT study. There is a mismatch between the smaller core of infarcted tissue seen on the CBV study and the larger penumbra, or tissue at risk, as identified on the TTP map, suggesting that the lesion may be amenable in the acute setting to therapy.

peduncle, the anterior pons, and extending into the medulla, where 80% of the fibers cross to the contralateral side. Dystrophic calcification, sometimes gyriform in pattern, can also be seen in chronic infarcts on CT.

1.8.8 Hemorrhagic Transformation

Hemorrhagic transformation can be seen with ischemic infarcts in up to one-quarter of cases. This is observed more commonly on MR than on CT, with MR more sensitive to blood products. Deoxyhemoglobin will be visualized on sequences sensitive to T2*, whereas methemoglobin—which is seen at a slightly later stage—is well visualized on T1-weighted sequences. Petechial hemorrhage is much more common than a parenchymal hematoma. Hemorrhage occurs when ischemic brain, with vessels in which the vascular endothelium is damaged, is reperfused. Predisposing factors include lysis of an embolus, opening of collaterals, restoration of normal blood pressure following hypotension, hypertension, and anticoagulation.

1.8.9 Periventricular Leukomalacia

Periventricular leukomalacia (PVL) is also referred to by the terms white matter injury of prematurity and hypoxic-ischemic encephalopathy and is the result of infarction of periventricular white matter in the premature infant. This disease is most commonly encountered on CT and MR in its end stage manifestation, in older infants and young children. Many PVL patients develop cerebral palsy or epilepsy. Premature infants are at greatest risk, with hypoxia or ischemia (decreased oxygen or blood flow) leading to white matter ischemia in watershed areas. In the neonatal time period, ultrasound is the modality of choice for screening, with MR also quite sensitive (due to restricted diffusion and the presence of hemorrhage). Late (chronic) findings in PVL include decreased quantity of periventricular white matter and abnormal increased signal intensity on T2-weighted scans in that remaining (gliosis) (▶ Fig. 1.79). The area most often affected is that adjacent to the lateral ventricles posteriorly. There may be focal dilatation of the ventricular system adjacent to the area of damage, depending on the extent of involvement. In most instances, the involvement is symmetric. Thinning of the corpus callosum is seen in more severe cases, which also typically involve the periventricular white matter both anteriorly and posteriorly. Although PVL is generally a diagnosis made on MR, gross structural changes may be seen in part on CT.

1.9 Dementia and Degenerative Disease

1.9.1 Alzheimer Disease

Alzheimer disease is today the most common diagnosed cause of dementia. Histology is nonspecific. CT and MR imaging signs are nonspecific, with generalized brain atrophy seen in advanced cases. Accentuated temporal lobe atrophy may be present.

1.9.2 Frontotemporal Dementia

This heterogeneous group of disorders is characterized by selective frontal and temporal lobe atrophy (▶ Fig. 1.80). Less common than Alzheimer disease, it also has a younger mean age of onset. The term Pick disease is today used for a distinct

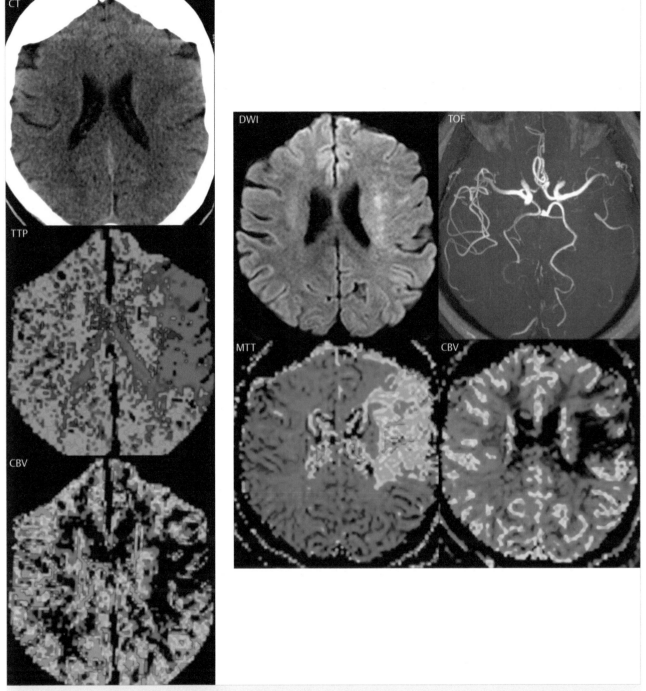

Fig. 1.76 Hyperacute middle cerebral artery infarct, CT, MR, and DSA (with diffusion perfusion mismatch and subsequent thrombectomy). Clinical presentation was within a few hours of symptom onset, with CT, MR and DSA performed in a rapid temporal sequence. Unenhanced CT was normal (**part 1**), specifically without evidence of parenchymal hemorrhage. The area of ischemia (involving a portion of the MCA distribution) is well identified on the TTP image, with a smaller region of reduced perfusion (CBV). On MR (**part 2**), only a small area of abnormality involving the white matter of the corona radiata is noted on diffusion weighted imaging (with restricted diffusion, confirmed on the ADC map, not shown). There is a paucity of left MCA branches on the TOF MRA, reflecting either occlusion or slow flow. MTT and CBV derived from the MR study demonstrate similar findings to CT, with a large diffusion perfusion mismatch ("penumbra" or tissue at risk).

(*Continued*)

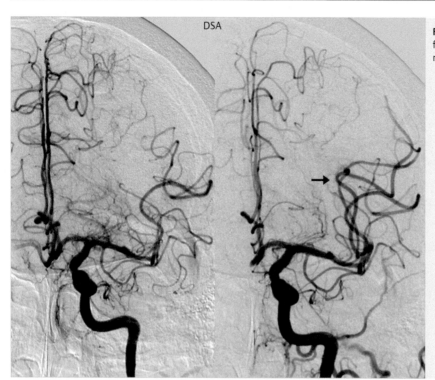

DSA

Fig. 1.76 (*Continued*) DSA performed prior to and following thrombectomy (**part 3**) demonstrates recanalization of the superior MCA trunk (*arrow*).

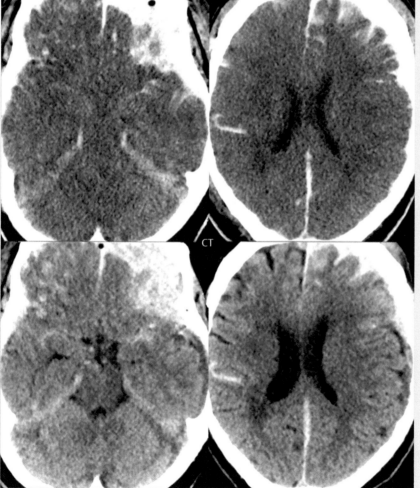

CT

Fig. 1.77 Brain death. An unenhanced CT at two anatomic levels reveals global loss of gray-white matter differentiation and generalized efface-ment of the sulci and cisterns, reflecting massive cerebral edema. There is prominent acute sub-arachnoid blood. The upper set of images is 24 hours subsequent to the lower set of images, with the patient now intubated and in a profound coma. The tips of the temporal horns, the sulci surrounding the brainstem, the cerebral sulci, and the lateral ventricles are normal on the immediate prior exam. Note the interval decrease in size of the lateral ventricles, more apparent by comparison with the prior exam, reflecting the markedly increased intracranial pressure. Bilateral uncal herniation is also present. This 88-year-old patient fell down a flight of stairs, with the clinical presentation including multiple skull fractures and widespread subarachnoid hemorrhage.

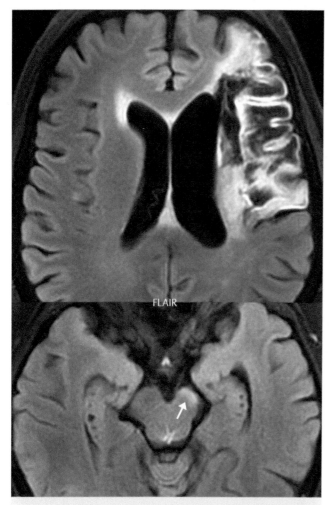

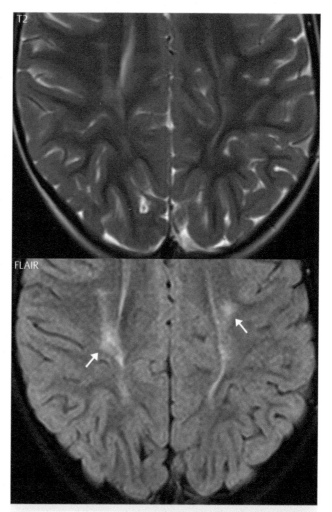

Fig. 1.78 Chronic MCA infarct, Wallerian degeneration. A large chronic left MCA distribution infarct is noted, with both gliosis (high signal intensity) and cystic encephalomalacia (low signal intensity) on FLAIR together with ex-vacuo dilatation of the adjacent lateral ventricle. In the brainstem, the left cerebral peduncle is small, with abnormal high signal intensity consistent with gliosis (*white arrow*), due to secondary anterograde degeneration of axons and accompanying myelin sheaths.

Fig. 1.79 Periventricular leukomalacia. There is loss of normal white matter adjacent to the ventricular system posteriorly, together with gliosis (*white arrows*) in the immediate periventricular white matter, the latter best seen on FLAIR.

neurodegenerative disease within this group, defined by the presence of Pick bodies (dark staining aggregates of proteins on histopathology).

1.9.3 Multisystem Atrophy

The most accepted classification of multisystem atrophy (MSA) considers symptomatology a key for diagnosis. The disease is designated as MSA-P if parkinsonism is the main symptom, whether associated or not with autonomic dysfunction. Striatonigral degeneration is the old term for the same disease. On the other hand, if cerebellar ataxia is the main symptom, once again whether associated or not with autonomic dysfunction, it is designated as MSA-C. Olivopontocerebellar atrophy/degeneration is the old term for this disease. MR imaging in Parkinson disease reveals loss of the substantia nigra pars compacta, with reduced width in a lateral to medial gradient (most prominently of the more lateral portion), best evaluated on dedicated inversion recovery T1-weighted sequences. In MSA-C, there is atrophy of the pons, middle cerebellar peduncles, olives (which lie along and form the anterolateral margin of the medulla), and cerebellar hemispheres. The "hot cross bun" sign is also described in MSA-C, with cruciform high T2 signal intensity on axial imaging within the pons, reflecting selected loss of myelinated transverse fibers and neurons in the pontine raphe (▶ Fig. 1.81). MR findings may appear many years after clinical findings, and alone cannot confirm the diagnosis.

Atrophy of the vermis, most commonly, but often including the cerebellar hemispheres also occurs in up to 40% of chronic alcoholics. It is irreversible. Cerebellar atrophy is known as well to be associated with the chronic use of Dilantin (phenytoin) for treatment of seizures (▶ Fig. 1.82).

1.9.4 Small Vessel White Matter Ischemic Disease

Patients with chronic small vessel white matter ischemic disease, an extremely common entity in the elderly patient population, demonstrate multiple, nonspecific, patchy foci of

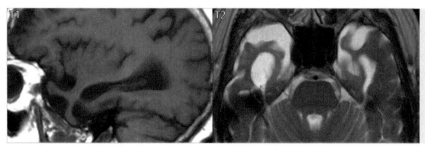

Fig. 1.80 Frontotemporal dementia. There is marked, disproportionate atrophy of the anterior temporal lobes, reflected by loss of brain substance, prominent sulci, and dilatation of the tip of the temporal horns. The degree of frontal involvement in this patient was less.

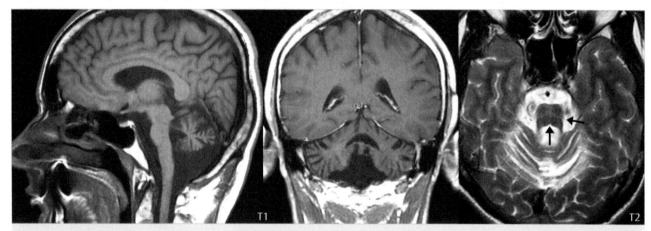

Fig. 1.81 Multisystem atrophy (MSA-C). Sagittal and coronal T1- and axial T2-weighted scans reveal atrophy of the vermis, cerebellar hemispheres, and pons. Also noted is the hot cross bun sign, with cruciform high signal intensity in the pons on the T2-weighted axial scan (*arrows*).

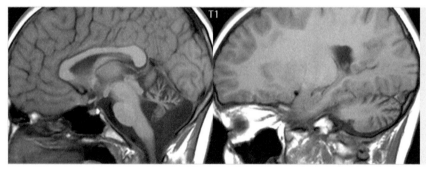

Fig. 1.82 Cerebellar atrophy. Both the vermis and cerebellar hemispheres are atrophic, with loss of brain substance and prominent sulci. The etiology in this pediatric patient was chronic high-dose Dilantin administration.

increased signal intensity on T2-weighted scans in the periventricular white matter, centrum semiovale, and subcortical white matter (▶ Fig. 1.83). The involvement is usually relatively symmetric when comparing the right and left hemispheres. The foci seen on MR correspond pathologically to areas of necrosis, small infarcts, demyelination, astroglia proliferation, and arteriolosclerosis. In long standing advanced disease, the lesions may appear confluent. Progression with age is seen, and in personal experience correlated with smoking, granted that there are many possible etiologies and risk factors. Although seen in advanced disease as generalized periventricular low density, CT poorly visualizes the disease process. On MR, FLAIR is the sequence of choice for best disease visualization.

1.10 Vasculitis and Vasculitides

1.10.1 Sickle Cell Disease

There is a high incidence of infarcts in patients with sickle cell disease, with these commonly watershed in distribution.

Clinically silent lesions, ischemic in etiology, are noted in deep white matter, with the MR appearance consistent with gliosis (▶ Fig. 1.84).

1.10.2 Moyamoya Disease

In Moyamoya disease there is marked stenosis and/or occlusion of the terminal internal carotid arteries, together with the proximal anterior and middle cerebral artery branches. An extensive network of small collateral arterial vessels develops at the base of the brain, involving the lenticulostriate and thalamoperforating arteries (the "cloud of smoke" on angiography). Moyamoya is predominantly a disease of children, with an increased incidence in the Japanese and Korean populations, and relentless progression. MR reveals the multiple tiny collaterals, as flow voids, both in the basal ganglia and within enlarged CSF spaces (▶ Fig. 1.85). MRA and CT angiography (CTA) reveal the narrowing of the supraclinoid internal carotid arteries, and preferential vascular disease involving the anterior circulation. Collateral vessels from the extracranial circulation (external carotid

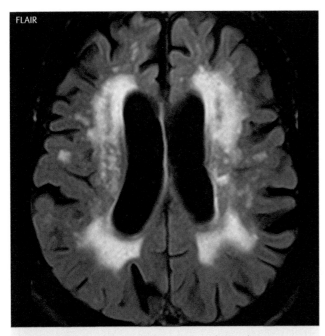

Fig. 1.83 Chronic small vessel white matter ischemic disease. There is prominent, symmetric, and partially confluent abnormal high signal intensity in the periventricular and more distal white matter that is best visualized on FLAIR. Note the accompanying mild ventricular enlargement and sulcal prominence in this elderly patient.

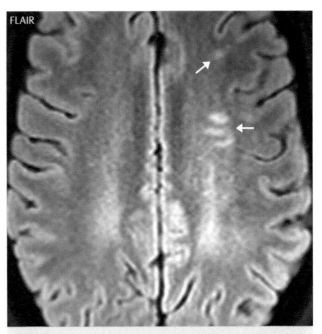

Fig. 1.84 Sickle cell disease. Although distinct infarcts may be seen early in childhood, the most common presentation is that of small, focal, nonspecific white matter hyperintense lesions (*arrows*) on FLAIR, and thus could potentially be confused with multiple sclerosis. To some extent these may lie within the watershed territory in the deep white matter.

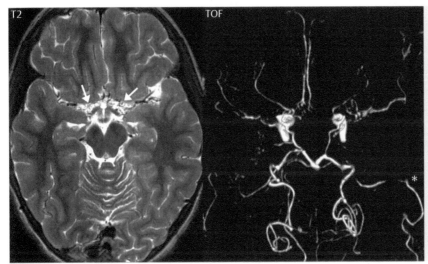

Fig. 1.85 Moyamoya. On the axial T2-weighted image, the visualized portions of the middle cerebral arteries are thin in caliber and threadlike. In the cisterns there is a myriad of tiny collaterals, seen as a tangle of small flow voids (*white arrows*). The time of flight MRA demonstrates predominantly anterior circulation disease, with abrupt narrowing/stenosis of the supraclinoid internal carotid arteries, small MCA branches bilaterally, collateral flow from the posterior circulation, and collaterals from the extracranial to intracranial circulation (*asterisk*).

artery) may also be visualized. Multiple, bilateral hemispheric and deep white matter infarcts may be present, predominantly in the carotid distribution and in watershed regions. Surgical treatment of moyamoya includes both direct and indirect revascularization.

1.10.3 CADASIL and Behçet Disease

Two other vasculitides of note are CADASIL and Behçet disease. The most common imaging presentation for CADASIL, an acronym for cerebral autosomal dominant arteriopathy with subcortical infarcts and leukoencephalopathy, is that of multiple bilateral lesions involving the basal ganglia and white matter.

Behçet disease is characterized by skin lesions, with CNS involvement in 25%, notably of the brainstem and in particular the cerebral peduncles.

1.10.4 Systemic Lupus Erythematosus

Systemic lupus erythematosus (SLE) is multisystem autoimmune disease characterized by vasculitis, with CNS disease seen in 40% of patients. The most common imaging finding is that of multiple small subcortical and deep white matter lesions, which are hyperintense on FLAIR (▸ Fig. 1.86). As with most brain parenchymal disease, CT is relatively poor for lesion visualization, with MR the imaging exam of choice. Discrete infarcts

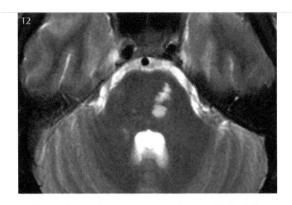

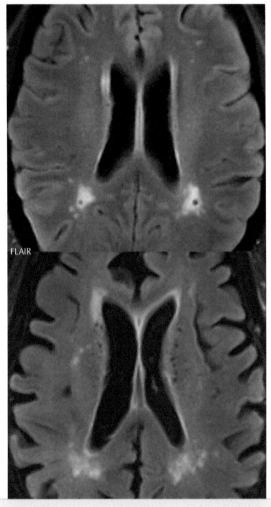

Fig. 1.86 Systemic lupus erythematosus (SLE). **Part 1:** As with sickle cell, distinct arterial territory infarcts can be seen, but are not common. A chronic unilateral pontine infarct is noted in this 35-year-old woman with SLE. **Part 2:** The most common imaging appearance in SLE is however that of nonspecific focal white matter lesions, best seen on FLAIR. The first image in part 2 presents a scan from the same patient (as part 1), with the more common and very nonspecific findings of mild focal periventricular and deep white matter disease. The second image in part 2 is presented for comparison, from a different patient, with—on first glance—a similar appearance within white matter. But this simply represents chronic small vessel white matter ischemic disease, in an elderly patient, with the correct diagnosis more evident upon recognition of the accompanying findings of prominence of the sulci and ventricular system, due to atrophy.

are less common, but occur, and scans may reflect either an acute presentation or simply the chronic residual of such an infarct. Volume loss, focal or generalized, is seen long term in SLE. The differential diagnosis, strictly on an imaging basis, includes MS, chronic small vessel white matter ischemic disease, and other vasculitides.

1.11 Vascular Lesions

1.11.1 Aneurysms

By definition, an aneurysm is an abnormal dilatation, typically saccular or fusiform in shape, of an artery. Intracranial aneurysms are thought to result from hemodynamic stress, abnormal remodeling, and inflammation. Saccular aneurysms are generally found at arterial branch points, although many are not clearly associated with branch vessels. Multiple lobes and daughter sacs ("Murphy's tit") are common in ruptured aneurysms. Rupture is typically at the apex. Although variable percentages in terms of sites of occurrence are published in the scientific literature, for unruptured aneurysms without subarachnoid hemorrhage, MCA (▶ Fig. 1.87), cavernous carotid, and distal internal carotid are the most common (about 20% each), followed by PCOM and ACOM (▶ Fig. 1.88, including ACA) aneurysms (about 10% each). Posterior circulation aneurysms are least common (▶ Fig. 1.89), with about 5% vertebrobasilar/PCA and 5% basilar tip. The prevalence of aneurysms in the general population, without subarachnoid hemorrhage, is about 3%. The prevalence is higher in patients with atherosclerosis and also increases with age.

Multiple aneurysms are found in about 20% of all aneurysm cases. Risk factors for multiple aneurysms include smoking and hypertension (which are felt to be risk factors as well for simply aneurysm formation and subarachnoid hemorrhage). Infundibula, conical dilatations at an artery origin, are benign incidental findings not to be confused with an aneurysm. Intracranially, an infundibulum is most common at the PCOM origin.

There are several medical conditions well known to be associated with aneurysms. The two most important are polycystic kidney disease and a familial disposition. Estimates of prevalence of intracranial aneurysms in autosomal dominant polycystic kidney disease (ADPKD) range widely (up to 40%). The risk of aneurysm rupture with subarachnoid hemorrhage appears to be higher than in the general population, with presentation at a younger age. Twenty-five percent of patients with ADPKD and an aneurysm develop a second aneurysm within 15 years. Screening by noninvasive imaging is reasonable in ADPKD patients with a known aneurysm or prior subarachnoid hemorrhage or in patients who have a familial history.

In considering familial aneurysms, specifically when at least two first-degree relatives are affected, assessments of prevalence range widely, with 10% likely a reasonable estimate. There is a predilection for the middle cerebral artery, as well as for multiple aneurysms and subarachnoid hemorrhage at a younger age. Screening of such patients, if pursued, should be by noninvasive imaging. Other less common conditions with an increased incidence of intracranial aneurysms include Ehlers-Danlos syndrome type IV, α1-antitrypsin deficiency, fibromuscular dysplasia, and in association with an arteriovenous malformation.

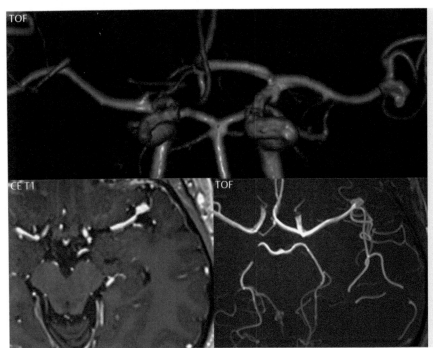

Fig. 1.87 MCA bifurcation aneurysm. A small multilobulated aneurysm is noted on the left, visualized on TOF MRA and on planar imaging post-contrast as well as.

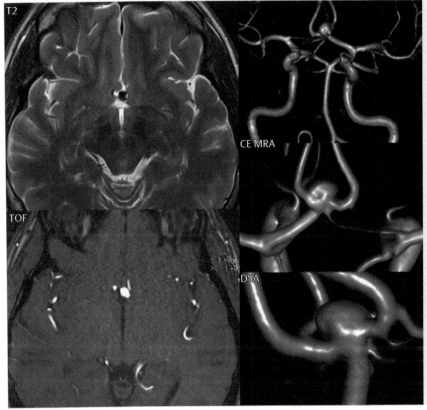

Fig. 1.88 ACOM aneurysm. A flow void is noted in the region of the anterior communicating artery (ACOM) on an axial T2-weighted image, with signal intensity corresponding to arterial flow on an axial source image from a 3D TOF MRA. CE MRA images further confirm the aneurysm, with the right A1 segment of the ACA noted to be very small in diameter. DSA confirms that the aneurysm has a wide neck, an important finding for treatment planning.

The natural history of unruptured intracranial aneurysms is controversial. The overall risk of rupture is likely 1 to 2% per year. The rate of rupture appears to be lower for small anterior circulation aneurysms. Larger aneurysms are at greater risk for rupture. If an aneurysm ruptures (with subarachnoid hemorrhage), the mortality rate is very high, greater than 50%.

Although a small saccular aneurysm may be visualized on a conventional MR or CT scan, 3D time of flight (TOF) MR angiography (MRA) and CT angiography (CTA) are specifically employed for detection and delineation. CTA is the modality of choice in the acute presentation with subarachnoid hemorrhage, while 3D TOF MRA is often used for detection and

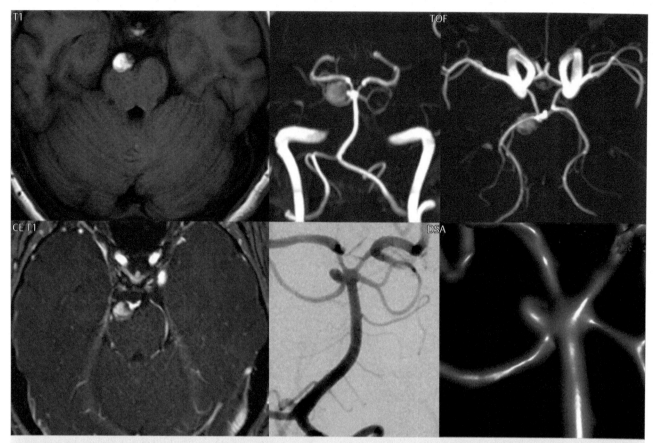

Fig. 1.89 Superior cerebellar artery aneurysm. A predominantly hyperintense lesion is noted on the right, anterior to the pons on an axial T1-weighted image, causing mild adjacent deformity. Additional scans identify the abnormal high signal intensity to represent methemoglobin, in a SCA aneurysm that is predominantly thrombosed and has only a small residual patent component (medially). The TOF exams, with thick coronal and axial MIPs illustrated, visualize both the methemoglobin (with slight hyperintensity) and the small patent portion of the aneurysm. DSA identifies the patent lumen of the aneurysm, but not the much larger thrombosed component.

evaluation of asymptomatic aneurysms, as well as for correlation and further definition of lesions in the acute setting and on follow-up. Modern scanners easily detect aneurysms as small as 2 mm in diameter. Treatment of intracranial brain aneurysms that have bled, or are deemed to present a significant risk to the patient because of potential bleeding in the future, is by either surgical clipping or endovascular occlusion. Surgery is much less common today, although not all aneurysms can be treated by an endovascular approach.

Surgical treatment was considered in the past to be the gold standard for treatment; however, complication rates are high. In surgical treatment of unruptured aneurysms, the mortality rate is about 3%, with permanent morbidity seen in up to 20%. In surgical treatment of ruptured aneurysms, the mortality rate is about 15%, with substantial, permanent morbidity in an additional 15%. The frequency of a residual aneurysm is 4 to 8%.

The complication rate with endovascular treatment of an unruptured brain aneurysm is approximately 10%. The rate of permanent complications is less than half this figure. Repeat hemorrhage is uncommon, seen in 3%. The advent of detachable coils, led by the development of the Guglielmi detachable coil (GDC) conceived in the early 1980s, enabled development of the field of aneurysm coiling as we know it today. With this system, until the coil is in satisfactory position, it remains attached to the pusher wire. Detachment is achieved by application of a low-amplitude electrical current, causing electrolysis of the connection between the coil and the wire. Numerous technical refinements have followed, with an array of shapes and sizes available. Wide-neck aneurysms present an additional challenge, with one current approach being deployment of a thin wire mesh stent across the neck, within the parent vessel. Coils can then placed via a microcatheter that enters the aneurysm through the interstices of the stent, with the latter acting as a scaffold to hold the coils within the aneurysm. Recurrence after coiling (defined as recanalization sufficiently large to allow retreatment, either surgical or endovascular) is seen in about 20% of patients 1 to 2 years following initial treatment.

Most cavernous carotid aneurysms are discovered incidentally. Large aneurysms within the cavernous sinus can cause symptoms due to compression of the cranial nerves that run therein (▶ Fig. 1.90). The most common symptoms are diplopia, due to involvement of the oculomotor nerves, and pain, due to involvement of the trigeminal nerve. Rupture is seen in well less than 10%. Rupture often produces a carotid-cavernous fistula. Subarachnoid hemorrhage is rare.

Paraclinoid ICA aneurysms arise between the distal dural ring and the origin of PCOM. There are three major types: aneurysms that arise from the ophthalmic or superior hypophyseal artery origins and carotid cave aneurysms. Carotid cave aneurysms arise from the clinoid segment of the ICA (proximal to the

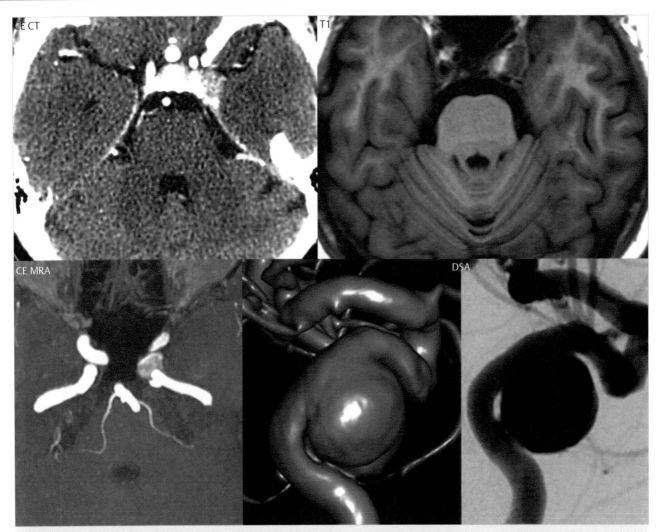

Fig. 1.90 Aneurysm, cavernous carotid artery. A small mass lesion is noted within the left cavernous sinus on both CT and MR (axial imaging), with CT revealing enhancement therein. MRA confirms this to be an aneurysm, with the DSA provided for comparison (from an initial balloon test occlusion study). This 12 mm aneurysm of the cavernous segment of the internal carotid artery was subsequently coiled, without complication.

origin of the ophthalmic artery) and project medially. These are not infrequently noted incidentally on TOF MRA of the circle of Willis. Ophthalmic artery aneurysms typically project superiorly and medially. Of symptomatic lesions, half present with visual symptoms (due to impingement on the optic nerve) and half with subarachnoid hemorrhage. Coiling is preferred due to the risk of visual loss with surgery. Superior hypophyseal artery aneurysms arise from inferomedial aspect of the ICA, projecting also in this direction. This vessel arises just distal to the ophthalmic artery.

PCOM aneurysms, the most common supraclinoid ICA aneurysm, typically project inferiorly and laterally. A small percentage (< 10%) of all unruptured intracranial aneurysms present with mass effect, typically cranial nerve palsy. Of these, oculomotor palsy due to impingement on the third cranial nerve by a PCOM aneurysm is the most common. Rupture of a PCOM aneurysm is a common cause of subarachnoid hemorrhage. In this instance, the epicenter of acute subarachnoid blood is typically located laterally in the suprasellar and ambient cisterns. At the carotid terminus, the internal carotid artery branches into the MCA and ACA. Aneurysms here are not uncommon and tend to be large.

As with all intracranial aneurysms, screening MR is very effective for diagnosis/visualization of nonruptured anterior communicating artery (ACOM) aneurysms. Attention to the characteristic areas where aneurysms occur intracranially is mandatory in exam interpretation. Rupture of an ACOM aneurysm, like that of a PCOM aneurysm, is a common cause of subarachnoid hemorrhage (▶ Fig. 1.91). With acute rupture, hemorrhage occurring in the pericallosal cistern is somewhat specific, with hemorrhage inferomedially in the frontal lobe less so. Anterior cerebral artery aneurysms arising distal to the anterior communicating artery are much less common, but still compose a significant percentage (perhaps 5%) of all intracranial aneurysms. Most are small and occur at the A2–A3 junction, being referred to as pericallosal artery aneurysms. Although an azygos ACA (azygous A2 segment) is uncommon, this anatomic variant is strongly associated with aneurysms, specifically at the termination of the A2 segment.

Middle cerebral artery aneurysms are the third most common cause of aneurysmal subarachnoid hemorrhage, in incidence behind ACOM and PCOM artery aneurysms. Acute subarachnoid hemorrhage in the sylvian fissure can occur with internal carotid,

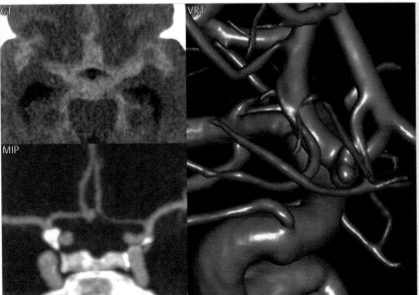

Fig. 1.91 Acute subarachnoid hemorrhage from a small ACOM aneurysm. The images presented include an axial unenhanced CT, a coronal MIP from the CTA, and a 3D magnified view of the aneurysm from the CTA, obtained using volume rendering technique (VRT). The latter shows the distal internal carotid artery, the two anterior cerebral arteries, and the small multi-lobulated aneurysm originating from the ACOM, near its origin from the anterior cerebral artery on one side. There is diffuse acute subarachnoid hemorrhage, symmetric in distribution (thus favoring the diagnosis of an ACOM aneurysm), filling the suprasellar cistern and sylvian fissures.

PCOM, or MCA aneurysms. Eighty-five percent of MCA aneurysms occur at the bifurcation/trifurcation. More distal aneurysms are likely to be infectious or inflammatory in origin.

Half of all posterior circulation aneurysms are located at the basilar tip. Surgery is difficult in this location, with endovascular treatment (coiling) the technique of choice. The most characteristic distribution of blood is that of perimesencephalic or interpeduncular cisternal hemorrhage in combination with midbrain hemorrhage. Aneurysms at the origin of the posterior inferior cerebellar artery (PICA), from the vertebral artery, account for about 2% of all intracranial aneurysms. Due to this incidence, acquisition of time of flight MRA exams in all cases to include the origin of PICA is strongly suggested, with one major purpose of this exam being screening for aneurysms.

About 80% of nontraumatic subarachnoid hemorrhage (SAH) occurs due to a ruptured aneurysm. Thus 20% of patients with spontaneous SAH will have a negative angiographic workup. Within this latter category of patients, there are two important entities to remember. The first is perimesencephalic nonaneurysmal subarachnoid hemorrhage. In this entity, subarachnoid hemorrhage is present anterior to the pons, often in an asymmetric pattern and within the ambient cistern as well. The bleed is thought to be venous in origin. Neurologic changes are uncommon and the clinical outcome excellent. The second entity is reversible cerebrovascular constriction syndrome, seen primarily in women. Presentation with a thunderclap headache is common. Up to a third of patients with this syndrome will have SAH. On angiography, whether DSA or MRA, pathognomonic segmental vasoconstriction is seen. Prognosis is very good, with symptoms and angiographic findings resolving within a week. Other important, though much less common, causes of SAH include AVM, dural AVF, disorders of coagulation, cocaine, vasculitis, and venous sinus thrombosis. In addition, it should always be kept in mind that the most common cause of SAH is trauma.

The classic clinical presentation of aneurysmal subarachnoid hemorrage is sudden onset of "the worst headache of my life." Other characteristic symptoms that should raise the suspicion of acute SAH from an aneurysm include nausea and vomiting, diminished consciousness, and focal neurologic findings. The presentation on CT is that of prominent hyperdense blood in the subarachnoid space, commonly also intraventricular. CTA assumes today the primary role in the workup of spontaneous SAH, having replaced catheter angiography. The latter is still indicated in cases of acute SAH not explained by CTA.

In the acute setting, with a small ruptured aneurysm, it is well known that a small percentage of patients can have a normal X-ray angiogram. This is presumed to be due to vasospasm, thrombosis, or mass effect, with nonfilling of the aneurysm, despite the abundant subarachnoid blood. It stands to reason that MRA and CTA can also be negative in this instance. Regardless, for angiogram-negative SAH, MR remains a diagnostic option. Repeat angiography (DSA) is indicated if a ruptured aneurysm remains clinically suspect, with the yield of a second such exam as high as 15%.

Up to one third of patients presenting with a ruptured intracranial aneurysm will die within the first month. Most deaths occur within 2 weeks, and over half occur within 48 hours. Long-term morbidity is substantial. The highest risk of rebleeding occurs within the first 24 hours (up to 20%). Half of all patients re-bleed within 6 months. Patients with more severe symptoms upon admission and those with larger aneurysms are at greater risk for re-bleeding. Early treatment of an aneurysm, within 24 hours (prior to the onset of vasospasm), by either surgery or coiling is indicated in order to minimize the risk of re-hemorrhage and possible complications from treatment. After treatment, the risk of recurrent SAH continues to be substantially higher than in the general population.

Hydrocephalus is common following SAH. When evaluating a scan, close inspection of the tips of the temporal horns can be particularly helpful in diagnosing ventricular enlargement. Chronic shunt-dependent post-SAH hydrocephalus is also common, occurring in up to half of patients. Seizures, in the acute time period, as well as chronically, are not uncommon (occurring in <10%).

Symptomatic vasospasm, seen in approximately one fourth of patients, is the major cause of mortality and morbidity following SAH. Angiographically, it is defined as a greater than 50%

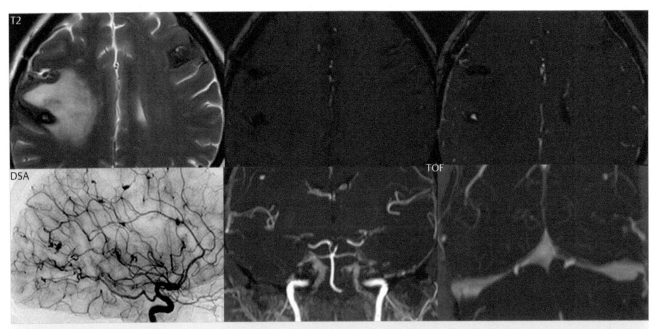

Fig. 1.92 Multiple cerebral aneurysms, due to myxomatous emboli. Several small lesions with peripheral hemosiderin are noted on the axial T2-weighted scan, one with marked associated vasogenic edema. Comparison of axial source images from a TOF exam both prior to and following contrast enhancement reveals a small focus of enhancement within one of the previously noted lesions. A lateral projection from DSA confirms multiple peripheral cerebral aneurysms, with several visualized (as small, round enhancing foci) in the presented thick section, coronal MIP images from an enhanced TOF MRA.

reduction in arterial caliber and involves both large and small intracranial arteries. Vasospasm rarely occurs prior to day 3, is maximal at 1 week, and resolves in most patients by 2 weeks. The presence of red blood cells (RBCs) is necessary for vasospasm to occur, and the timing of the onset of vasospasm correlates with that of RBC lysis. Clinical features include confusion and a decline in consciousness. The more blood present on the CT at presentation, the greater are the likelihood and severity of vasospasm. Catheter angiography remains the gold standard for diagnosis. CTA is excellent for detection of significant vasospasm involving large intracranial vessels. Regional areas of decreased CBF indicative of symptomatic vasospasm can be detected by CT perfusion studies.

The term mycotic aneurysm is used colloquially for all infectious aneurysms, although strictly the term mycotic refers to fungal. Infectious aneurysms are uncommon, accounting for less than 1% of all intracranial aneurysms. Most mycotic aneurysms are caused by septic emboli. The majority of patients have endocarditis. Most present with rupture, and the majority are within the MCA territory. Multiple lesions occur in 20% (▶ Fig. 1.92). Streptococcus and Staphylococcus are the most common causes, with intracranial fungal aneurysms actually rare. Infectious aneurysms and their adjacent vessels are fragile. First-line therapy for unruptured infectious aneurysms is antibiotics. Surgery is reserved for hemorrhagic lesions or lesions that enlarge despite antibiotic therapy. Historically, the mortality rate was high, up to 40%, although recent reports describe good outcomes in 80%. Mycotic aneurysms are usually peripheral in location, in distinction to saccular aneurysms. Conventional CT and MR imaging is nonspecific in regard to appearance, demonstrating a small enhancing lesion with surrounding cerebral edema.

A giant aneurysm by definition is one that is ≥25 mm in diameter. These can be saccular or fusiform in shape and are more common in the posterior circulation (with other frequent locations including the cavernous and supraclinoid internal carotid artery). They comprise 5% of all intracranial aneurysms and occur in older patients. Intraluminal thrombus is common. The annual rate of rupture is high. Clinical presentation may be due to mass effect (cranial nerve palsies) or rupture (subarachnoid hemorrhage). Giant aneurysms may not be depicted in their entirety on 3D TOF MRA due to slow flow within the aneurysm, and in this instance, correlation with 2D TOF and conventional (non-flow-related) images, or additional contrast-enhanced 3D MRA, can be helpful in delineating the true luminal extent. Comparison of conventional MR scans with source images from the MRA exam improves recognition of thrombus. On rare occasion, with giant aneurysms, layered thrombus is present.

Dolichoectatic and fusiform aneurysms are uncommon, accounting for < 2% of all intracranial aneurysms. Compression of adjacent structures (brainstem, cranial nerve) is a common cause of symptoms. Rupture is less frequent than with saccular aneurysms. Intraluminal thrombus can be present (▶ Fig. 1.93). Vertebrobasilar dolichoectasia is generally included within this category.

1.11.2 Vascular Malformations

An arteriovenous malformation (AVM) consists of a nidus (tangle) of tightly packed, dilated, tortuous arteries and veins, without an intervening capillary network, with the result being arteriovenous shunting. It is the most common symptomatic vascular malformation of brain. The risk of hemorrhage is 2 to 4% per year, with each episode having a 30% risk of

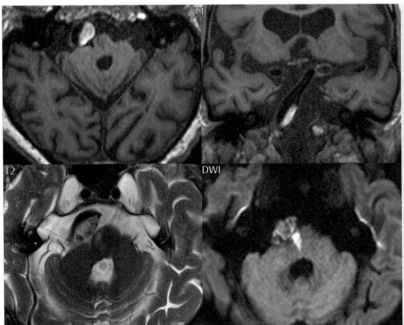

Fig. 1.93 Non-obstructing clot/thrombus in the basilar artery. Methemoglobin clot is visualized medially within a focal aneurysmal dilatation of the basilar artery (dolichoectasia) on axial and coronal T1-weighted scans. Evaluation of axial T2-weighted and DWI scans reveals a small acute infarct, located within the brainstem just medial to the clot, and presumed to be secondary to occlusion of small paramedian penetrating branches from the basilar artery.

death. Most lesions present clinically between 20 and 40 years of age, and involve peripheral branches of the ACA or MCA. Aneurysms of the feeding arteries (perinidal aneurysms), due to high flow, are seen in less than 10% of cases. AVMs are considered to be congenital in origin; they are one tenth as common as aneurysms. Hemodynamically, AVMs have high flow and low resistance.

AVMs are well depicted on conventional, cross-sectional MR imaging (due to flow phenomena), with TOF MRA used to better demonstrate the nidus, enlarged arterial feeding vessels, and enlarged draining veins (▶ Fig. 1.94). On occasion, a small AVM will be visualized only on MRA and not well seen on other MR sequences. On precontrast conventional MR scans, multiple serpiginous vessels, most with low signal intensity (SI) due to rapid flow, are typically visualized. Contrast enhancement often provides improved visualization of the nidus, together with the enlarged draining veins.

Between the large draining veins there will be preserved normal brain parenchyma. Gliosis is uncommon. There is usually little mass effect, with vasogenic edema unusual. Acute hemorrhage is well visualized on unenhanced CT; however, on such scans, even large AVMs may not be detected. Calcification is seen in the minority of cases (▶ Fig. 1.95). Enhancement on CT (together with CTA) provides visualization of the nidus and large draining veins. DSA remains the gold standard for evaluation of an AVM, with one major advantage being the clarification of feeding vessels and draining veins. For example, for a convexity lesion, contributions from the ACA and MCA can be distinguished. This can also be done currently by MR, but requires specialty expertise.

The risk of hemorrhage from an AVM is 2 to 4% per year (▶ Fig. 1.96). The risk of re-bleeding is increased for several years following a prior hemorrhage. Hemorrhage is the most common presenting symptom (seen in half of all cases), followed by seizures (seen in one quarter).

Treatment includes surgery, radiosurgery, and embolization. Asymptomatic lesions, difficult to treat lesions, and patients at high risk for complications warrant conservative treatment. Lesions are stratified according to surgical risk by

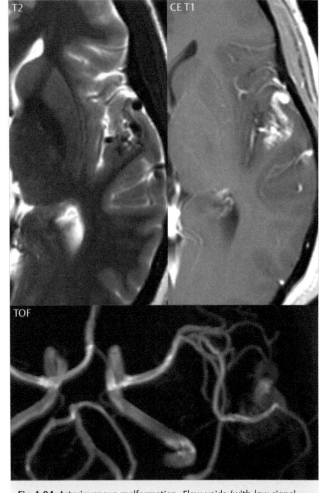

Fig. 1.94 Arteriovenous malformation. Flow voids (with low signal intensity) are demonstrated on the T2-weighted scan, with enhancement post-contrast of both the lesion nidus and a large draining vein, in this temporal lobe lesion. The 3D TOF MRA demonstrates flow in both of these components, together with enlargement of feeding branches from the middle cerebral artery.

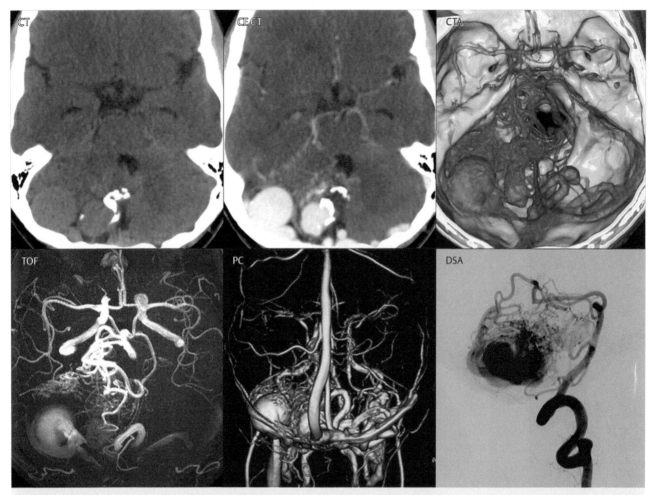

Fig. 1.95 Posterior fossa arteriovenous malformation. Although AVMs can be difficult to detect on unenhanced CT, calcifications – as present with this lesion – are not uncommon and can be a key for diagnosis. There is prominent mass effect upon the adjacent cerebellum, together with mild compression of the fourth ventricle. Both the CTA and the TOF exam demonstrate the arterial inflow to be primarily from the PCA, SCA, AICA, and PICA on the right. The venous outflow is predominately via the right and left transverse sinuses, with a giant venous varix seen on the right.

the Spetzler-Martin grading system, which assigns points relative to size, location, and venous drainage. Lower grade lesions have lower permanent morbidity and mortality following surgery (for example, with permanent morbidity < 5% and mortality < 4% in Spetzler-Martin grades I-III).

Radiosurgery delivers a high radiation dose to the isocenter, with a substantially lower dose to nontargeted structures. Radiotherapy causes endothelial damage, leading eventually to stenosis of the vessels in the treated area and subsequent occlusion. This approach is minimally invasive, low risk (but specifically not free of complications, with permanent neurologic deficits seen in 5%), and effective for smaller lesions (≤ 3 cm). Its disadvantage is that obliteration is delayed, occurring over 2 to 3 years following treatment.

Embolization can be performed for palliation (treatment of part of the lesion) or prior to surgery. The latter is performed to reduce the volume of the nidus and to occlude feeders that might be difficult to reach by surgery. Cure rates (complete obliteration) are low for treatment of AVMs with embolization alone (5–10%).

The vein of Galen aneurysmal malformation is easily recognized on MRI or enhanced CT due to the presence of a large midline varix in the neonate or infant (▸ Fig. 1.97). The

epicenter of the varix is in the quadrigeminal plate cistern. Presenting symptoms are due to high-output cardiac failure, with embolization the treatment of choice.

A dural arteriovenous fistula (AVF) is an acquired vascular malformation of the brain that is most commonly seen in the posterior fossa. The etiology is believed to be occlusion of a venous sinus, with recanalization along the walls of the sinus leading to numerous direct connections between small feeding arteries and venous drainage. Clinical complications include venous infarction, parenchymal hemorrhage, and subdural hematoma. On MR and enhanced CT large superficial dural-based veins may be identified, without a parenchymal nidus (▸ Fig. 1.98).

There are two types of carotid-cavernous fistulas (CCFs): direct and indirect. Most direct CCFs are traumatic in etiology, secondary to skull base fracture. These are high flow lesions. Indirect CCFs are low flow, nontraumatic acquired lesions, representing an AVF of the cavernous sinus with branches either of the external carotid artery or the cavernous carotid artery. With direct CCFs, findings include proptosis, dilatation of the superior ophthalmic vein(s), and enlargement of the cavernous sinus(es) (▸ Fig. 1.99). Prominent flow voids will be present in the cavernous sinus on MR. DSA is the definitive exam for

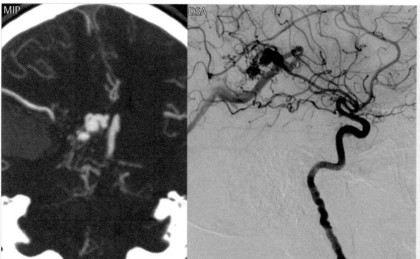

Fig. 1.96 Acute parenchymal hemorrhage, from an underlying AVM, in a patient with fibromuscular dysplasia (FMD). Intracranial aneurysms are a well-known associated finding in FMD, with the occurrence of intracranial arteriovenous malformations less common. The coronal thick MIP CTA demonstrates a portion of the nidus, medial to an acute parenchymal hemorrhage, together with midline shift and prominent midline draining veins. Both the nidus and draining veins are well visualized on the lateral DSA projection. Fibromuscular dysplasia within the distal internal carotid artery is easily identified on the DSA, with a "string of beads" appearance. This finding was somewhat subtle, but recognizable, on TOF MRA (not shown).

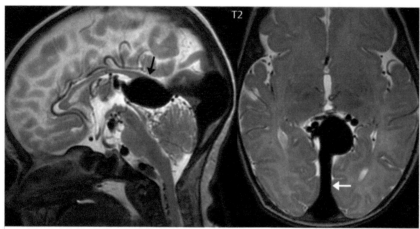

Fig. 1.97 Vein of Galen aneurysmal malformation. On sagittal and axial images (**part 1**), the anterior cerebral arteries and the basilar artery are enlarged, with a markedly dilated median prosencephalic vein (MPV, *black arrow*) forming a large pouch behind the third ventricle. In this instance, further drainage is through a vein (*white arrow*) that lies in location somewhat between a classic falcine sinus and the straight sinus. Two views (**part 2**) from the TOF MRA depict the enlarged arteries of both the anterior and posterior circulations draining into the dilated MPV, with subsequent venous drainage as described.

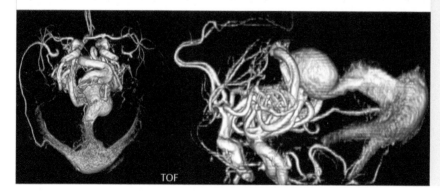

diagnosis. On DSA, early filling of the cavernous sinus, together with retrograde filling of the superior ophthalmic vein, can be seen. There may be reduced flow in the internal carotid artery beyond the fistula.

Detection of an indirect CCF on MR and CT can be difficult. Enlargement of the superior ophthalmic vein(s) is perhaps the most consistent and earliest finding. As with other AVFs, post-contrast imaging may demonstrate increased vascularity surrounding one or both cavernous sinuses. Unlike direct CCFs, the cavernous sinuses are typically not as prominent with an indirect CCF. Indirect CCFs are rarely detected by non-DSA imaging before symptoms are observed clinically.

A cerebral cavernous malformation (CCM, previously known as a cavernous angioma) histologically consists of a honeycomb of vascular spaces, separated by fibrous strands, without intervening normal brain parenchyma (▶ Fig. 1.100). Seventy-five percent are supratentorial, with multiplicity common (25%) (▶ Fig. 1.101). They are prone to spontaneous hemorrhage and, for symptomatic lesions in at risk patients, are treated by surgical resection (▶ Fig. 1.102).

As with almost all brain disease (in particular parenchymal lesions), MR is the modality of choice for detection, differential diagnosis, and evaluation. A CCM will have mixed low and high SI on both T1- and T2-weighted images (a "popcorn ball"

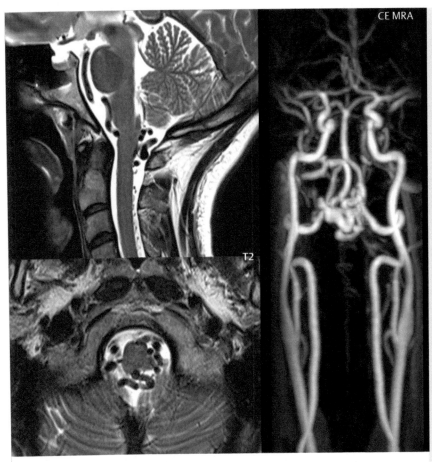

Fig. 1.98 Dural arteriovenous fistula. Sagittal and axial T2 weighted scans (**part 1**) reveal multiple serpiginous flow voids at the level of the foramen magnum, with contrast-enhanced MRA confirming these to be early filling, dilated, draining veins. Both early and late arterial phases from DSA, with a vertebral artery injection, are also illustrated (**part 2**). A dural shunt is identified supplied by the posterior meningeal branch of the vertebral artery. The perimedullary veins are grossly dilated (*large white arrow*). The late arterial phase reveals venous drainage of the shunt both via the contralateral superior petrosal sinus (*small white arrows*) and downward to the spinal perimedullary venous system (*asterisk*).

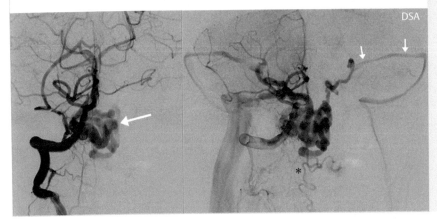

appearance), with a complete hemosiderin rim. The latter is best visualized on gradient echo (GRE) T2-weighted images, as low signal intensity. Susceptibility weighted imaging (SWI) provides a further improvement in visualization of the hemosiderin rim, as well as improved detection of very small lesions. Mild heterogeneous contrast enhancement is common with all but the smallest lesions. On CT, large CCMs can be visualized, and present as focal high-density lesions, with associated calcification (▶ Fig. 1.103). They may be associated with a developmental venous anomaly (DVA).

The more descriptive term developmental venous anomaly (DVA) is now used in place of the older term venous angioma. In this entity, a stellate collection of peripheral veins (the "caput medusae") lying in white matter converge to a dilated central draining vein, an appearance well visualized on contrast-enhanced MR. Supratentorial DVAs typically drain toward the wall of the lateral ventricle whereas infratentorial lesions may drain into the sigmoid sinus (▶ Fig. 1.104). DVAs are usually solitary, are commonly visualized incidentally on contrast-enhanced MR, and are the most common asymptomatic vascular malformation of brain.

A capillary telangiectasia is histologically a cluster of enlarged, dilated capillaries interspersed with normal brain parenchyma. These are rare, clinically benign, lesions with the most common site being the pons (often centrally) (▶ Fig. 1.104). MR imaging characteristics include a size < 1 cm,

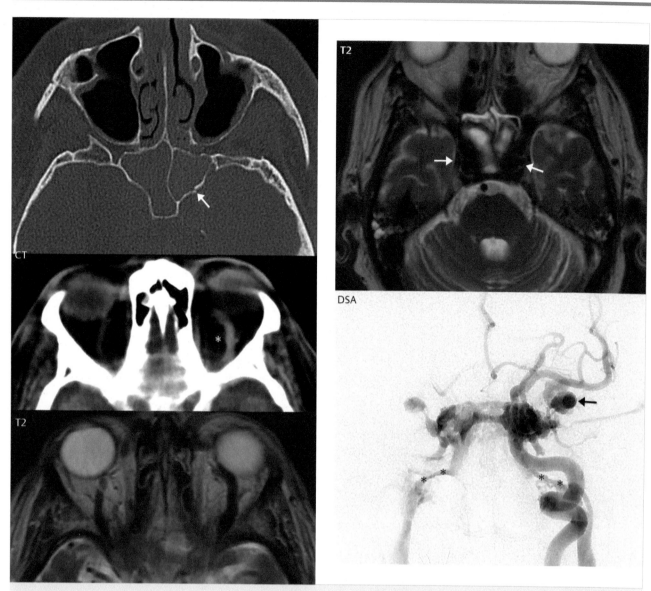

Fig. 1.99 Carotid cavernous fistula, traumatic. The images are all from a single patient. In **part 1**, the axial CT reconstructed with a bone algorithm reveals complete opacification of the sphenoid sinus (by blood in this instance) in this trauma patient, together with a fracture of the wall of the sinus on the left (*white arrow*). Fractures were also noted of the left occipital bone and petrous apex (not shown). The axial CT and MR through the orbits demonstrate an enlarged superior ophthalmic vein (*white asterisk*) on the left. This is seen as a flow void (dark) on the MR. In **part 2**, prominent flow voids are seen within, together with engorgement of, both cavernous sinuses (*white arrows*). The frontal DSA projection from a left internal carotid artery injection reveals the shunt into the left cavernous sinus, with filling as well of the contralateral cavernous sinus and retrograde filling of the left superior ophthalmic vein (*black arrow*). There is prominent filling of the inferior petrosal sinuses bilaterally (*black asterisks*).

faint contrast enhancement, hypointensity on GRE and SWI, and in about half of cases faint hyperintensity on FLAIR. These are usually visualized incidentally, typically being quiescent without symptoms.

Vertebrobasilar dolichoectasia by definition involves both an increase in length ("dolicho") and diameter ("ectasia") of the involved vessels (▶ Fig. 1.105). This entity is seen in the elderly with hypertension and atherosclerotic disease. Regarding the basilar artery, elongation results in the artery lying lateral to the clivus or dorsum sellae, or terminating above the suprasellar cistern. A diameter > 4.5 mm on CT is considered to be ectatic. Cranial nerve deficits may occur. There can be marked (long standing) deformity of the pons. However, vertebrobasilar dolichoectasia by itself is typically asymptomatic.

1.11.3 Sinus Thrombosis

Dural venous sinus thrombosis has many etiologies, and can be the result of infection, dehydration, trauma, neoplasia, oral contraceptives, pregnancy, or hematologic abnormalities. Patients present with signs of increased intracranial pressure, including specifically headache, nausea, papilledema, and lethargy. Venous infarction, specifically including hemorrhagic infarction, is a known complication (▶ Fig. 1.106). Sinus thrombosis is treated medically with anticoagulants, with recanalization of the sinus in most instances long-term (usually verified by follow-up MR). On CT, the sinus will be hyperdense precontrast, and post-contrast an "empty delta sign" will be seen, due to enhancement of venous collateral channels that surround the thrombosed sinus.

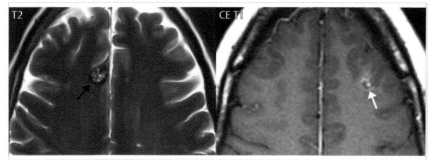

Fig. 1.100 Cavernous malformation. Lesions in two different patients are illustrated, showing classic imaging appearances of this vascular malformation. On a T2-weighted scan, a "popcorn ball" appearance is seen (*black arrow*), with diagnosis also requiring the presence of a complete low signal intensity hemosiderin rim (which will be more apparent on a T2* GRE scan). On a post-contrast scan, heterogenous, spotty focal enhancement is seen within a different cavernous malformation (*white arrow*).

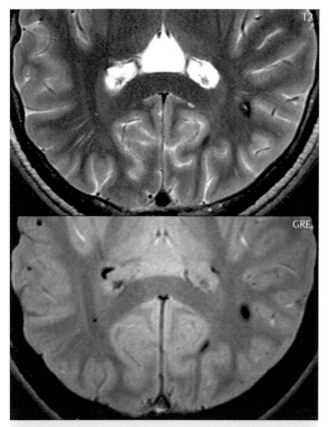

Fig. 1.101 Multiple cavernous malformations. A few, small, focal low signal intensity lesions are seen on the T2-weighted scan. These are much more evident on the gradient echo T2*-weighted scan, which identifies multiple additional lesions.

On MR, the venous clot early on may be composed of deoxyhemoglobin, with low SI therein on T2-weighted scans. This presentation is less common than that of a methemoglobin subacute clot; however, deoxyhemoglobin clots can be difficult to recognize and demand close inspection of images. Most visualized clots within the dural sinuses are methemoglobin in composition and easily recognized due to the high signal intensity within the clot on T1-weighted scans. Imaging of the dural sinus in two planes is recommended, to avoid confusion with flow phenomena. Post-contrast on MR there may be enhancement of small venous collaterals immediately surrounding the sinus. MR venography (MRV) is used to confirm the absence of flow within the sinus, most often with 2D TOF MRA techniques (which are sensitive to the slower flow within the dural sinuses) (▶ Fig. 1.107).

One caveat is the high signal intensity of methemoglobin on certain MRA sequences. Phase contrast MRA techniques can also be used, and do not suffer from this potential pitfall.

1.12 Infection and Inflammation

1.12.1 Parenchymal Abscess

The typical appearance on MR and CT of a brain abscess is that of a round mass lesion with central necrosis, demonstrating a distinctive uniform thin rim of contrast enhancement. On T2-weighted scans, the abscess capsule may also demonstrate slight low signal intensity. There will be prominent accompanying vasogenic edema. The area of central necrosis may be heterogeneous. Although not entirely specific for an abscess (this finding can also be seen, rarely, in brain metastases), restricted diffusion on MR of the central fluid collection is characteristic for an abscess (▶ Fig. 1.108). The most common location is at the gray-white matter junction. Differential diagnostic considerations include a glioblastoma and a solitary necrotic metastasis. Glioblastomas, however, are typically much larger lesions, with the rim of contrast enhancement notable for its irregularity and of varying thickness.

Early in bacterial infection, prior to the formation of a distinct abscess, cerebritis will be present, with a somewhat nonspecific imaging appearance on MR. There will be focal vasogenic edema, with or without patchy contrast enhancement. Secondary findings may provide important clues to the diagnosis, including meningitis and lesion location (e.g., with the area of cerebritis adjacent to an infected frontal or mastoid sinus) (▶ Fig. 1.109).

1.12.2 Epidural and Subdural Abscesses

MR is superior to CT for identification and definition of epidural and subdural abscesses, due both to its soft tissue sensitivity and the lack of artifact from the calvarium. In epidural lesions, close inspection should also be made of the adjacent bone for possible disease extension (osteomyelitis). On FLAIR, infected fluid collections, regardless of location, will have increased signal intensity, distinct from normal CSF (with very low SI). The displaced dura may be recognizable in epidural abscesses as a low signal intensity interface on a T2-weighted scan (▶ Fig. 1.110).

As with brain abscesses, DWI is invaluable, permitting differentiation of infected (with restricted diffusion) and sterile fluid collections. Abnormal contrast enhancement of the lesion margins will be seen, increasing conspicuity, but not

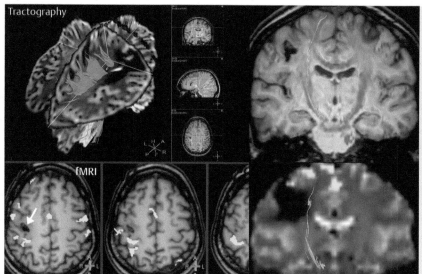

Fig. 1.102 Cavernous malformation, tractography and functional MRI (fMRI). Preoperative assessment of the corticospinal tract can be accomplished in patients on MR by integrating fMRI data with diffusion tensor tractography. In this patient with a cavernous malformation (*arrow*) in the right pre-central gyrus, activation due to finger and thumb opposition is noted both posterior and lateral to the lesion, with fibers of the corticospinal tract demonstrated medial to the lesion on coronal images.

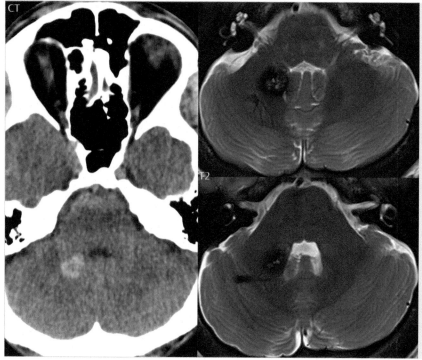

Fig. 1.103 Cavernous malformation, with an associated developmental venous anomaly. On CT, a small, well delineated, hyperdense, round, focal lesion is seen pre-contrast, to the right and posterior to the fourth ventricle. On axial T2-weighted scans, a complete hemosiderin rim is demonstrated, together a "popcorn ball" appearance centrally, with mixed high and low signal intensity – all characteristic for a cavernous malformation. Just lateral and posterior to the lesion is an additional finding, a large flow void and associated caput medusa, consistent with an associated developmental venous anomaly.

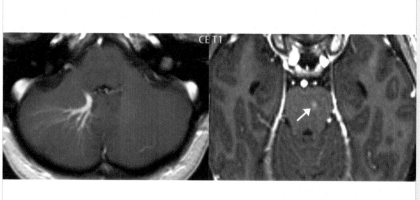

Fig. 1.104 Developmental venous anomaly, capillary telangiectasia. These two incidental vascular lesions are both seen best on post-contrast MR, often being undetected on precontrast scans. A classic caput Medusa, composed of multiple, small veins draining into a single large vein, is well seen in the first patient. In the cerebellum, as illustrated, drainage is usually into the sigmoid sinus. In the second patient, a small lesion with mild contrast enhancement (*white arrow*) is seen on thin section imaging in the pons. This appearance, together with low signal intensity on T2*-weighted scans, is characteristic of a capillary telangiectasia, a much less common entity. Developmental venous anomalies are seen not infrequently in daily clinical practice, assuming post-contrast imaging is performed.

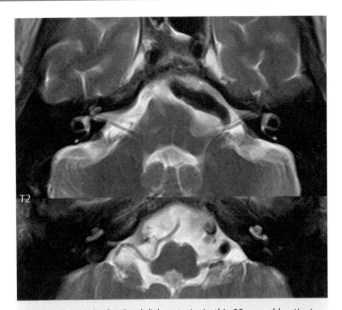

Fig. 1.105 Vertebrobasilar dolichoectasia. In this 66-year-old patient, there is an increase in length and diameter of the vertebrobasilar system, visualized in part on two axial images. The basilar artery is markedly enlarged and irregular in cross-section, with both vertebral arteries also large in diameter (with atherosclerotic plaque nearly occluding one vertebral artery).

entirely specific for infection. Use of fat saturation with post-contrast scans can markedly improve lesion depiction, and recognition of abnormal contrast enhancement, due to the suppression of high signal intensity in the fat of the diploic space and extracranial soft tissues. Recognition of adjacent osteomyelitis, accompanying an epidural abscess, is also markedly improved by the use of fat suppression, both on precontrast T2-weighted scans, and post-contrast. Depending on the location of a lesion, imaging planes other than the axial may markedly improve visualization of the lesion (e.g., coronal images in a lesion near the vertex), due to less partial volume imaging.

1.12.3 Meningitis

Common organisms responsible for bacterial meningitis in the general adult population include *Streptococcus pneumoniae,* group B *Streptococcus,* and *Neisseria meningitidis.* In the neonate, the common organisms are *Escherichia coli,* other gram-negative rods, and group B *Streptococcus.* Bacterial meningitis is rapidly lethal without treatment and, despite treatment, often complicated by infarction, sensorineural hearing loss, epilepsy, and intellectual impairment. CT is very insensitive to meningitis. On MR, FLAIR may demonstrate hyperintense signal, in areas of involvement, within sulci and cisterns, with

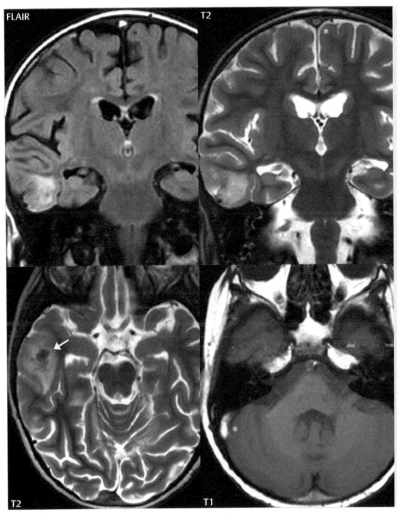

Fig. 1.106 Venous infarction. Vasogenic edema is noted in the right temporal lobe (*arrow*), but specifically not in an arterial vascular distribution. There is a small parenchymal hemorrhage, with low signal intensity on the T2-weighted scan, seen within the infarct on the axial image. This venous infarct was the result of dural sinus thrombosis, with clot (*asterisk*) well depicted on multiple images, including specifically within the superior sagittal sinus on coronal images and the right transverse sinus on the axial T1-weighted scan.

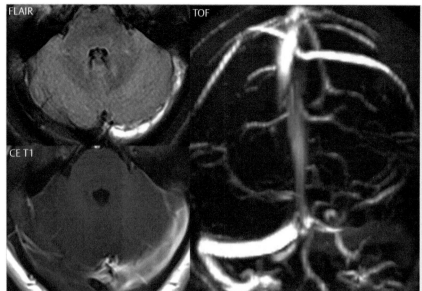

Fig. 1.107 Venous sinus thrombosis. There is abnormal hyperintensity on FLAIR in the left transverse sinus, consistent with methemoglobin. On sagittal and axial precontrast T1-weighted scans (not shown, but the primary scans one would acquire to identify methemoglobin), the clot was hyperintense as well. Post-contrast, there is enhancement along the walls of the expanded sinus, which is of slightly higher signal intensity than the methemoglobin clot therein. Two-dimensional TOF MRA confirms occlusion, with the shadow of the left transverse sinus that is visualized corresponding to methemoglobin clot.

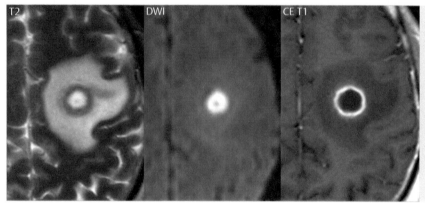

Fig. 1.108 Cerebral abscess. All three imaging sequences demonstrate characteristic findings of a brain abscess. There is a mass lesion (in the left frontal lobe) on the T2-weighted scan, with extensive surrounding edema, with the most characteristic finding on this sequence being the slight low signal intensity, round, abscess capsule. The abscess contents are high signal intensity on DWI. And, there is a thin uniform rim of abnormal enhancement post-contrast.

this finding however nonspecific. Abnormal contrast enhancement occurs within the leptomeninges (▶ Fig. 1.111) and any accompanying purulent exudate. Such an exudate may be present covering the cerebral hemispheres, along the base of the brain, and around the intracisternal segments of the cranial nerves. Imaging findings correlate with the severity of involvement. Mild cases of meningitis may have no abnormality on MR. Subdural empyemas can also be seen (with *Streptococcus pneumoniae* typically the organism) but are not common. Epidural empyemas are even less common. Diagnostic clues for a subdural or epidural empyema include restricted diffusion within the fluid collection and an enhancing rim. Sterile subdural effusions are also associated with meningitis. These however follow CSF on all MR pulse sequences.

Viral meningitis has no specific treatment, with most patients recovering on their own by 7 to 10 days. As with milder cases of bacterial meningitis, findings on MR may be subtle or the scan may be normal. Findings include mild leptomeningeal enhancement and loss of cortical sulci due to generalized mild brain swelling.

1.12.4 Ventriculitis

Ventriculitis is inflammation of the ependymal lining of a ventricle, and can be seen as a complication of meningitis, following surgery, or due to contiguous extension of infection. As with meningitis, findings on MR may be subtle or not present. CT is rarely abnormal. Two findings are characteristic for ventriculitis on MR: increased signal intensity within the immediate periventricular white matter on FLAIR and enhancement of the ependymal lining (▶ Fig. 1.112). Ependymal spread of neoplastic disease is the primary differential diagnosis, with nodularity (if present) favoring tumor.

1.12.5 Encephalitis

In older children and adults, herpes simplex virus (HSV) type 1 is the most common cause of viral encephalitis. The disease is caused by reactivation of virus in the trigeminal ganglion, with spread via the fifth cranial nerve to the meninges of anterior and middle cranial fossa. Thus, the disease most commonly affects the temporal and inferior frontal lobes (▶ Fig. 1.113). The clinical presentation includes headache, fever, seizures, confusion, and behavioral changes. HSV encephalitis is a devastating disease with early empiric therapy strongly advocated, specifically intravenous (IV) acyclovir. T2 and FLAIR hyperintensity is noted in areas of involvement, together with restricted diffusion. Disease may be unilateral or bilateral. In some instances, involvement is initially unilateral with progression to bilateral disease. Mild patchy contrast enhancement is noted early in the disease process. There is cortical and subcortical involvement, with early, partial sparing of white matter. CT once again is relatively insensitive to disease. Hemorrhage is a late feature.

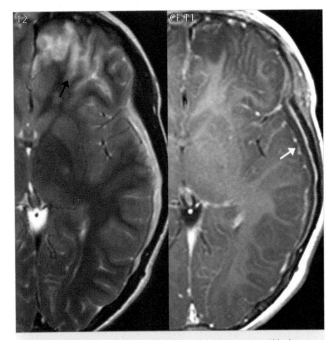

Fig. 1.109 Meningoencephalitis. Ill-defined hyperintensity (*black arrow*), consistent with vasogenic edema (and encephalitis in this instance) is seen on the T2-weighted scan in the left frontal lobe, involving both gray and white matter, in a nonvascular distribution. In addition, there is diffuse mild enhancement post-contrast within the cerebral sulci, consistent with meningitis, together with enhancement of the pia-arachnoid overlying the convexity and the dura, with an intervening fluid collection (*white arrow*). The latter was hyperintense on DWI (not shown), consistent with a subdural empyema. Infection in this instance spread from the frontal sinus.

In the neonate, herpes simplex encephalitis type 2 is the disease of relevance. Transmission is most commonly due to exposure at birth during vaginal delivery, with development of the disease by 2 to 4 weeks of age. On MR, early in the disease process, edema and restricted diffusion will be seen in patchy regions of the brain (predominantly white matter) (▶ Fig. 1.114), followed in time by atrophy and cystic changes. Focal low attenuation is noted on nonenhanced CT. The initial patchy areas of brain involvement can rapidly increase in size leading to generalized edema/brain involvement. Long-term sequelae include extensive cystic encephalomalacia, cortical atrophy, ventriculomegaly, and calcification (involving white matter, cortical gray matter, and gray matter nuclei).

1.12.6 Toxoplasmosis

Toxoplasmosis is a ubiquitous obligate intracellular protozoan that causes mild self-limited infection with lymphadenopathy and fever in normal adults. Approximately 50% of the U.S. population has been exposed and has antibodies, with the mode of transmission being insufficiently cooked meat and cat feces. Toxoplasmosis is an important pathogen in the fetus and in immunocompromised patients. Acute infection of the mother can lead to transmission to the fetus, with the result being focal or diffuse encephalitis. Scattered intracranial calcifications are seen on CT throughout the brain (in distinction to congenital infection with cytomegalovirus [CMV], which demonstrates predominantly periventricular calcifications).

Toxoplasmosis is the most common intracranial opportunistic infection in AIDS. As with many opportunistic infections, appropriate specific prophylaxis and antiretroviral therapy has resulted in a marked change in outcome of the disease. With appropriate therapy, lesions resolve within a time frame of weeks. Focal lesions located in the basal ganglia or at the gray-white matter junction are characteristic, with nodular or ring enhancement, and often prominent vasogenic edema (▶ Fig. 1.115). In immunosuppressed patients, the degree of contrast enhancement of lesions is often mild (faint), less then what might be otherwise anticipated.

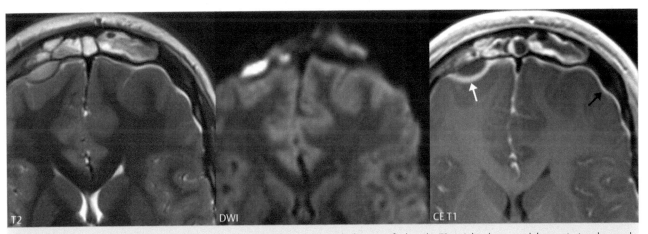

Fig. 1.110 Epidural abscess. Inflammatory disease is seen in the frontal sinus, which is opacified on the T2-weighted scan, and demonstrates abnormal contrast enhancement—neither sign is specific however for infection versus simple inflammatory changes. On DWI, a hyperintense small extra-axial fluid collection is noted (consistent with an abscess, due to extension of infection from the frontal sinus), just posterior to the right frontal sinus. This can be seen to be epidural in location on the T2-weighted scan. Post-contrast there is striking enhancement of the inflamed/infected leptomeninges medial to the fluid collection (*white arrow*), as well as along the entire anterior surface of the brain (*black arrow*).

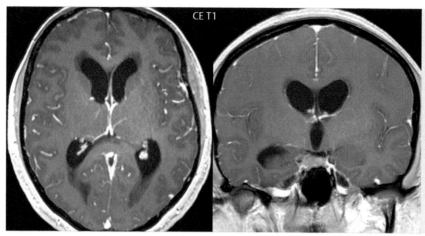

Fig. 1.111 Meningitis, causing extraventricular obstructive hydrocephalus. The ventricles are prominent, with a generalized absence of sulci. The abnormal low signal intensity in the immediate periventricular region reflects interstitial edema due to increased ventricular pressure. On the post-contrast scans there is diffuse mild enhancement of the leptomeninges, consistent with meningitis.

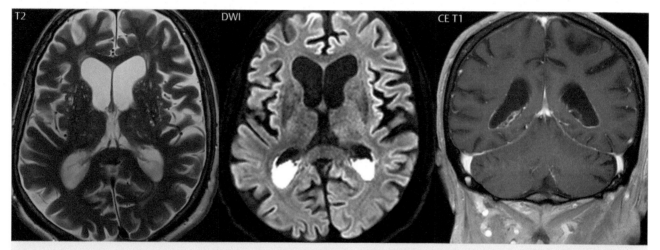

Fig. 1.112 Ventriculitis. On the T2-weighted scan there is subtle abnormal signal intensity (slightly less than normal CSF) in the posterior portion of the atria of the lateral ventricles. Abnormal high signal intensity (restricted diffusion) is present in this area on the diffusion-weighted scan, with ependymal enhancement post-contrast, both findings consistent with infection.

1.12.7 Neurocysticercosis

Neurocysticercosis is infection of the CNS by the larval stage of the pork tapeworm *(Taenia solium)*. Viable larvae survive for 4 to 5 years, with a pronounced host inflammatory reaction upon parasite death. Clinical presentation includes seizures (due to parenchymal cysts) and obstructive hydrocephalus (due to intraventricular cysts). On CT, calcifications (subarachnoid in location, or at the gray-white matter junction) can be seen in end stage disease, with few other findings. Four distinct temporal stages are recognized, and can be differentiated on MR (▶ Fig. 1.116). In the vesicular stage, the larva is still viable and a cyst without accompanying edema or enhancement is seen. In the colloidal vesicular stage, the larva is dying, inciting an intense inflammatory reaction, with ring enhancement and prominent edema. In the subsequent granular nodular stage there may be faint rim enhancement, with the edema decreasing. The nodular calcified stage is the end result, with dense focal calcification seen on CT and hypointensity on MR.

1.12.8 Tuberculosis

Two main patterns of brain involvement occur in tuberculosis: parenchymal lesions (tuberculoma) and meningitis. In developing countries, up to 40% of all parenchymal mass lesions in the brain are tuberculomas. These can demonstrate ring or nodular enhancement, with the capsule often thicker than for pyogenic infection. Unlike a bacterial abscess, the center of the lesion may be either hypoor hyperintense on T2-weighted scans. Basilar exudates (meningitis) are more common than parenchymal lesions in tuberculosis (▶ Fig. 1.117). Complications include communicating hydrocephalus due to blockage of CSF flow by the inflammatory exudate and infarction due to thrombosis of vessels coursing through the basal cisterns. Most commonly affected are the small penetrating arteries to the basal ganglia. MR is superior to CT for disease detection and evaluation, in particular for basal meningitis.

1.12.9 Creutzfeldt-Jakob Disease

Creutzfeldt-Jakob disease is a fatal neurodegenerative disease caused by prions—infectious proteins that propagate by transmitting a misfolded state. Brain biopsy is required for definitive diagnosis. MR is frequently performed and reveals typical findings. High signal intensity is seen in the cortex on FLAIR in half of cases, with the sensitivity of DWI substantially higher (80%)—with cortical areas demonstrating restricted diffusion (▶ Fig. 1.118). The basal ganglia, predominantly the

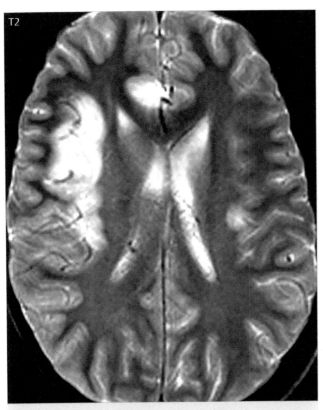

Fig. 1.113 Herpes encephalitis type 1. Abnormal high signal intensity is noted predominantly unilaterally in the right medial temporal lobe and insula. This appearance alone is extremely characteristic. However, in this patient, there is additional involvement of the low frontal lobe medially (cingulate gyrus) on the right, as well as subtle involvement of the contralateral temporal lobe, further suggesting by pattern of involvement (limbic system) the diagnosis of herpes encephalitis type 1.

caudate nucleus and putamen, are abnormal on MR in about half of cases. DWI demonstrates restricted diffusion in the involved basal ganglia, and is equivalent or superior in sensitivity to any other pulse sequence.

1.12.10 Neurosarcoidosis

Both leptomeningeal and parenchymal disease can be seen in neurosarcoidosis, a multisystem inflammatory disease of unknown etiology characterized by noncaseating granulomas. The most common presentation is that of a granulomatous leptomeningitis involving the skull base (▶ Fig. 1.119). Clinical findings include cranial nerve palsies, meningeal signs, and hypothalamic dysfunction. Parenchymal involvement is thought to be the result of spread of leptomeningeal disease via the Virchow-Robin spaces. Ophthalmic changes are seen in up to 60% of patients, with the lacrimal gland most frequently involved. Differential diagnostic considerations, for the leptomeningeal presentation, include tuberculosis, bacterial meningitis, and leptomeningeal carcinomatosis.

1.12.11 HIV/AIDS

HIV encephalitis is due to a direct neurotrophic effect of the virus. In early disease involvement, patchy abnormal areas of high signal intensity are seen within white matter on FLAIR (▶ Fig. 1.120). Treatment at this stage with antiretroviral therapy can result in marked improvement, as assessed by MR imaging. With more extensive longstanding disease, there is ventriculomegaly, prominence of the cerebral sulci, diffuse periventricular white matter high signal intensity on FLAIR, and loss of gray-white matter differentiation (▶ Fig. 1.100). The latter is often striking on T1-weighted scans.

Progressive multifocal leukoencephalopathy (PML) is a viral demyelinating disease, caused by the JC (John Cunningham) virus. PML is most commonly seen in HIV infection, but can be seen in any immunosuppressed patient. With the introduction of highly active antiretroviral therapy (HAART), there has been a marked decrease in incidence of PML. The MR imaging appearance of PML is that of focal areas of abnormal white matter with high signal intensity on T2-weighted scans, often in an asymmetrical distribution (▶ Fig. 1.121). The cortex is spared. There is involvement of subcortical U-fibers, a differentiating point from HIV encephalitis.

Immune reconstitution inflammatory syndrome (IRIS) is a diagnosis of exclusion, with identification of atypical MR or CT findings in an immunosuppressed patient pivotal for early recognition. The disease occurs when the immune system begins to recover and then manifests an overwhelming inflammatory response to a previously acquired infection. Diagnostic clues on imaging include abnormal contrast enhancement, transient increase in parenchymal high signal intensity FLAIR abnormalities, mass effect, restricted diffusion, and meningitis.

1.13 Demyelinating Disease

1.13.1 Multiple Sclerosis

MS is still a disease of unknown pathogenesis, although generally viewed as autoimmune in type. Incidence is higher in women, and in Caucasians of Northern European descent living in temperate zones. Most patients are 20 to 40 years of age at diagnosis, although presentation in older patients occurs. Although four major clinical subtypes are recognized, 85% of patients fall into the *relapsing-remitting MS* subtype in which relapses of disease alternates with periods of remission.

Dissemination of lesions in space and time is required for diagnosis. The revised McDonald criteria requires for disease diagnosis two focal, hyperintense lesions seen on T2-weighted scans, with one each in any of the following four areas: periventricular, juxtacortical, infratentorial, and spinal cord. A new lesion on follow-up scan or the presence on a single scan of asymptomatic enhancing and nonenhancing lesions fulfills the temporal requirement. MS plaques are poorly visualized on CT, with MR the definitive imaging modality.

The hallmark of MS is punctate white matter lesions (plaques), in particular in the immediate periventricular region (and, specifically, perivenular in location). Chronic lesions tend to be small, with active lesions larger, with less well-defined margins. Acute lesions may evoke mild vasogenic edema. Disease involvement is typically asymmetric in nature, when comparing the right and left sides of the brain, one of many differentiating features from chronic small vessel white matter ischemic disease. There is a predisposition for the occurrence of lesions in characteristic areas (▶ Fig. 1.122). These include the immediate periventricular white matter, the corpus callosum

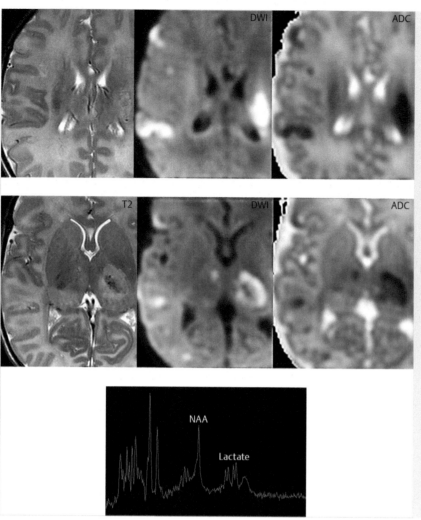

Fig. 1.114 Herpes encephalitis type 2. This 2-week-old infant demonstrates multiple focal abnormalities, best seen on diffusion-weighted imaging, in the white matter of the left corona radiata, left thalamus, two areas of cortical gray matter on the right, and other scattered small areas within the brain (**parts 1** and **2**). Abnormal high signal intensity is seen on diffusion-weighted images, confirmed on the ADC maps to represent restricted diffusion (low ADC), consistent with cytotoxic edema. These abnormalities represent early ischemic lesions, in congenital herpes infection. Hemorrhage (deoxyhemoglobin) is also seen within the left thalamic lesion. Note that the abnormalities are poorly visualized on the T2-weighted FSE scans, although some vasogenic edema is present. Single voxel spectroscopy (**part 3**) of the white matter lesion demonstrates decreased NAA, and the presence of lactate (note the classic "doublet"). NAA is a marker of axonal and neuronal viability, with a decrease in NAA reflecting neuronal loss. Lactate is generated by anaerobic metabolism (and is usually absent in spectra of the normal brain), and is seen in hypoxia and ischemia.

(with even greater specificity for lesions that have a flat ependymal margin, or lesions that radiate along the white matter tracts from the ventricular surface), immediately adjacent to the temporal horns (an unusual area for lesions in chronic small vessel white matter ischemic disease), the colliculi, middle cerebellar peduncles, pons, and medulla (► Fig. 1.123). Optic nerve lesions also occur, and can be the reason for initial clinical presentation. Rarely, a solitary giant lesion can be seen, mimicking primary neoplasm, metastatic disease, or infection.

MS plaques in general are best visualized on FLAIR (as focal high signal intensity lesions), with high-resolution 3D scan acquisition at 3 T preferred. Callosal lesions are often best detected in the sagittal plane. MS plaques also demonstrate low signal intensity on T1-weighted scans, another minor differentiating point from chronic small vessel white matter ischemic disease in which the lesions are typically poorly visualized on T1-weighted scans. Some chronic plaques demonstrate very low signal intensity, with these referred to in the literature as "black holes." Diffusion weighted scans may depict active lesions as hyperintense (another distinctive imaging feature), which in the majority of cases is due to "T2 shine through" (the T2-weighting of the sequence), rather than representing true restricted diffusion. Gray matter lesions do occur, but are not well seen in general on conventional MR pulse sequences. Use

of newer MR scan techniques such as MP2RAGE and double inversion recovery (DIR) can further improve detection of lesions (► Fig. 1.124), including those within cortical gray matter. Although not readily evident on clinical scans, there also is a more generalized involvement of white matter, with otherwise normal appearing white matter distinctive by MR parameters from that in the normal population by quantitative measures. Nonspecific findings in chronic disease include ventricular enlargement, cerebral atrophy, and thinning of the corpus callosum. The absence of lesions in the brain does not rule out the diagnosis of MS, with a complete evaluation including imaging of the cervical and thoracic cord, and the conus.

The majority of visualized lesions are chronic in nature and do not demonstrate contrast enhancement. Lesion enhancement is transient, exists for less than 4 weeks in most cases, correlates with active disease, and is a marker for new lesions (► Fig. 1.125). Both punctate and ring enhancement occur, and are common. An incomplete arc of enhancement adjacent to a lesion can also occur. Neurologists consider contrast administration to be a mandatory part of the exam, to assess active disease. In patients evaluated by MR during quiescent periods of the disease clinically, few if any enhancing lesions will be seen. When lesion enhancement is seen, it typically involves only a few lesions, although in rare instances, particularly with initial

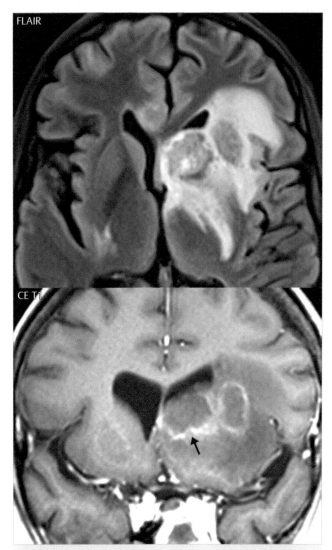

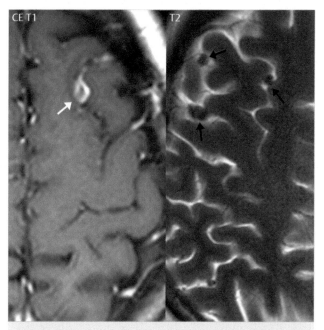

Fig. 1.116 Neurocysticercosis. The imaging appearance in this disease is varied, dependent on stage and lesion location. Subarachnoid lesions, which are the most common, in the intermediate to late stages of the disease enhance (*white arrow*). Chronically, these lesions demonstrate dense calcification, seen as a signal void (*black arrows*) in distinction to the adjacent high signal intensity CSF on T2-weighted MR scans.

Fig. 1.115 Toxoplasmosis. Focal lesions with associated edema are seen most commonly in the basal ganglia, as illustrated (in this instance, the caudate and lentiform nuclei). Peripheral enhancement is characteristic, often mild in degree, due to the immunocompromised patient status.

MP2RAGE and 3D double inversion recovery, MS lesions can, as well, be more correctly localized as cortical, subcortical, or mixed in location (▶ Fig. 1.127).

1.13.2 Neuromyelitis Optica

This disease entity, once considered a form of MS, is defined by optic nerve (one or both) and spinal cord involvement. With the latter, long segments of involvement (more than three segments) dominate. Important to note is that nonspecific white matter lesions in the brain do not exclude this diagnosis.

1.13.3 Acute Disseminated Encephalomyelitis

The typical clinical presentation of acute disseminated encephalomyelitis (ADEM) is in a child, following a mild viral illness or vaccination. In decades past, two events led to large numbers of cases: measles epidemics and the small pox vaccination. Clinical presentation includes confusion, somnolence, coma (in severe cases), convulsions, headache, fever, and ataxia. The disease is generally monophasic. The imaging appearance is that of multifocal white matter lesions (involving both deep and peripheral white matter), hyperintense on FLAIR (▶ Fig. 1.128). In many instances, the lesions are somewhat large, with ill-defined margins. Lesions in the brainstem and cerebellum are common. Contrast enhancement of lesions is common in the acute presentation, with the majority of lesions demonstrating enhancement. CT, despite the presence of severe disease, can be

symptomatic presentation, there may be a large number of enhancing white matter plaques.

The severity of disease involvement varies widely. Early in the disease course, few plaques may be seen. In late stage involvement, the periventricular plaques may become confluent. There can be some overlap in imaging appearance, in any single patient exam, with SLE (in which multiple small subcortical and deep white matter lesions can be seen) and acute disseminated encephalomyelitis. Lesions in SLE, however, are usually not immediate periventricular in location.

MRI at 7 T offers improved confidence in comparison to 3 T for the diagnosis of demyelinating disease. Small structures and subtle disease involvement are better depicted, due principally to the higher achievable spatial resolution (▶ Fig. 1.126). At 7 T there is also better characterization of white matter lesions, specifically those with central veins and iron content (using SWI), and higher detection rates for cortical MS plaques. Using

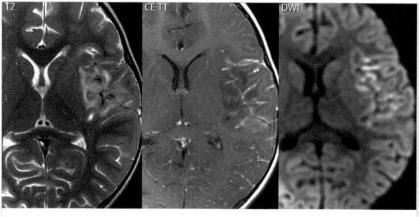

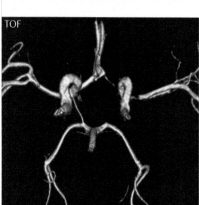

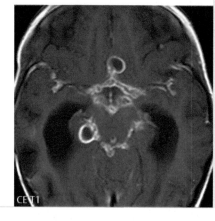

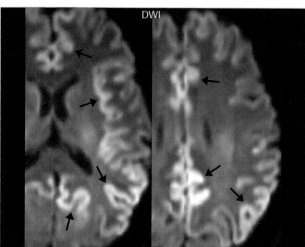

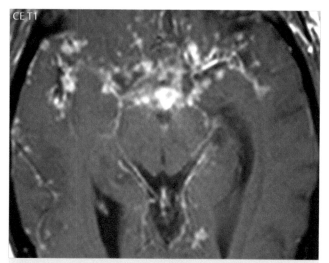

Fig. 1.117 Tuberculous meningitis. In **part 1**, there is extensive vasogenic edema in the left insula and temporal lobe, with leptomeningeal enhancement post-contrast Only a small portion of this lesion demonstrates restricted diffusion, as reflected by high SI on the diffusion-weighted image. These findings are consistent with a meningoencephalitis, with an accompanying but substantially smaller area of infarction. In **part 2**, the same patient, TOF MRA reveals an arteritis with severe stenosis of the proximal left MCA. In **part 3**, a different patient, there is marked enhancement of the basal cisterns consistent with meningitis, encasing the major arteries, the classic presentation for tuberculosis. Also noted are two ring-enhancing lesions, representing abscesses (tuberculomas), despite their extra-axial location.

Fig. 1.118 Creutzfeldt-Jakob disease (CJD). Both FLAIR and DWI abnormalities are the most characteristic in this disease process, with (classic) striking cortical hyperintensity (*black arrows*) on DWI (typically asymmetric from side to side) illustrated in this patient. These areas may also be high signal intensity on FLAIR, together with the basal ganglia.

Fig. 1.119 Neurosarcoidosis. Leptomeningeal infiltrates, often with nodularity, are the most common imaging finding in CNS sarcoid. Abnormal contrast enhancement is the most easily recognized feature, as illustrated in a case of very extensive disease. Note the diffuse enhancement of the leptomeninges, with prominent nodularity, involving the brainstem and the intracisternal portion of multiple cranial nerves.

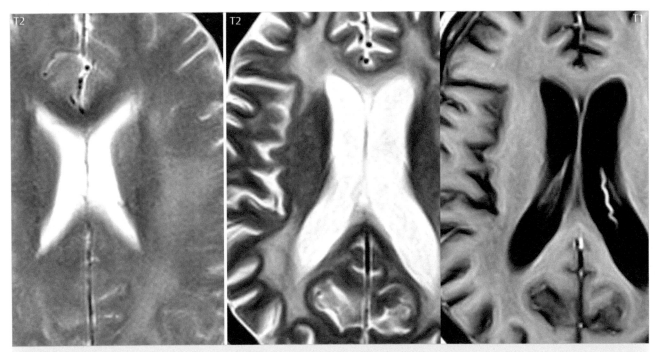

Fig. 1.120 HIV encephalitis. Scans from two different patients are presented. Ill-defined abnormal hyperintensity within white matter is seen on T2-weighted imaging in the first patient, at presentation with initial neurologic manifestations without prior known disease. These findings regressed with antiretroviral therapy. T2- and T1-weighted scans are illustrated in the second patient, a young adult with long standing disease, with striking diffuse hyperintensity within white matter on the T2-weighted scan, loss of gray-white matter differentiation on the T1-weighted scan, and diffuse marked cerebral atrophy reflected by prominence of the sulci and enlargement of the lateral ventricles.

normal. Although complete lesion resolution is seen on MR in the majority of patients, 20% are left with disabilities and mortality is high (up to 20%).

1.14 Neoplasms

1.14.1 Pilocytic Astrocytoma

This benign, World Health Organization (WHO) grade I, tumor occurs in the cerebellum, optic pathway (optic nerve, chiasm), thalamus/hypothalamus, and brainstem (pons). It is the most common posterior fossa tumor of childhood (although close in incidence to medulloblastoma). Pilocytic astrocytomas are slow growing and typically large at diagnosis. In the cerebellum a lesion in the hemisphere (laterally located) is more common than in the vermis (medially located). The classic presentation is that of a cystic posterior fossa lesion, with an enhancing mural nodule, extrinsic to and causing mass effect upon the fourth ventricle (▶ Fig. 1.129). The cystic component will be hyperintense to CSF on FLAIR, due to protein content. A pilocytic cerebellar astrocytoma can thus present with obstructive hydrocephalus. Solid pilocytic astrocytomas also occur in the cerebellum, but like their cystic counterpart, are typically well circumscribed. Lesions involving the optic chiasm and optic nerve (optic glioma) are not uncommon in neurofibromatosis type 1 (NF1); however, many such lesions are found in patients who do not have NF1. Enhancement of an optic tract lesion is variable, and can be absent. In the pons, a relatively large lesion is the most common presentation (with the lesion limited to the pons). Contiguous involvement of other portions of the brainstem (and thus a rather extensive lesion extending superiorly and/or inferiorly) occurs, but is rare.

Tectal (quadrigeminal plate) gliomas are included here for discussion due to their indolent nature. This is a subtype of brainstem glioma, presenting in childhood and young adults. Features include periaqueductal location, lack of contrast enhancement, and long-term stability. Tectal gliomas present as a small bulbous mass lesion, hyperintense on T2-weighted scans, and often narrow the cerebral aqueduct causing obstructive hydrocephalus (and thus clinical presentation). These are considered to be very low-grade lesions, with histology usually not available, and conservative management recommended. The main differential diagnostic consideration is benign aqueductal stenosis. The latter however can be distinguished by the presence of only a thin rim of periaqueductal T2 high signal intensity, without an associated mass.

1.14.2 Low-grade Astrocytoma

This WHO grade II tumor is infiltrative in nature, histologically well differentiated, and demonstrates slow growth with time. On imaging, its presentation is that of a focal mass lesion with its epicenter in white matter. Low-grade astrocytomas on MR are well-defined, homogeneous, non-enhancing mass lesions, with little mass effect and minimal vasogenic edema. They are hypointense on T1- and hyperintense on T2-weighted images. The appearance of this lesion on MR, as a seemingly well-defined mass, is somewhat misleading relative to its infiltrative nature (▶ Fig. 1.130). The most common location is that of the frontal or temporal lobe. A rather characteristic location is in the insula extending medially to lie adjacent to the MCA trifurcation. Low-grade astrocytomas are poorly visualized on CT (they are often isodense with brain). Calcifications are noted in 25%. Clinical

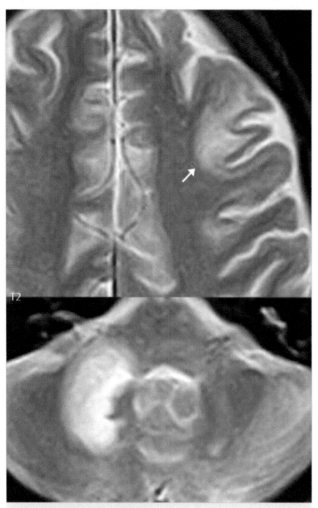

Fig. 1.121 Progressive multifocal leukoencephalopathy (PML). The supratentorial lobar white matter (*arrow*) is most commonly involved, although the imaging presentation is quite varied. A single lesion is not uncommon. There is typically preservation of the overlying cortex, as noted in the presented case. Mass effect and abnormal contrast enhancement are usually absent, with PML best seen on T2-weighted scans as a focal area of abnormal high signal intensity white matter. The second most common location is the middle cerebellar peduncle, with a lesion in this location also illustrated from a different patient.

presentation is generally in the third to fifth decades of life, and they are a common primary tumor of adults. About half of pontine gliomas (▶ Fig. 1.131) are low-grade astrocytomas, as distinguished from pilocytic (WHO grade I) astrocytomas.

A general comment about astrocytomas is in order. On biopsy, different portions of a lesion commonly display different histology (and a different grade). Lesions are also not static histologically with time, with eventual progression in grade seen (from low-grade to anaplastic to a glioblastoma multiforme).

1.14.3 Anaplastic Astrocytoma

As with almost all features, this tumor is intermediate between a low-grade astrocytoma and a glioblastoma multiforme in histology (this is a WHO grade III tumor), imaging appearance, and

prognosis. On MR, in distinction to a low-grade astrocytoma, an anaplastic astrocytoma is typically less well defined, mildly heterogeneous, often exhibiting some contrast enhancement, and displays mild to moderate mass effect and accompanying vasogenic edema (▶ Fig. 1.132). Intravenous contrast administration on MR is important for identification of recurrent or residual tumor (both with anaplastic astrocytomas and glioblastomas), with enhancement however correlating more closely only with the higher grade portions of the lesion. Recurrent tumor usually enhances, even if preoperatively it did not. One caveat is important about abnormal enhancement following surgery. A follow-up exam should always be obtained within 24 hours after resection, at which time any abnormal enhancement (along or adjacent to the resection margin) will be due to residual tumor, with postoperative changes causing abnormal enhancement only in subsequent days. Abnormal contrast enhancement does not differentiate between radiation necrosis (which usually occurs more than 1 year following treatment) and recurrent tumor. Perfusion (CBV) studies, either by CT or MR, however permit this differentiation. Diffusion also plays a role both in assessing tumor grade (▶ Fig. 1.133) and in the identification following treatment of recurrent tumor. Histologic tumor grade (for glial tumors) correlates inversely with the minimum ADC. ADC maps provide information analogous to FDG-PET, allowing an approximation of tumor grade. And, for differentiation from chemoradiation injury, a reduction in ADC generally correlates with recurrent tumor. Radiation and chemotherapy reduce tumor cellularity, and thus usually lead to an increase in ADC.

1.14.4 Glioblastoma Multiforme

When considering astrocytomas of all grades, a glioblastoma multiforme (GBM) is the most common tumor (▶ Fig. 1.134). It is also the most common of all primary intracranial tumors. The hallmark on histology of this lesion is necrosis. When compared to lower grade astrocytomas, patients with a GBM are older, have a shorter duration of preoperative symptoms, and have a shorter survival. This highly malignant, WHO grade IV, widely infiltrative lesion grows along white matter tracts, with extension histologically of tumor beyond any border marked on imaging by high signal intensity on T2-weighted images or abnormal contrast enhancement. The typical location is in the cerebral hemisphere, with a frontal lobe location slightly more common than other lobes. Multiple lobe involvement and spread via the corpus callosum to the opposite hemisphere are not uncommon (▶ Fig. 1.135). The prognosis is poor, with survival of 1 to 2 years. Treatment includes surgical resection (with the greater the extent of tumor removed, the better prognosis), followed by radiotherapy and chemotherapy (temozolomide and bevacizumab).

The appearance of a glioblastoma multiforme on MR (and on CT, although lesions are less well depicted with this modality) is distinctive, being a large lesion with a thick irregular enhancing ring, gross central necrosis, substantial mass effect, and extensive vasogenic edema in the adjacent white matter. The white matter tracts of the corpus callosum are very compact, thus high signal intensity extending along the corpus callosum

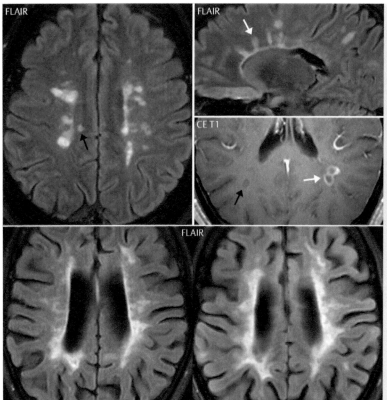

Fig. 1.122 Multiple sclerosis (MS). Scans from four patients are presented. In the first, an axial FLAIR image reveals multiple, focal, high signal intensity periventricular white matter plaques, with one lesion (*black arrow*) medial to the ventricular system, and thus in the corpus callosum. A sagittal FLAIR scan in a second patient demonstrates multiple immediate periventricular lesions, but in this plane the ovoid shape (*white arrow*) of the lesions is evident, extending along white matter tracts, together with the characteristic flat ependymal border at the ventricular surface. Both enhancing and nonenhancing (*black arrow*, in the third patient) plaques may be seen, with rim enhancement (*white arrow*) common. In the fourth patient, FLAIR scans are illustrated several years apart, demonstrating a temporal progression in cerebral atrophy (note the increase in size of the sulci) together with a greater number of, and more confluent, periventricular lesions.

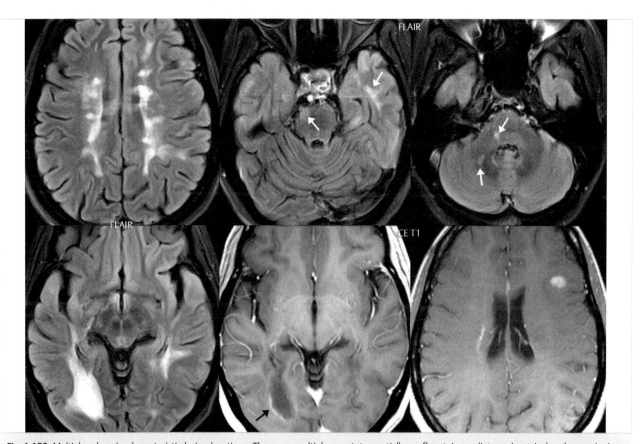

Fig. 1.123 Multiple sclerosis, characteristic lesion locations. There are multiple punctate, partially confluent, immediate periventricular plaques. Lesions are also noted in the more peripheral periventricular white matter. Additional small focal lesions are seen in the pons, anterior temporal lobe, middle cerebellar peduncle, and cerebellar white matter (*white arrows*). Two enhancing lesions are noted, with that of the left frontal lesion homogeneous in character. The large lesion in the right occipital lobe has partial rim enhancement (*black arrow*), an uncommon but also characteristic appearance.

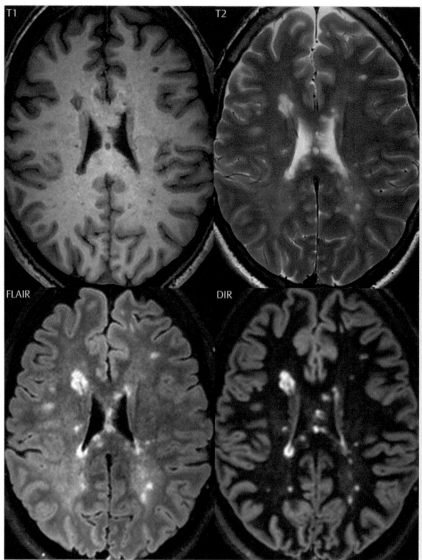

Fig. 1.124 Multiple sclerosis, visualization of plaques with differing MR techniques. As with most brain lesions, MS plaques demonstrate low signal intensity on T1- and high signal intensity on T2-weighted scans. Of note is that some MS plaques manifest very low signal intensity on T1-weighted scans relative to normal appearing white matter, so called "Black Holes". These are felt to represent areas of irreversible demyelination and axonal damage. FLAIR scans are invaluable for identification of MS plaques, and represent the clinical mainstay technique, in particular for lesions immediately adjacent to the ventricular system. On heavily T2-weighted scans such lesions may be poorly depicted, due to the high signal intensity of adjacent CSF. Double inversion recovery (DIR) is a newer scan technique, with higher lesion-white matter contrast, and improved sensitivity dependent upon lesion location.

on T2-weighted scans represents tumor extension, not edema. In a small percent of patients, on additional focus of tumor may be visualized distant from the primary lesion with apparent intervening normal brain.

1.14.5 Gliomatosis Cerebri

By definition, this diffusely infiltrating glial tumor involves three or more lobes of the brain. Although it infiltrates, and enlarges the involved brain, the underlying brain architecture is largely preserved. Gliomatosis cerebri has abnormal high signal intensity on T2-weighted scans, (▶ Fig. 1.136) where the involvement is best depicted, and typically displays no abnormal contrast enhancement.

1.14.6 Oligodendroglioma

This is a well differentiated, slowly growing cortical and subcortical, typically WHO grade II tumor, most commonly located in the frontal lobe, presenting in young to middle-aged adults. Oligodendrogliomas arise in white matter, and are usually

peripherally located. Calcification is common, about half of all lesions mildly enhance, and there is rarely substantial associated edema. Due to their slow growth and location, they can cause calvarial erosion/ remodeling (▶ Fig. 1.137). Fifty percent of oligodendrogliomas are mixed lesions (oligoastrocytoma). Although often seemingly well-defined on imaging, oligodendrogliomas are infiltrating lesions histologically. Treatment is by surgical excision and radiation. As with all suspected brain tumors, MR spectroscopy can be useful for further lesion evaluation (▶ Fig. 1.138). Functional MRI (fMRI) is an important additional pre-surgical tool, providing the ability to localize eloquent areas of the brain, such as that for movement and language.

Higher grade tumors do occur, specifically anaplastic (WHO grade III) oligodendrogliomas and mixed lesions (▶ Fig. 1.139). Lesion perfusion is commonly assessed on imaging, typically by MR. As a general rule, higher grade gliomas demonstrate higher CBV, although oligodendrogliomas can have foci of high CBV, irrespective of grade. The most common benign tumor of the brain, a meningioma, also can have high CBV. With MR, there are two different techniques to acquire perfusion information,

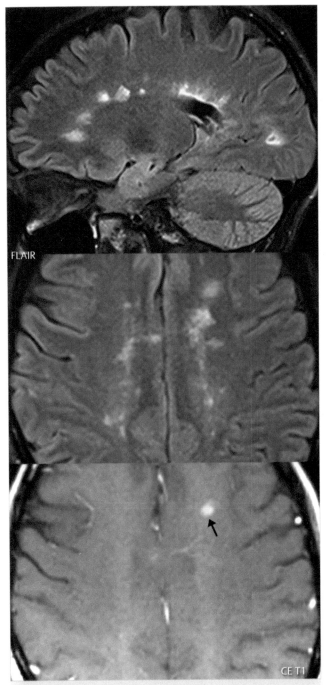

Fig. 1.125 Multiple sclerosis, active disease. This 28-year-old woman with a history of relapsing-remitting MS underwent a follow-up MR, which demonstrated progression of disease both in the brain and spinal cord (the latter not shown). Multiple punctate high signal intensity periventricular plaques, reflecting chronic lesions, are noted on sagittal and axial FLAIR images. Multiple enhancing lesions, indicative of active disease, were seen both in the brain and cord, with a moderate in size homogeneously enhancing left frontal plaque illustrated (*arrow*).

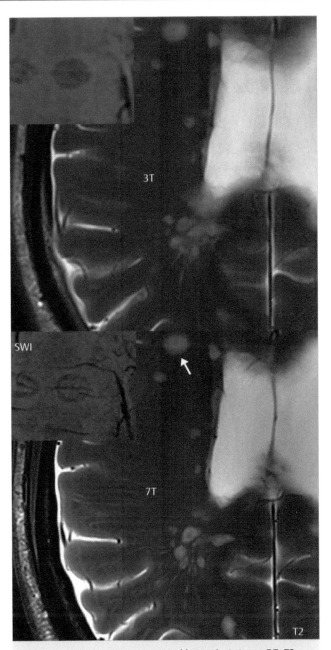

Fig. 1.126 Multiple sclerosis, improved lesion depiction at 7 T. T2-weighted images demonstrate the achievable higher spatial resolution at 7 T, with improved delineation of MS lesions posterior to the right lateral ventricle as compared to the image acquired at 3 T. On SWI (image inserts), there is higher diagnostic confidence at 7 T for identification of the central vein and iron deposition (rim of low SI) involving the large MS plaque on the right (*arrow*). Springer E, Dymerska B, Cardoso PL, et al. Comparison of Routine Brain Imaging at 3 T and 7 T. Invest Radiol. 2016;51(8):469–482.

echoplanar dynamic imaging during bolus intravenous contrast administration and arterial spin labeling (ASL)—the latter not requiring contrast administration. The spatial resolution of ASL is however lower, and only CBF measurements can be obtained (not mean transit time) (▶ Fig. 1.140).

1.14.7 Ganglioglioma

The temporal lobe is the most frequent location for this slow growing, well demarcated, lower grade tumor (80% are grade I). The frontal and parietal lobes are the next most common locations. Gangliogliomas can be solid (▶ Fig. 1.141) or cystic with a mural nodule, the latter being the most common presentation. Additional imaging characteristics include little or no associated edema, calcifications (in about half of cases), and contrast enhancement (in about half). Treatment of this tumor, which occurs in older children and young adults, is by surgical resection, which carries a relatively good prognosis.

1.14.8 Hemangioblastoma

This is the most common primary cerebellar tumor in an adult (and are classified as WHO grade I), although it should be kept in mind that the most common posterior fossa neoplasm in an adult is a metastasis. This highly vascular tumor is most commonly located in the cerebellar hemisphere. Most cases are sporadic, with von Hippel-Lindau disease patients predisposed to development of hemangioblastomas, both in the cerebellum and spine. The classic presentation is that of a well-defined cystic mass with a peripheral enhancing mural nodule (▶ Fig. 1.142). The signal intensity of the cyst on MR will be readily differentiable from CSF on FLAIR. One-third of lesions are solid. Multiple tumors are almost always associated with von Hippel-Lindau disease (▶ Fig. 1.143). Enlarged associated blood vessels are often noted (▶ Fig. 1.144).

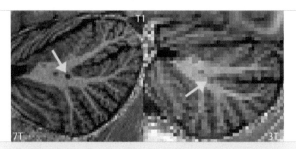

Fig. 1.127 Misclassification of cerebellar MS lesions at 3 T. The lesion (*arrow*) was correctly classified at 7 T to be within pure white matter, and incorrectly classified at 3 T as leukocortical in location. The difference is due to spatial resolution, 0.58 mm isotropic at 7 T vs 1 × 1 × 1.2 mm² at 3 T. The scans were obtained with MP2RAGE. Fartaria MJ, O'Brien K, Şorega A, et al. An Ultra-High Field Study of Cerebellar Pathology in Early Relapsing-Remitting Multiple Sclerosis Using MP2RAGE. Invest Radiol. 2017;52(5):265–273.

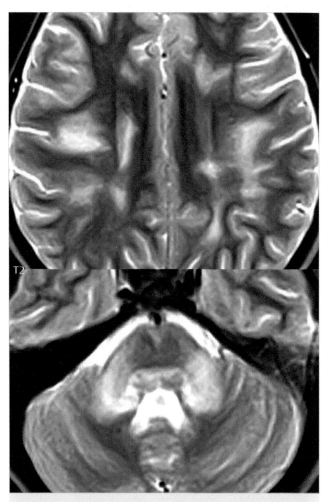

Fig. 1.128 Acute disseminated encephalomyelitis (ADEM). This pediatric patient demonstrates large poorly defined white matter lesions in the corona radiata and the bilateral middle cerebellar peduncles. The imaging appearance of prominent focal white matter lesions, together with clinical presentation (these children are usually quite ill), leads to high confidence in diagnosis of this fortunately rare disease entity.

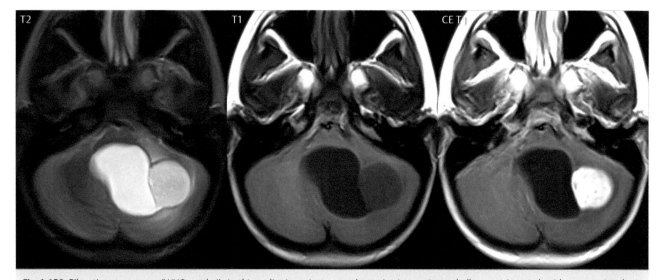

Fig. 1.129 Pilocytic astrocytoma (WHO grade I). In this pediatric patient, a moderate in size cystic cerebellar mass is noted, with an associated enhancing mural nodule laterally within the cerebellar hemisphere.

1.14.9 Primary CNS Lymphoma

Lymphoma is the one diagnosis often not included in the differential (for lesions that subsequently prove to be lymphoma), so an important entity to keep in mind. Lymphoma carries a poor prognosis. The classic imaging description follows, although many lesions do not have this appearance. The presentation is that of an enhancing mass lesion, within the basal ganglia or periventricular white matter (▶ Fig. 1.145), often involving the corpus callosum. The common misconception is that this tumor is always or most often located in central white matter. In one clinical series, this was true in only 30% of cases. Lymphoma tends to be hyperdense on CT, and exhibit restricted diffusion on MR due to its high cellularity, the latter an important differential diagnostic point. On T2-weighted scans lymphoma may appear slightly hypointense to brain, another somewhat characteristic feature. The lesion is usually large at presentation (>2 cm), in immunocompetent patients. There is usually prominent peritumoral edema. In immunocompromised patients (with this patient population having an increased incidence of lymphoma) there may be central necrosis with peripheral enhancement.

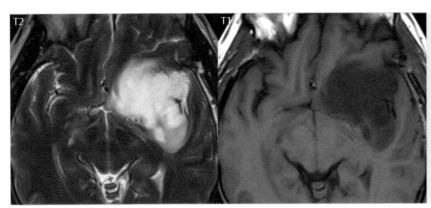

Fig. 1.130 Astrocytoma (WHO grade II). A fairly well defined large focal lesion is noted, with its epicenter in the insula. This grade II astrocytoma demonstrates characteristic, relatively uniform, high and low signal intensity on precontrast T2- and T1-weighted scans, without abnormal contrast enhancement (scan not shown). There is mild local mass effect without definite accompanying vasogenic edema.

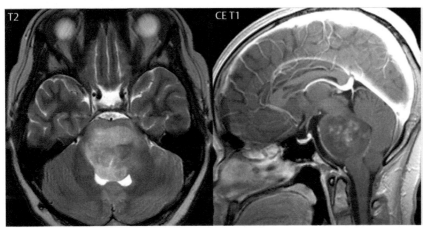

Fig. 1.131 Brainstem astrocytoma. In this pediatric patient, the pons is diffusely involved and markedly enlarged, with heterogeneous abnormal high signal intensity on the T2-weighted scan and compression of the fourth ventricle. Lesion enhancement, if present, will typically be heterogeneous and mild in degree, as illustrated in the sagittal post-contrast image.

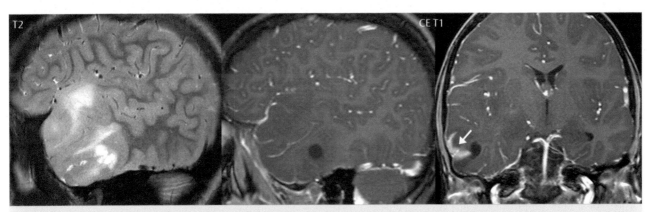

Fig. 1.132 Anaplastic astrocytoma (WHO grade III). A mass lesion with heterogeneous signal intensity and relatively poor definition of extent is noted within the temporal lobe of this pediatric patient on a sagittal T2-weighted image. Post-contrast, on the coronal scan, a small area of enhancement (*arrow*) is seen laterally within the lesion, together with slight pial enhancement on the sagittal scan. There is mild deformity of the ventricular system, reflecting mild mass effect.

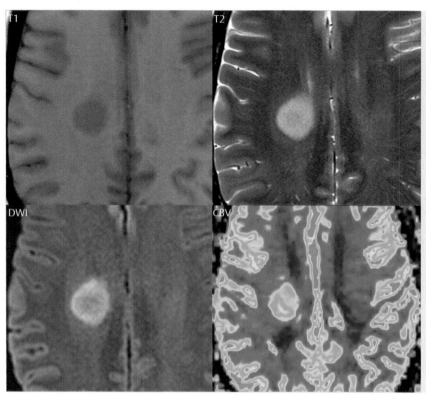

Fig. 1.133 Anaplastic astrocytoma (WHO grade III). A relatively well-defined, homogeneous lesion is noted in the right centrum semiovale, with restricted diffusion and mildly elevated rCBV. There was no abnormal contrast enhancement (image not shown). The diffusion restriction (confirmed on the ADC map, not shown) and elevated rCBV correctly suggest a higher-grade lesion, with the lesion falsely appearing on other image sequences to be of lower grade.

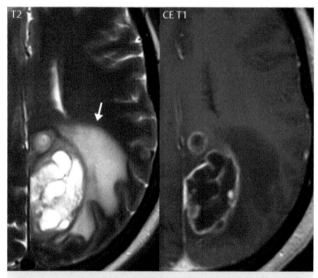

Fig. 1.134 Glioblastoma multiforme (WHO grade IV). A large mass lesion, with central necrosis (high and low signal intensity, respectively, on T2- and T1-weighted scans) is present in the left parietal lobe. The epicenter of the lesion is in white matter, with involvement of both gray and white matter. There is extensive accompanying vasogenic edema (*white arrow*), and irregular rim enhancement.

1.14.10 Medulloblastoma

The alternative term for medulloblastoma is a posterior fossa primitive neuroectodermal tumor (PNET). This is the second most frequent brain tumor of childhood after pilocytic astrocytoma, and the most common malignant lesion (it is WHO grade IV). Medulloblastomas are tumors of childhood and young adults, although predominantly occurring in the first decade of life. Histologically, this embryonal tumor is a heterogeneous disease with distinct subtypes, felt to originate from neuronal stem cells. These tumors most commonly arise from the roof of the fourth ventricle (the superior medullary velum). The tumor may either encroach upon or fill the fourth ventricle, with normal brain displaced (▶ Fig. 1.146).

In older patients medulloblastomas may arise in the cerebellar hemispheres. This highly cellular tumor is hyperdense on CT, demonstrates restricted diffusion, may appear relatively isointense with brain on T1- and T2-weighted sequences, and most commonly demonstrates intense enhancement. Abnormal contrast enhancement is however not always seen with medulloblastomas, and the enhancement can be heterogeneous. Small cystic or necrotic areas are noted in about half of all cases. Clinical presentation is often with increased intracranial pressure due to rapid tumor growth and obstructive hydrocephalus. Dissemination at the time of presentation in the CSF is common. Medulloblastomas are treated by surgical resection followed by chemotherapy and craniospinal radiation. The primary differential diagnoses include pilocytic astrocytoma, ependymoma, choroid plexus papilloma, and atypical teratoid/rhabdoid tumor.

1.14.11 Supratentorial PNET

As with medulloblastoma, this highly malignant WHO grade IV lesion demonstrates restricted diffusion and is prone to CSF dissemination. The latter characteristic mandates screening (with contrast-enhanced MR) of the entire neural axis. The most common imaging presentation is that of a large, complex hemispheric mass with little associated vasogenic edema, in a young child (▶ Fig. 1.147). Calcification is seen in about half. Contrast enhancement is typically heterogeneous. Hemorrhage, a cystic component, and necrosis within the lesion are common.

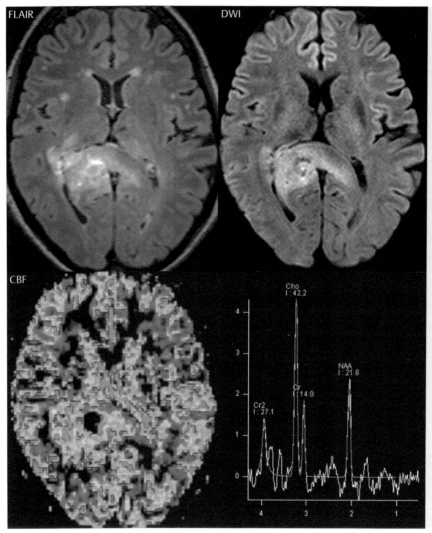

Fig. 1.135 Glioblastoma multiforme: MR diffusion, perfusion, and spectroscopy. An axial FLAIR image depicts a mass lesion with its epicenter in the right splenium of the corpus callosum, in a 79-year-old woman. There is extension of the lesion (through the splenium) across the midline to the left. Slight high signal intensity within portions of the lesion on the diffusion-weighted scan corresponded to areas of restricted diffusion (confirmed on the ADC map, not shown), a finding that correlates clinically with higher tumor grade and poorer prognosis. CBV and CBF also correlate well with histopathologic grade, and can be used to differentiate a low-grade glioma from an anaplastic astrocytoma and from a glioblastoma, being highest in the latter (with high CBF seen within portions of the lesion). On MR spectroscopy there is decreased NAA (a marker of neuronal integrity) and increased choline (a marker of increased cellular turnover), consistent with neoplastic disease (and seen in glioblastomas, but not specific for the diagnosis).

1.14.12 Dysembryoplastic Neuroepithelial Tumor

This rare WHO grade I tumor characteristically presents as a well-demarcated, "bubbly," wedge-shaped cortical/ subcortical mass. The lesion will be very hyperintense on T2-weighted scans, with no associated edema, and typically no enhancement. Clinical presentation is usually a child or young adult with partial complex seizures.

1.14.13 Choroid Plexus Papilloma

This highly vascular WHO grade I tumor occurs most often in either a lateral ventricle or the fourth ventricle. On CT and MR intense homogeneous enhancement is seen. Choroid plexus papillomas are typically well-circumscribed, lobulated lesions (▶ Fig. 1.148). Both communicating and noncommunicating (obstructive) hydrocephalus can occur, the first due to overproduction of CSF, the latter due to outlet obstruction. Presentation is more common under the age of two. In the differential for this tumor is a choroid plexus carcinoma, which is less common, and prone to CSF spread.

1.14.14 Ependymoma

Two-thirds of ependymomas are located in the fourth ventricle. One-third are supratentorial in location, arising adjacent to the lateral ventricles. The latter often have a cystic component. Calcification and CSF spread are common features. Ependymomas are usually lobulated, heterogeneous lesions, with variable enhancement (▶ Fig. 1.149). This is a tumor of children and adolescents. When located in the fourth ventricle, this soft tumor may squeeze ("creep") through the outlet foramina.

1.14.15 Pituitary Microadenoma

Prolactinomas are the most common secretory lesion of the pituitary, with 90% found in women. Clinical symptoms include irregular menses, amenorrhea, and galactorrhea. A serum prolactin level >300 µg/L is considered diagnostic, a level >100 µg/L indeterminate. Due to these tumors being hormonally active, they present as microadenomas. Dopamine agonist drugs (e.g., bromocriptine and cabergoline) are the treatment of choice. Less common functional lesions include adenomas that secrete either growth hormone or ACTH.

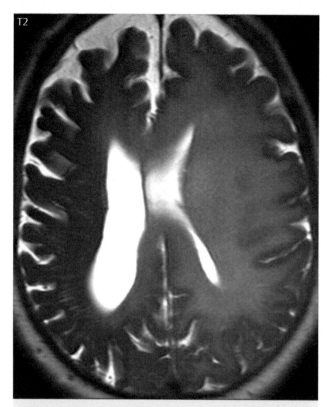

Fig. 1.136 Gliomatosis cerebri. In this entity, there is widespread tumor growth, infiltrating and expanding the involved regions but with preservation of underlying architecture. T2-weighted scans, as illustrated, show diffuse hyperintensity with accompanying mass effect, with ventricular and sulcal effacement. The lesion shown involves the left hemisphere diffusely, with extension to the right both anteriorly and posteriorly through the corpus callosum.

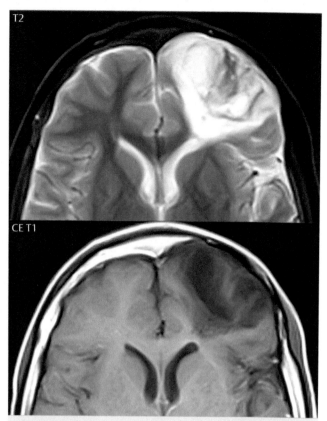

Fig. 1.137 Oligodendroglioma. A focal lesion, involving both gray and white matter but not in a vascular territory, is seen the frontal lobe (the most common location) demonstrating mild mass effect. There is thinning and remodeling of the overlying calvarium, consistent with a long standing, slow growing, lesion. There is no abnormal contrast enhancement.

CT is poor for evaluation of the pituitary, due to both beam hardening artifact and poor soft tissue contrast, and is no longer so used. Findings on CT historically described include asymmetry of the pituitary gland and abnormality of the sellar floor. Deviation of the infundibulum was also described, but was unreliable.

On MR, following bolus intravenous contrast injection, there is immediate, prominent enhancement of infundibulum, anterior pituitary, and cavernous sinus. Pituitary adenomas (both macro- and microadenomas) demonstrate a later peak of enhancement with slower washout. Thus, early postcontrast scans have substantial utility for lesion identification, with greater relative enhancement of the normal pituitary as compared to an adenoma. Most microadenomas however can be identified on precontrast images alone, with slight hypointensity on T1-weighted scans and hyperintensity on T2-weighted scans, relative to the normal pituitary (▶ Fig. 1.150).

Evaluation of the pituitary gland on MR should include thin section (≤3 mm) imaging in the coronal and sagittal planes, with both T2- and T1-weighted scans acquired along with dynamic and subsequent high-resolution post-contrast scans (or alternatively high-resolution scans acquired immediately following bolus contrast administration). Small cysts are not uncommon in the pituitary, mandating distinction between a cystic lesion and a small soft tissue mass, together with clinical correlation. Rathke cleft cysts are the most common type, with this benign (and typically asymptomatic) lesion found in the posterior portion of the anterior pituitary.

1.14.16 Pituitary Macroadenoma

The distinction between a micro- and macroadenoma is made on the basis of size, with the latter defined as a lesion > 10 mm in diameter. Macroadenomas are usually nonsecretory, with clinical symptoms caused by pressure on adjacent structures, most commonly hypopituitarism and visual loss. When very large, these lesions can compress and splay the optic chiasm, producing bitemporal hemianopsia (loss of vision in the outer half of both visual fields, due to compression of the optic chiasm). Excision is by transsphenoidal surgery, which in the past was performed via an incision under the upper lip, but which today can be performed by an endonasal approach.

On MR, macroadenomas are isointense with brain on both T1- and T2-weighted scans, and demonstrate predominantly uniform moderate contrast enhancement (▶ Fig. 1.151). The normal pituitary is typically compressed against the walls of the sella, and difficult to identify. Careful inspection of coronal images, both pre- and post-contrast, is important for detection of cavernous sinus invasion. Post-contrast scans can be particularly valuable for the differentiation between enhancing tumor

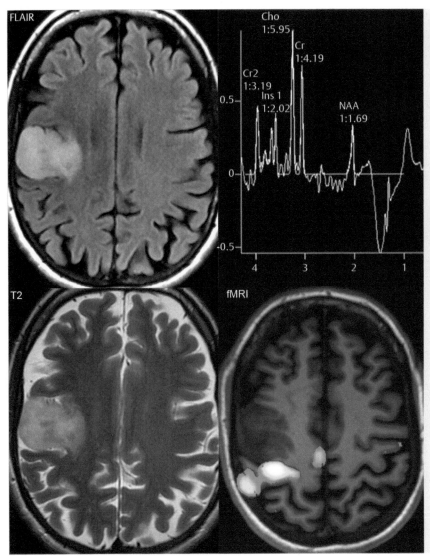

Fig. 1.138 Oligodendroglioma, WHO grade II. A mass lesion is noted on the right, in the posterior frontal lobe, somewhat peripherally located and expansile in nature. The lesion is hyperintense on T2-weighted scans, and fairly homogeneous in nature. There was no abnormal contrast enhancement (image not shown). In neoplastic disease, choline is increased and NAA decreased, relative to normal brain, a finding well illustrated by the proton spectra from within the lesion. Lactate (an inverted peak) is seen at about 1.4 ppm, with an additional lipid peak to the right. Higher-grade glial tumors tend to have lipid and lactate, as a result of necrosis. Lactate, which results from anaerobic metabolism, can also be seen in infarction. Left hand movement (fMRI) induces activation in the right primary sensorimotor cortex and in supplementary motor areas, which are shown to lie posterior and medial to the lesion.

and blood within the cavernous sinus. With pituitary macroadenomas, suprasellar extension is usually preceded by sella expansion. Large tumors are often dumbbell in shape, when there is substantial suprasellar extent, with constriction of the tumor at the level of the diaphragma sellae. The differential diagnosis for a large mass lesion with expansion of the sella includes intrasellar meningiomas and pituitary metastases, both of which are much less common.

Pituitary apoplexy is acute bleeding into either the normal pituitary or a pituitary tumor. Rapid enlargement of the gland, due to such a bleed, causes symptoms due to compression of adjacent structures (▶ Fig. 1.152). Treatment with bromocriptine can cause intratumoral hemorrhage in some instances, both with microadenomas and macroadenomas. Visualization of a fluid collection with high signal intensity on T1-weighted scans, reflecting methemoglobin, should raise the question of a treated lesion.

1.14.17 Craniopharyngioma

A craniopharyngioma is a slow growing, benign, well encapsulated, WHO grade I tumor arising from remnants of Rathke pouch. There are several age peaks, with one group in children and one to two in adults. Clinical symptoms vary with size of the lesion and patient age. The most common symptoms are due to compression, specifically of the optic chiasm (bitemporal hemianopsia) and of the pituitary (endocrine abnormalities, specifically growth hormone deficiency in a child). Seventy percent have both intrasellar and suprasellar components, whereas 20% are solely suprasellar. A craniopharyngioma is the most common suprasellar tumor and in pediatrics the most common nonglial intracranial tumor.

The tumor itself is usually heterogeneous, with both cystic and solid components (▶ Fig. 1.153). The cystic component is usually high signal intensity on T2-weighted scans and may be high signal intensity as well on T1-weighted scans. Protein, cholesterol, and methemoglobin content contribute to the latter signal intensity. In the adult the appearance on T1-weighted scans may be that of only slightly higher signal intensity when compared to normal brain, whereas in a child the lesion may be very high signal intensity similar to fat. The solid components and the rim of the lesion display contrast enhancement, which assists in differential diagnosis and in defining lesion margins. Calcification is seen on CT in 80% of cases in children, and in 40% of cases in

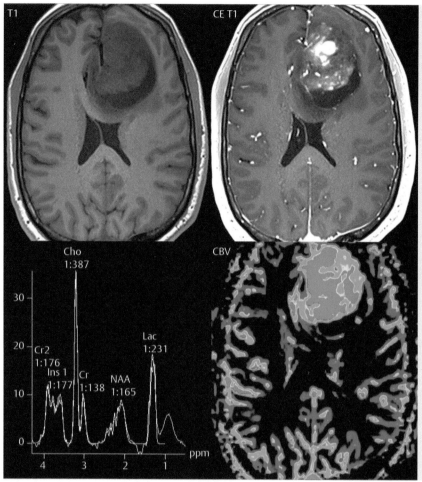

Fig. 1.139 Anaplastic oligoastrocytoma (WHO grade III). A large mass lesion is noted with its epicenter in the left frontal lobe, with mild accompanying vasogenic edema. Despite the extensive mass effect, on the basis of the precontrast exam alone a lower grade glial cell tumor might be questioned. The degree of enhancement of the lesion is however not consistent with this diagnosis. On MR spectroscopy, choline is elevated and NAA decreased, consistent with neoplastic disease. Lactate, present in this lesion, results from anaerobic metabolism and can be seen in necrotic tumors and cerebral ischemia. The high CBV of the lesion further suggests a higher grade tumor.

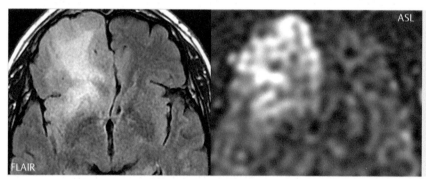

Fig. 1.140 Oligodendroglioma (presumptive diagnosis), arterial spin labeling (ASL). A somewhat ill-defined right frontal lesion with abnormal high signal intensity is noted on the axial FLAIR image. The lesion is likely long standing, with thinning and remodeling of the adjacent calvarium. ASL demonstrates marked high signal intensity within the lesion, consistent with higher vascular density and thus suggesting a higher grade tumor.

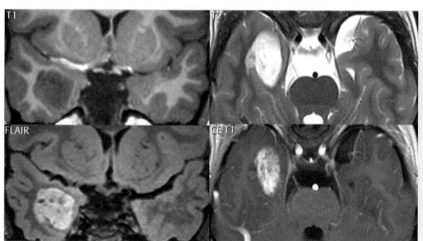

Fig. 1.141 Ganglioglioma. A relatively well defined intraaxial mass lesion is noted in the right temporal lobe, with respectively low- and high signal intensity on T1- and T2-weighted scans, and prominent enhancement. There is only mild accompanying vasogenic edema. Location in the temporal lobe is characteristic for this diagnosis, as was the patient's age (13 years), with this tumor seen in children and young adults.

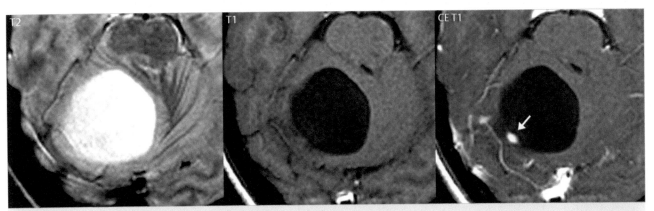

Fig. 1.142 Hemangioblastoma. A large cystic cerebellar lesion is noted, with mass effect upon the pons. Post-contrast there is enhancement of a small nidus (*arrow*) along the cyst wall, together with a suggestion of prominent associated vessels.

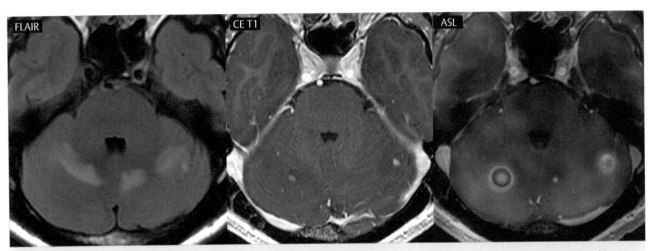

Fig. 1.143 Multiple cerebellar hemangioblastomas on MR, perfusion imaging (ASL). At least two small nodular enhancing lesions, with mild accompanying vasogenic edema and high CBF, are noted within the cerebellum in this patient with von Hippel Lindau disease. Arterial spin labeling (ASL) is an alternative technique to first pass perfusion MR, the latter acquired during bolus gadolinium chelate administration typically using echoplanar technique. The advantages of ASL include the lack of intravenous contrast administration and that the exam can be repeated. Disadvantages include low SNR (and thus typically lower spatial resolution) and limited anatomic coverage (and thus long scan times to acquire sufficient slices to cover the entire brain). Also, the technique is limited to acquisition only of CBF, with MTT not assessed. CBF and CBV can be used for improved differential diagnosis of brain tumors, with hemangioblastomas demonstrating the highest rCBV of all common lesions (including glial tumors, metastases, and lymphoma).

adults. Although the differential for lesions in this region is somewhat broad, in terms of imaging similarities only a hypothalamic glioma and a Rathke cleft cyst bear any resemblance.

1.14.18 Pineal Region Neoplasms

Tumors of the pineal region divide easily into two general groups, those of pineal parenchymal origin and germ cell tumors. These are uncommon tumors, making up about 5% of childhood intracranial tumors and 1% of adult tumors. Clinical presentation is often due to obstructive hydrocephalus. There can be paralysis of upward gaze, a distinctive clinical finding, due to compression of the tectum. Germ cell tumors can also have endocrine abnormalities.

Germ cell tumors make up 95% of all tumors arising from the pineal gland itself, occur in the first three decades of life, have a male predominance, and are all prone to CSF seeding. Due to

the latter, contrast administration is critical, together with imaging (screening) of the entire neural axis. Germ cell tumors can also arise in the hypothalamus and suprasellar region. The major differential for a suprasellar germinoma is Langerhans cell histiocytosis. A germinoma is the most common pineal tumor. These tumors are markedly radiosensitive. On MR, germinomas demonstrate homogeneous prominent enhancement. Due to their high cellularity, there may be restricted diffusion. The next most common tumor following a germinoma is a mixed germ cell tumor (▶ Fig. 1.154). Much less common, pineal region germ cell tumors include teratoma, yolk sac tumor, embryonal carcinoma, and choriocarcinoma.

Pineal parenchymal tumors are divided into three types, which from most malignant to least are pineoblastoma, pineal parenchymal tumor of intermediate differentiation (PPTID), and pineocytoma. Pineoblastomas are highly malignant, WHO grade IV lesions, and occur in the first two decades of life. These are typically large bulky tumors, heterogeneous in appearance,

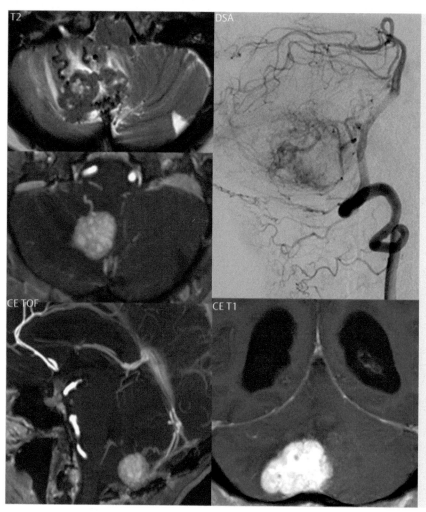

Fig. 1.144 Hemangioblastoma with a prominent vascular supply. A cerebellar mass lesion is seen on the axial T2-weighted scan, with mild accompanying vasogenic edema. A distinctive additional finding is the many prominent associated vascular structures (flow voids). TOF MRA performed with contrast administration reveals a highly vascular lesion, with prominent early enhancement, and tortuous feeding vessels both anteriorly and posteriorly. There is prominent homogeneous enhancement on the coronal post-contrast T1-weighted scan. DSA reveals a vascular mass, with prolonged staining (confirmed by later temporal series images), and A-V shunting.

with necrotic areas, restricted diffusion due to high cellularity and prominent enhancement. CSF spread is common. PPTIDs (▸ Fig. 1.155) occur in middle-aged adults and are an intermediate grade lesion, with an intermediate imaging appearance (between the two extremes). A pineocytoma is a benign, well-demarcated, noninvasive, slow growing tumor that presents in adults. These appear as small mass lesions on MR, without distinctive signal characteristics, and display prominent enhancement, which may be solid or rim like. On CT, pineal calcifications tend to be displaced by a pineocytoma, rather than engulfed—a pattern seen in germinomas.

As discussed elsewhere in this text, a pineal cyst is a common normal variant, and should not be confused for a pineal region tumor. These are typically ovoid, smoothly marginated, with a thin cyst wall, homogeneous contents, and slightly hyperintense to CSF on FLAIR. They may demonstrate a thin, uniform rim of enhancement (specifically without nodularity).

1.14.19 Brain (Parenchymal) Metastases

MR is the imaging modality of choice for screening and follow-up for brain metastases. Treatment options depend on the number of detected lesions. Surgical resection combined with radiotherapy for single brain metastases prolongs survival and improves quality of life. Single lesions are thus today treated by

surgical resection, if in an amenable area of the brain. Stereotactic radiation is used for multiple lesions, with variable cut offs in lesion number but often about five. Otherwise, the only option for treatment is whole brain radiation. It should be noted that whole brain radiation is palliative only. In patients with multiple metastases, whose only option is whole brain radiation, median survival is in the range of 1 year. Given that half of metastases to the brain are solitary and that another 20% of patients have only two metastases, MR plays an important role in choice of treatment. Lung carcinoma, breast carcinoma, and renal cell carcinoma are common cancers that metastasize to the brain. Most cases of adenocarcinoma, a type of non-small-cell lung carcinoma, and small-cell lung carcinoma are associated with smoking. Lung cancer in general has early preferential metastasis to the brain.

Although metastases occur in all areas of the brain, a frequent location is the gray-white matter junction (▸ Fig. 1.156). Prominent associated vasogenic edema is common; however, many metastases have no associated edema.

Intravenous contrast enhancement using the gadolinium chelates is mandatory, markedly increasing lesion detectability. Many small metastases may not manifest sufficient edema or T2 abnormality to be recognized otherwise. On post-contrast scans metastases may be solid or ringlike, the latter with central necrosis. In clinical practice, for practical purposes, it is

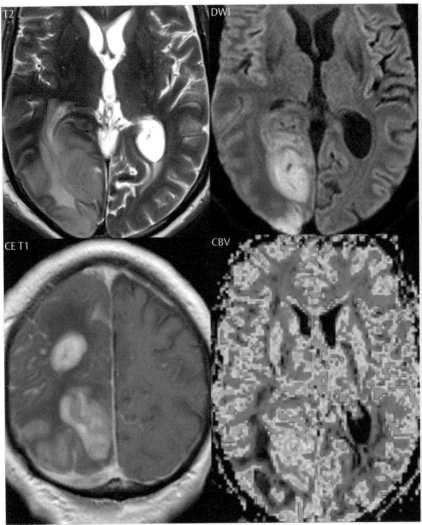

Fig. 1.145 B cell lymphoma. A hyperintense periventricular mass lesion with accompanying vasogenic edema is noted in the right occipital lobe on the T2-weighted scan, with contrast enhancement seen on the coronal T1-weighted scan. The mass had restricted diffusion (reflected by the high SI on DWI), which is compatible with primary CNS lymphoma, a diagnosis confirmed at surgery. rCBV is elevated, but not to the degree expected for a glioblastoma, favoring again the diagnosis of primary CNS lymphoma.

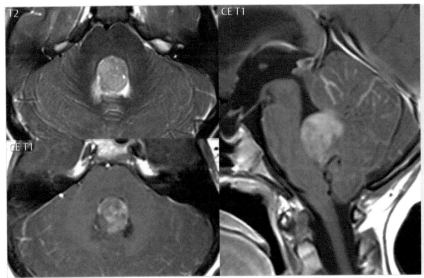

Fig. 1.146 Medulloblastoma. An enhancing lesion is noted filling the fourth ventricle on axial images, mildly displacing adjacent brain. The mass causes obstructive hydrocephalus, with enlargement of the third and lateral ventricles seen on the midline sagittal image. Contrast enhancement along the cerebellar folia reflects leptomeningeal carcinomatosis, seen in up to one-third of patients at presentation.

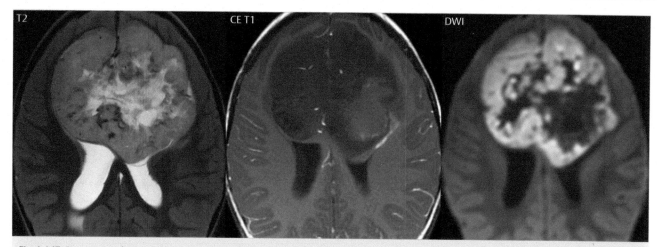

Fig. 1.147 Supratentorial primitive neuroectodermal tumor(PNET). A large bilateral frontal mass lesion, with little accompanying vasogenic edema, is noted in this 2.5-year-old patient. The lesion is relatively well demarcated, with little abnormal contrast enhancement. The T2-weighted scan demonstrates abnormal high signal intensity centrally within the mass, likely reflecting necrosis. Small hypointense foci consistent with hemorrhage are also noted within the mass on this sequence. On the diffusion-weighted scan, the mass is predominantly hyperintense, reflecting restricted diffusion due to the dense cellularity of this tumor type.

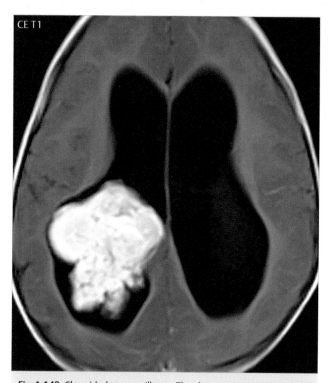

Fig. 1.148 Choroid plexus papilloma. The characteristic appearance of this benign entity is illustrated in an infant, with a large, sharply marginated, lobulated lesion noted within the lateral ventricles, with intense relatively homogeneous contrast enhancement. There is accompanying dilatation of the ventricular system (longstanding, without interstitial edema).

accepted standard. There are many caveats, however, with both gradient echo and fast spin echo 3D T1-weighted scan types available, and further optimization in terms of sensitivity to contrast media possible. Recent publications have demonstrated fast spin echo 3D T1-weighted scans such as SPACE to be markedly superior, although the gradient echo technique MP-RAGE with lower sensitivity is commonly used due mainly to a lack of dissemination of this knowledge. Detectability of brain metastases is further improved by the use of high contrast dose, specifically 0.3 mmol/kg as opposed to 0.1 mmol/kg. Today, only the macrocyclic gadolinium chelates have approval for administration at high dose, advocating further their use. In summary, to maximize detection of brain metastases, scans should be acquired with high contrast dose (0.3 mmol/kg), at 3 T, using optimal imaging techniques (3D techniques with high sensitivity to contrast media), with a slight time delay (a few minutes) following contrast injection (due to the temporal course of lesion enhancement) and with the latest, highest SNR, dedicated brain coil.

Hemorrhage is not uncommon, de novo, in parenchymal metastases (▶ Fig. 1.157). Hemorrhage may also be seen following radiation therapy. Renal cell carcinoma, melanoma, choriocarcinoma, thyroid carcinoma, lung carcinoma, and breast carcinoma are the common primary tumor types associated with hemorrhagic metastases. Melanotic melanoma metastases also demonstrate high signal intensity precontrast on T1-weighted images (due to the paramagnetic effect of metals, predominantly iron, bound by melanin), with this appearance dependent on a sufficient percentage of melanotic cells being present (▶ Fig. 1.158).

1.14.20 Leptomeningeal Metastases

Contrast-enhanced MR is markedly superior to CT for the detection of leptomeningeal metastases. However, detection of this disease principally relies clinically on CSF cytology, which requires large volumes and multiple samples but is superior to both MR and CT. Imaging may be negative despite positive

assumed that essentially all metastases demonstrate enhancement. However, experimental studies have shown that very small, early metastases may not have sufficient disruption of the blood-brain barrier to be so visualized. The choice of imaging technique is crucial for high lesion sensitivity, with high spatial resolution 3D techniques acquired at 3 T the current

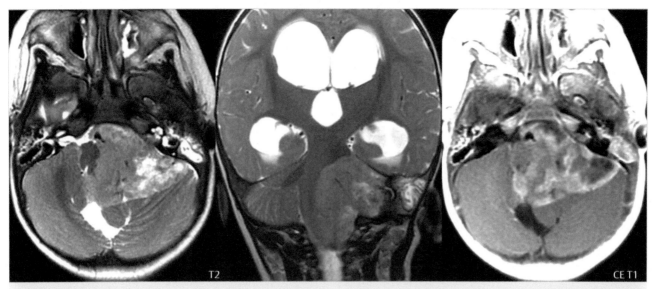

Fig. 1.149 Ependymoma. A large infratentorial extraaxial mass lesion, involving the fourth ventricle, foramen of Luschka, and cerebellopontine angle on the left, is seen on axial and coronal images. Obstructive hydrocephalus is present, with enlargement of the third and lateral ventricles, together with interstitial edema—the latter best seen immediately superior to the lateral ventricles and inferior to the temporal horns on the coronal image. The medulla is displaced to the right, and the basilar artery encased by tumor. Cystic portions of the lesion are present, reflected in part by mixed signal intensity, with prominent heterogeneous enhancement.

cytology. Leptomeningeal spread of neoplastic disease portends a poor prognosis. Primary neoplasms with a propensity for leptomeningeal spread include high-grade astrocytoma, medulloblastoma, and ependymoma. Secondary (metastatic) tumors with a propensity for leptomeningeal spread include breast and lung carcinoma and melanoma. Abnormal contrast enhancement is seen on MRI of the leptomeninges, commonly with both nodular and smooth linear components (▶ Fig. 1.159).

1.14.21 Calvarial Metastases

Large calvarial metastases are well seen on CT due to focal bone destruction (involving the outer or inner table). If attention is paid to evaluation of the diploic space on MR, this modality is exceedingly sensitive to diploic space metastases (▶ Fig. 1.160). On unenhanced T1-weighted scans, diploic space lesions are easily recognized, appearing as small focal masses distinct from normal high signal intensity fatty marrow. Confirmation of a metastasis can be made by comparison with the T2-weighted scan. On postcontrast scans, the majority of diploic space metastases enhance, with the exception of some osteoblastic lesions. By far the best scan for lesion detection is a post-contrast, thin section, fat saturation sequence.

1.14.22 Langerhans Cell Histiocytosis

This is a disease of childhood, previously referred to by the term eosinophilic granuloma (of bone). The unifocal form is male predominant, presents with a solitary osteolytic lesion, and is treated by excision. The classic presentation is that of a solitary skull lesion (not to be confused with a metastasis), well visualized by either CT or MR (▶ Fig. 1.161). On CT the lesion will be lytic and sharply marginated. The multifocal form presents with multiple bony lesions and in one-third of patients with diabetes

insipidus due to hypothalamic involvement, the correlate on MR being a thickened enhancing pituitary infundibulum.

1.14.23 Calvarial Hemangioma

This benign intraosseous skull lesion is most often solitary. Typically asymptomatic, they can present as a palpable mass. On CT a calvarial hemangioma appears as a sharply marginated expansile lesion, with the inner and outer tables intact and the outer table often more expanded (▶ Fig. 1.162). Trabecular thickening with radiating spicules of bone is also characteristic. The lesion is predominantly vascular, with resulting diffuse, heterogenous enhancement on MR (▶ Fig. 1.163).

1.14.24 Fibrous Dysplasia

This developmental skeletal disease occurs in both monostotic and polyostotic forms, with craniofacial involvement seen in 10 to 25% and 50%, respectively, of cases. Lesions are generally well vascularized. Other than the expansile nature, the appearance on CT is variable ("ground glass," sclerotic, cystic, or mixed). On MR, in active disease, intense enhancement can be seen.

1.14.25 Meningioma

Meningiomas are common "incidental" findings (unexpected findings in patients with clinical symptoms related to other disease processes), in particular when considering lesions < 1 cm in lesion diameter. Symptoms generally occur due to mass effect on adjacent vital structures. They are the most common benign intracranial tumor (15% of all intracranial tumors in adults), and the most common extraaxial adult tumor. Meningiomas are multiple in 8% of cases. The peak age of incidence is in older adults, and they are rare under age 30. They are 1.5 to 2 times

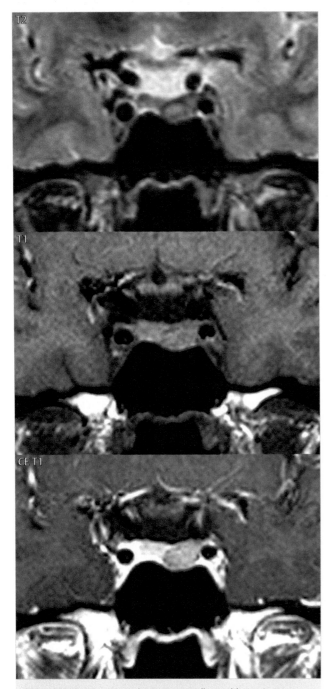

Fig. 1.150 Pituitary microadenoma. A small round lesion is seen within the pituitary, with only subtle differentiation on the basis of signal intensity precontrast from the normal pituitary gland (although the majority of microadenomas are well visualized precontrast). On the immediate post-contrast scan, the lesion is however well visualized, with lower enhancement compared to the normal, prominently enhancing, pituitary gland. Contrast enhancement is of substantial value for lesion identification in a small percentage of cases.

more common in women. Morphologically, meningiomas are usually globular in shape and well demarcated, often with a broad dural attachment. Much less common is the en plaque variant, with primary extension along the dura and without parenchymal invagination. Meningiomas are in general slow growing

tumors, which displace adjacent brain tissue. Although a benign tumor, they can invade the venous sinuses and bone (▶ Fig. 1.164 and ▶ Fig. 1.165). Histologically, there are several major subtypes. The meningothelial cell type is most common. Recurrence following resection is more common with the clear cell type.

Common locations for meningiomas include the falx (▶ Fig. 1.166), convexity (▶ Fig. 1.167), sphenoid wing, parasellar (cavernous sinus) (▶ Fig. 1.168) and suprasellar region, tentorium (▶ Fig. 1.169), and petrous ridge. Less common, yet characteristic, additional locations include the olfactory groove (▶ Fig. 1.170), cerebellopontine angle (where it is the second most common lesion following a vestibular schwannoma), and foramen magnum. It is important to consider the differential diagnosis for lesions in the suprasellar region, which includes pituitary macroadenoma, craniopharyngioma, optic nerve glioma, aneurysm, metastasis, chordoma, and hypothalamic glioma, although all—with the possible exception of metastasis—often have characteristic differentiating features. Intraventricular meningiomas are rare (1%), but do occur. A meningioma is the most common tumor of the atrium of the lateral ventricle. Meningiomas are frequently calcified. There is an increased incidence in neurofibromatosis type 2.

The typical imaging appearance of a meningioma is that of a well-circumscribed, extra-axial mass lesion with a flat dural interface. As with all extra-axial masses, multiplanar imaging is useful to confirm this location. On noncontrast CT, 25% are calcified and 75% appear hyperdense (with 25% isodense) (▶ Fig. 1.171). There can be adjacent bony hyperostosis.

Meningiomas are relatively isointense to brain on precontrast T2- and T1-weighted sequences. On a T1-weighted scan with good gray-white matter contrast, the gray matter can be seen displaced or "buckled" away from the lesion (confirming the extra-axial location). On T2-weighted sequences, a CSF cleft may be visualized between the lesion and adjacent brain. Enhancement, whether on CT or MR, is typically homogeneous and intense (▶ Fig. 1.172). Post-contrast, a dural tail (linear enhancing thickening of the meninges extending away from the tumor) is common, seen in about half of cases. However, this finding is not specific for a meningioma and can be seen with other extra-axial lesions. Vasogenic edema is not uncommon, and may be prominent. Although meningiomas are usually homogeneous lesions, necrotic areas, cysts, and hemorrhage can be seen. Densely calcified regions within a lesion are not uncommon, and on MR are visualized as a signal void on all pulse sequences.

An en plaque meningioma is a subtype that grows along the planes of the leptomeninges, in distinction to the typical globular lesion. Common locations are the sphenoid ridge and the convexity. These can be difficult to detect on CT, due to bone artifact, and somewhat surprisingly—even if quite large—may go unrecognized on unenhanced MR. Marked hyperostosis of adjacent bone is not uncommon, often disproportionate with tumor size. The differential diagnosis, both for an en plaque and a globular meningioma, includes a dural-based metastasis.

1.14.26 Hemangiopericytoma

Hemangiopericytomas arise from embryonic vascular elements (angioblasts), as do hemangioblastomas. These tumors have a higher cellularity, are extremely vascular, and are malignant

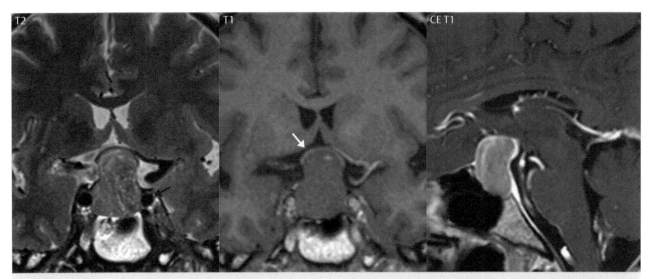

Fig. 1.151 Pituitary macroadenoma. A large mass lesion occupies and expands the sella, with marked suprasellar extension of the lesion. Characteristic mild heterogeneous high signal intensity on T2-, slight low signal intensity on T1-, and moderate enhancement (slightly heterogeneous in nature) on post-contrast T1-weighted scans are noted. The optic chiasm (*white arrow*) is thinned and splayed by the mass. The mass is slightly narrower in dimension at the level of the diaphragma sella (as if constricted here, a "figure of 8" appearance). On the T2-weighted scan, there is no abnormal soft tissue surrounding the cavernous carotid artery (*black arrow*), consistent with the lack of cavernous sinus invasion, a pertinent negative.

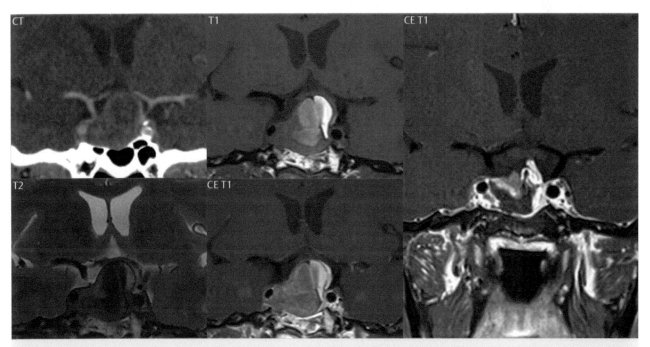

Fig. 1.152 Pituitary macroadenoma with hemorrhage. The sella is expanded by a mass lesion, which extends superiorly to compress the optic chiasm. There is extensive hemorrhage therein, representing a combination of intracellular and extracellular methemoglobin. Note post-contrast the enhanced pituitary infundibulum, draped over the left side of the mass. The coronal scan on the far right of the figure was obtained intraoperatively, and demonstrates residual tumor tissue both within the cavernous sinus on the right and superiorly to the right of the infundibulum (which is now more convoluted in shape).

(WHO grade II and III). They have a high rate of recurrence following resection. On imaging hemangiopericytomas present as lobular prominently enhancing extra-axial masses (most often supratentorial in location), and thus may be mistaken for a meningioma. Enhancement is often heterogeneous. Cystic and/or necrotic areas are common. Mass effect and associated vasogenic edema are common, as are signs of prominent vascularity such as flow voids. The peak incidence is in the fourth to sixth decades.

1.14.27 Radiation Injury

Following radiation therapy, whether focal or whole brain, changes can be observed in the white matter on MR (but

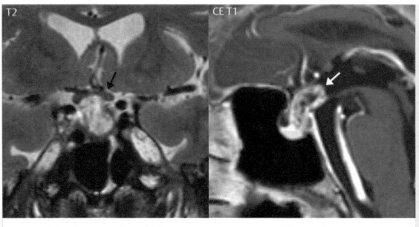

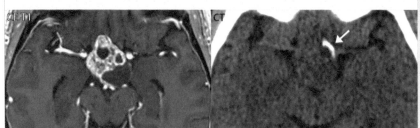

Fig. 1.153 Craniopharyngioma. **Part 1:** A mass (*white arrow*) with its epicenter in the suprasellar cistern is noted on the sagittal post-contrast image, with both enhancing and cystic components. This tumor also extends inferiorly into the sella itself. Mild compression of the optic chiasm (*black arrow*) above, and the pituitary gland below is seen on the coronal T2-weighted scan, although the margins of the lesion are poorly delineated due to near isointensity of the cystic portions with CSF. **Part 2:** In a second patient, the axial post-contrast MR identifies characteristic cystic and soft tissue components of this suprasellar lesion. In this instance, CT provides additional pertinent differential diagnostic information, specifically the calcification along a portion of the lesion (*white arrow*). The tumor itself is poorly delineated on CT, being isodense on this unenhanced scan.

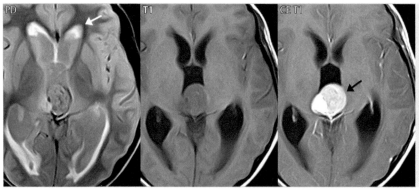

Fig. 1.154 Mixed germ cell tumor (pineal). A mass lesion of the pineal gland, with prominent enhancement (*black arrow*), is illustrated. Unfortunately, this appearance is not specific for any single tumor, although statistically a germinoma is most likely. There is acute obstructive hydrocephalus (caused by the lesion), identified by the slight prominence of the ventricular system in this pediatric patient, together with the periventricular high signal intensity (*white arrow*) seen on the proton density weighted scan, the latter consistent with interstitial edema.

limited to the area of radiation). Vasogenic edema is seen early following treatment, due to damage to capillary endothelium, with limited clinical consequences. This finding is rarely seen clinically, however, likely due to its low incidence and the timing of imaging exams relative to treatment. The late sequela of radiation therapy is that which is most often visualized, and is due to axonal demyelination with increased water content. The imaging appearance of these late changes on MR is that of diffuse, symmetric white matter hyperintensity on T2-weighted scans, involving the periventricular white matter but sparing the compact fibers of the corpus callosum (▶ Fig. 1.173).

The extent of involvement, and specifically the degree with which more peripheral white matter is involved, depends on many factors, including in particular radiation dose. The involvement of the white matter will be scalloped laterally, and in severe disease can extend to the cortical gray matter (but sparing the subcortical U-fibers). Radiation white matter changes are more common in elderly patients and with higher total radiation dose. The time of onset from treatment varies, and can be seen within the first year following a single radiation treatment. Clinically, radiation white matter changes are most often seen in patients given palliative whole brain radiation for metastatic disease. In this population, the early changes can be somewhat subtle and restricted to the more immediate periventricular white matter. Commonly with time this involvement will progress both in terms of the degree of abnormal high signal intensity on FLAIR and the extent of involvement of more peripheral white matter.

1.14.28 Radiation Necrosis

Radiation necrosis occurs in up to 25% of cases after conventional therapy. Both recurrent tumor and radiation necrosis present as a mass lesion with abnormal contrast enhancement and surrounding vasogenic edema, and thus cannot be differentiated on conventional pre- and postcontrast CT or MR

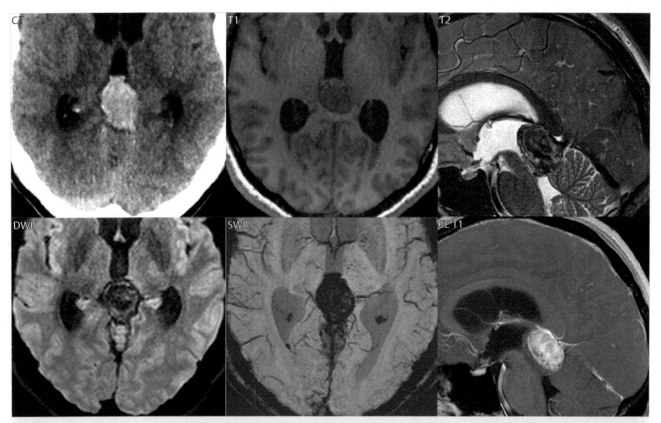

Fig. 1.155 Pineal parenchymal tumor (WHO grade III). An enhancing mass is noted with its epicenter in the region of the pineal gland. The ventricular system is enlarged, due to compression of the cerebral aqueduct. Hemorrhage is common with pineal parenchymal tumors, and is visualized in the current case (specifically hemosiderin, with low signal intensity) on the T2 FSE and DWI scans, but is best seen on SWI. On CT, these tumors are frequently hyperdense, as with this example. A pineal parenchymal tumor of intermediate differentiation (PPTID) – the specific diagnosis in this case – is an official WHO category, and is a neoplasm that is considered to be intermediate in biologic behavior between pineoblastoma and pineocytoma. Grade I pineal parenchymal tumors are pineocytomas, grade II and III PPTIDs, and grade IV pineoblastomas.

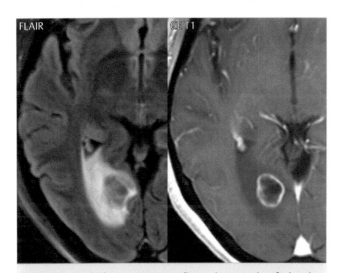

Fig. 1.156 Cerebral metastasis. A small mass lesion is identified at the gray-white matter junction (occipital in location in this instance), with a thin uniform rim of contrast enhancement and moderate associated cerebral edema (seen best on FLAIR), all common findings in intracranial metastatic disease.

(▶ Fig. 1.174). Diffusion-weighted scans are also of limited value, although restricted diffusion is seen much more frequently with recurrent tumor. Differentiating between these two entities is further complicated by the common existence of a mixture of tumor and radiation necrosis. Perfusion studies, which can be performed by either MR or CT, enable differentiation in many instances, with CBV decreased in radiation necrosis (and elevated in recurrent tumor). Often, a relative CBV (rCBV) value is reported, which can be obtained in the absence of measurement of the arterial input. MR spectroscopy has been used as well to improve the differentiation between radiation necrosis and recurrent tumor, with increased Cho/NAA and Cho/Cr ratios seen in recurrent tumor.

1.15 Nonneoplastic Cysts

1.15.1 Arachnoid Cyst

Arachnoid cysts are common, benign, CSF filled lesions. They represent 1% of all intracranial masses. In terms of etiology, they can be congenital, inflammatory, or posttraumatic. The most common location is the middle cranial fossa (▶ Fig. 1.175)

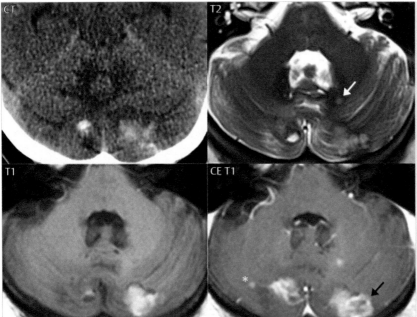

Fig. 1.157 Cerebellar metastases. Metastatic disease presents with a wide spectrum of imaging appearances, with MR markedly superior to CT. The latter modality may show associated hemorrhage, as in the current example, but otherwise reveal only large enhancing lesions. Regarding the appearance of intracranial metastatic disease on MR, a small lesion may be visible on T2-weighted scans with slight hyperintensity (*white arrow*), or may be undetectable without intravenous contrast administration (*asterisk*). Edema can vary from being absent to quite prominent. If there is hemorrhage (specifically methemoglobin, with high signal intensity on T1-weighted scans), close inspection of post-contrast images is mandatory to ensure that an enhancing lesion (*black arrow*) is not present immediately adjacent to the hemorrhage (being the source of bleeding).

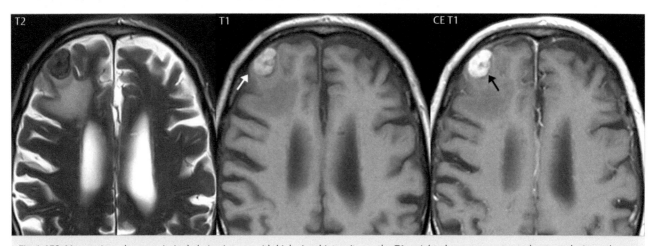

Fig. 1.158 Metastatic melanoma. A single lesion is seen with high signal intensity on the T1-weighted scan precontrast, due to melanin, and enhancement post-contrast (*black arrow*). Contrast enhancement of the lesion is easily identified, due to the further increase in signal intensity, by comparing similarly windowed and centered images, using the same imaging technique and plane, pre-and post-contrast. Whether a lesion like this is intraaxial (as in this instance) or extraaxial in location requires close inspection of the images, and is assisted by evaluation in all three orthogonal planes. Note the absence of a gray matter cortical ribbon medial to the lesion (which would be present in an extraaxial lesion), and that brain parenchyma extends lateral to the lesion posteriorly (*white arrow*), placing this metastasis within the brain parenchyma. T2* susceptibility effects (low signal intensity on T2) are also common in melanoma metastases, as illustrated, but unrelated to melanin content.

with other characteristic locations including overlying the brain convexity, in the perimesencephalic cistern, and posterior to the cerebellum. In the middle cranial fossa, arachnoid cysts can be accompanied by hypogenesis of the temporal lobe. The vast majority of arachnoid cysts are asymptomatic, although symptoms due to mass effect can occur. On CT, communication of these lesions with the subarachnoid space can be demonstrated, with filling by intrathecal contrast on delayed scans. On MR, arachnoid cysts will demonstrate CSF signal intensity on all pulse sequences. Although the appearance of an arachnoid cyst is characteristic, a consideration of two other entities that show some similarity on imaging is likely warranted. Epidermoid tumors on all scans other than diffusion are relatively

isointense to CSF, and like arachnoid cysts are space occupying masses. However, epidermoids are distinctive in having marked high signal intensity on diffusion weighted scans. Cystic neoplasms can be differentiated on the basis of demonstration of the cyst wall, abnormal contrast enhancement of a portion of the lesion, associated abnormal soft tissue, non-CSF signal intensity of the fluid, and accompanying vasogenic edema.

1.15.2 Epidermoid Cyst

These are rare, benign congenital lesions, resulting from incomplete cleavage of neural from cutaneous ectoderm at the time

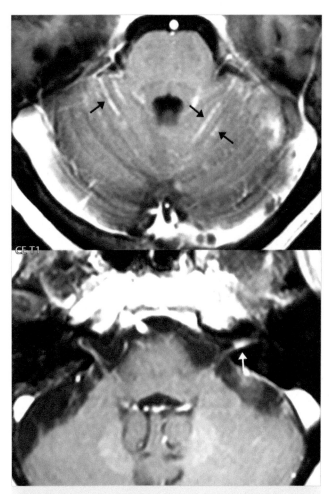

Fig. 1.159 Leptomeningeal carcinomatosis. There is abnormal enhancement involving the pia-arachnoid (*black arrows*) lining the surface of the cerebellum together with the seventh and eighth nerve complexes within the left internal auditory canal (IAC). Although this can be inflammatory in nature (due to infection or subarachnoid hemorrhage), the IAC involvement would be unusual. Leptomeningeal carcinomatosis is favored in this instance, and is the correct diagnosis in this patient with widely metastatic lung carcinoma.

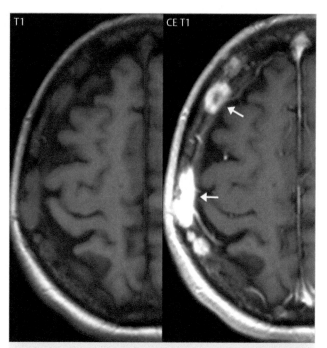

Fig. 1.160 Diploic space metastases. Multiple focal, mildly expansile, lesions of the diploic space (*arrows*) are noted. Enhancement is present post-contrast, which is critical for differential diagnosis as well as identification of lesions in patients with less prominent disease.

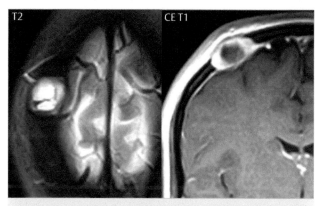

Fig. 1.161 Langerhans cell histiocytosis. On the axial image a small, well-defined calvarial (diploic space) lesion is visualized near the vertex. On the coronal post-contrast image the lesion demonstrates prominent enhancement, and is noted to be slightly expansile in nature.

of neural tube closure, with retention of ectopic ectodermal cells in the neural groove. Epidermoid cysts grow slowly by desquamation of epithelial cells from the lining and contain keratin and cholesterol. These lesions are thought of as pliable, extending into and conforming to the subarachnoid spaces. Thus, they are usually large at clinical presentation, which generally occurs in adults. Surgical resection is often incomplete. The classic location for an epidermoid cyst is the cerebellopontine angle. Here it is the third most common lesion after vestibular schwannoma and meningioma. Less common locations include the fourth ventricle (▶ Fig. 1.176) and the parasellar region/middle cranial fossa. On CT, these are round, lobulated lesions with low density. On MR, epidermoid cysts are very slightly greater than CSF in signal intensity on T1-weighted scans (rarely they can be hyperintense on T1), and on FLAIR are typically evident due to their slight hyperintensity. There is no abnormal contrast enhancement. Diffusion weighted imaging is critical, both for identification of the lesion and demonstration of the characteristic very high signal intensity (restricted

diffusion) – as well as for demonstration of recurrence or residual (▶ Fig. 1.177). MR is the imaging modality of choice for differentiation of this lesion from an arachnoid cyst, which has CSF signal intensity on all pulse sequences. Another differentiating feature between these two lesions is that an epidermoid encases nerves and vessels.

1.15.3 Dermoid Cyst

Like epidermoid cysts, these are rare, benign, congenital lesions. Both are considered "pearly" tumors, due to the glistening white appearance of the intact fibrous capsule at surgery. Dermoid cysts usually present in the first three decades of life, earlier than epidermoids. A dermoid cyst differs

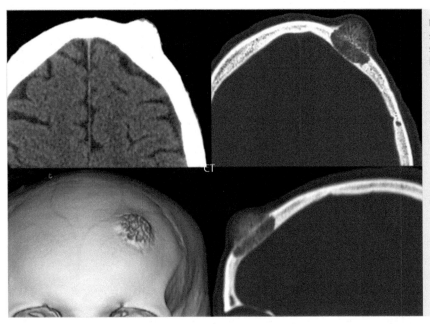

Fig. 1.162 Skull hemangioma, CT. A solitary, sharply marginated, expansile lesion with a sunburst pattern (on images reconstructed with a bone algorithm) is visualized on unenhanced CT.

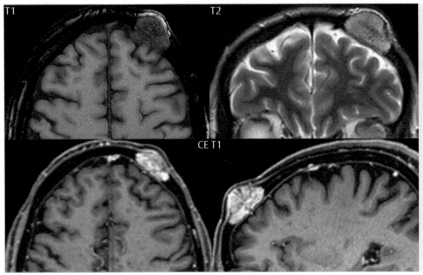

Fig. 1.163 Skull hemangioma, MR (same patient as ▶ Fig. 1.162). A large, well defined, expansile diploic space lesion is noted involving the left frontal bone, with slight hypo- and hyperintensity relative to brain on T1- and T2-weighted images. There is prominent enhancement, due to the presence of abundant vessels therein, which microscopically can be capillary, cavernous, or mixed in type.

pathologically from an epidermoid cyst due to the presence of skin appendages and hair follicles (dermal elements). They occur in the midline, with a suprasellar location most common, followed by the posterior fossa. Dermoid cysts can also originate in the spine, and then present clinically due to rupture, with fat globules seen distributed throughout the subarachnoid space of the brain (▶ Fig. 1.178). There is significant morbidity and mortality associated with rupture. Associated clinical symptoms include meningeal signs, seizure, and vasospasm. On CT, dermoid cysts are hypointense, due to the fat content. On MR, they demonstrate fat signal intensity, with chemical shift artifacts observed adjacent to the lesion on low bandwidth sequences. A scan with fat saturation is useful to confirm lesion composition (fat). There may be mild enhancement of the capsule with primary lesions.

1.15.4 Colloid Cyst

These are rare lesions of the anterosuperior third ventricle, round in shape, often found immediately adjacent to the foramen of Monro. The capsule is thin and fibrous, with the contents consisting of secretory and breakdown products, including fat, blood, cholesterol, and CSF. Colloid cysts are of congenital origin, and enlarge slowly. Their size ranges from millimeters to several centimeters. Half are incidental findings on imaging, without clinical symptoms. Colloid cysts are usually not symptomatic until adulthood, but when symptomatic can cause hydrocephalus (due to obstruction of the foramina of Monro), herniation, and death. On CT, the majority of colloid cysts are hyperdense (although they can be iso- to hypodense). The signal intensity on MR is variable, but most commonly

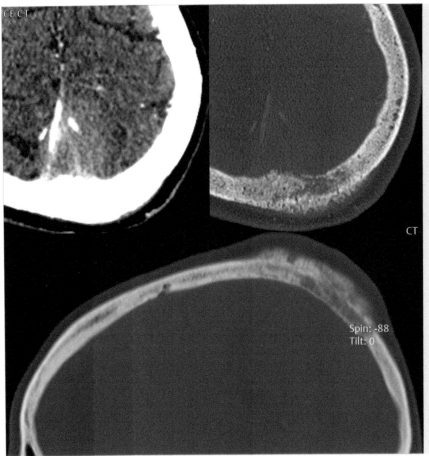

Fig. 1.164 Convexity meningioma with invasion of the superior sagittal sinus and the calvarium, CT. An enhancing lesion is identified along and to the left of the falx posteriorly, with occlusion of the superior sagittal sinus (diagnosed by the lack of enhancement). A portion of the sinus and adjacent draining cortical veins are identified along the anterior margin of the lesion. The calvarium is focally involved, with expansion, osteolysis and a suggestion of an extracranial component. The latter two features suggest a malignant (WHO grade III) meningioma.

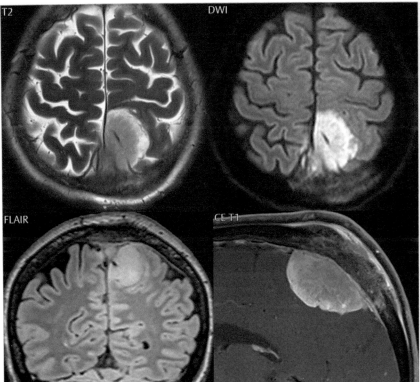

Fig. 1.165 Convexity meningioma with invasion of the superior sagittal sinus and the calvarium, MR (same patient as ▶ Fig. 1.164). An extra-axial mass lesion is noted, adjacent to and to the left of the falx. The superior sagittal sinus is occluded. Meningiomas with restricted diffusion (hyperintensity on DWI), as in this example, tend to be malignant or highly atypical. The sagittal post-contrast exam reveals the broad base of the lesion along the calvarium, with extension to involve both the skull and the subcutaneous tissue. Despite the extensive spread of disease, by histopathology this was a WHO grade II meningioma.

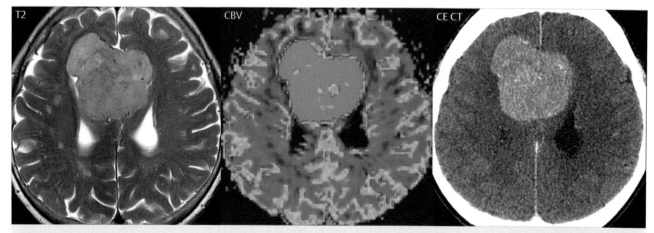

Fig. 1.166 Meningioma, along the falx. A large extra-axial lesion is noted along the midline, with displacement of adjacent brain well demonstrated on the axial T2-weighted scan. There is no associated vasogenic edema. On CT, there is homogeneous enhancement of the mass. High CBV, as in this lesion, correlates with histopathologic lesion vascularity. Most meningiomas have CBV higher than that of gray matter, with CBV very high in some cases. Both glioblastomas and metastases also have high CBV, with this measure thus of little value in differentiating a meningioma from the latter (e.g., a dural metastasis).

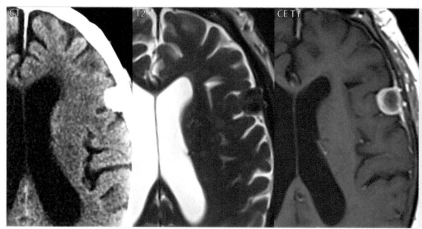

Fig. 1.167 Meningioma, along the cerebral convexity. A classic, densely calcified incidental small meningioma is well depicted on CT. The extremely dense calcification leads in MR to low signal intensity on the T2-weighted scan (due to the relative absence of soft tissue), and peripheral enhancement—as opposed to the more common homogeneous enhancement. The dural base and extra-axial location (with displacement of the adjacent gyrus) are readily evident.

increased signal intensity on T1- and isointense to brain on T2-weighted scans (▶ Fig. 1.179). The location and shape of the lesion are keys to diagnosis.

1.16 Cerebrospinal Fluid Disorders

1.16.1 Obstructive Hydrocephalus, Intraventricular

This entity is defined by obstruction proximal to the foramina of Luschka and Magendie. It can be acute or chronic (compensated) (▶ Fig. 1.180). The ventricular system proximal to the level of obstruction will be dilated, with the dilated portion more round in appearance ("ballooned"). In cases of acute obstruction there will also be abnormal high signal intensity on T2-weighted scans in the periventricular white matter (best seen on FLAIR, as a thick smooth hyperintense rim), representing interstitial edema. The sulci and cisterns will be effaced, and the corpus callosum thinned: the latter in cases where the lateral ventricles are both enlarged.

1.16.2 Obstructive Hydrocephalus, Extraventricular

In this entity, also known as communicating hydrocephalus, there is obstruction distal to the outlet foramina of the fourth ventricle. The lateral and third ventricles, and in most cases the fourth ventricle, will be enlarged without evidence of a specific (proximal) lesion causing obstruction. The enlargement of the ventricular system will be out of proportion to any enlargement of the subarachnoid space, the latter as assessed by prominence of the cortical sulci and the sylvian fissures. In some patients the fourth ventricle may appear near normal in size. Important differential diagnostic considerations include ventricular enlargement due to parenchymal atrophy and normal pressure hydrocephalus. The most common cause of extraventricular obstructive hydrocephalus is subarachnoid hemorrhage (▶ Fig. 1.181). Other etiologies include obstruction due to inflammatory or neoplastic exudates, and in this instance leptomeningeal enhancement will be demonstrated on contrast-enhanced MR.

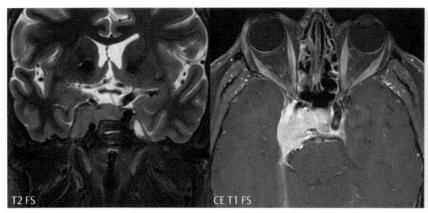

Fig. 1.168 Meningioma, cavernous sinus. On the coronal T2-weighted scan, a homogeneous soft tissue mass is seen within the right cavernous sinus, displacing the pituitary (and infundibulum) to the left. On the axial post-contrast scan, there is intense homogeneous enhancement, with convex outward bowing of the margin of the right cavernous sinus (consistent with a mass therein), encasement of the right internal carotid artery (seen also on the coronal scan), and a suggestion of extension of the lesion along the dural margin posteriorly (confirmed on scans not shown).

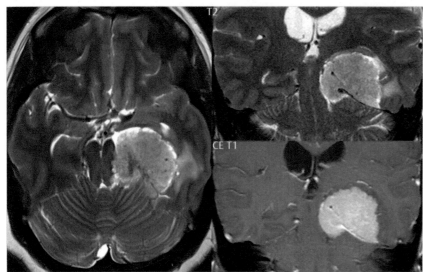

Fig. 1.169 Tentorial meningioma. A large extra-axial mass lesion is seen with a broad base along the tentorium. Note the compression of the cerebral peduncles, best seen on the axial exam. A classic finding is also seen, for the diagnosis of a meningioma, specifically a CSF cleft circumferential to the lesion (well visualized on the axial scan). Such a cleft is pathognomonic, although not common. There is mild accompanying vasogenic edema. This meningioma also demonstrates characteristic prominent, homogeneous contrast enhancement.

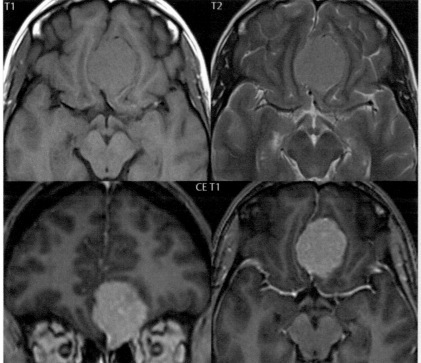

Fig. 1.170 Olfactory groove meningioma. A large, midline, extraaxial lesion is noted within the low frontal region, with homogeneous enhancement on post-contrast axial and coronal images. On the latter, the lesion is noted to extend inferiorly to the region of the left olfactory bulb.

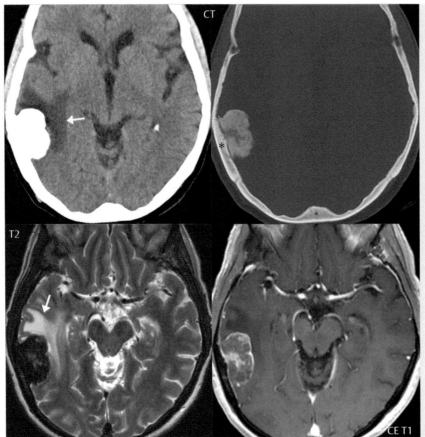

Fig. 1.171 Meningioma, densely calcified with moderate vasogenic edema. The dense calcification is well seen on both CT (with scans reconstructed using a soft tissue and a bone algorithm presented) and MR, the latter on the T2-weighted scan as a signal void (due to the absence of mobile protons). The lesion is moderate in size, with the accompanying vasogenic edema (*arrow*) seen as low attenuation on CT and high signal intensity on the T2-weighted scan. Note that despite the dense calcification, some enhancement can be seen within the lesion on MR. The mass is extraaxial, with a broad base along the convexity, and mild adjacent hyperostosis (*asterisk*), the latter best demonstrated on the unenhanced CT reconstructed with a bone algorithm.

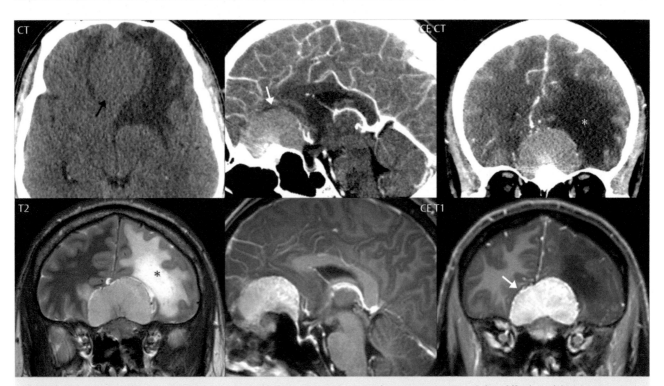

Fig. 1.172 Meningioma, planum sphenoidale. The mass (*black arrow*) is isodense on the precontrast CT, and thus difficult to delineate. On postcontrast sagittal and coronal scans, both on CT and MR, there is homogeneous enhancement of the lesion (*white arrows*). Substantial accompanying vasogenic edema (*asterisk*) is noted, with mass effect on the corpus callosum anteriorly well depicted on sagittal scans. There is prominent adjacent bony hyperostosis, visualized on both CT and MR.

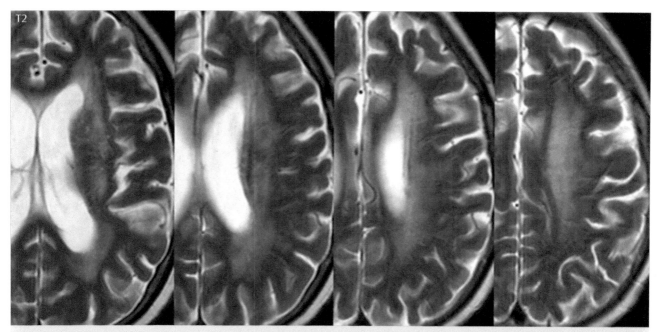

Fig. 1.173 Radiation white matter changes. There is diffuse abnormal increased signal intensity on T2-weighted images within the periventricular and supraventricular white matter, in this elderly patient who received whole brain radiation more than a year previous to the current exam. The abnormality extends from immediate periventricular in location toward the more peripheral white matter. These changes had progressed since the prior MR exam (not shown). Note that the corpus callosum (e.g., the genu and splenium, seen on the first image) is spared, being more resistant to injury due to the more compact nature of the white matter tracts.

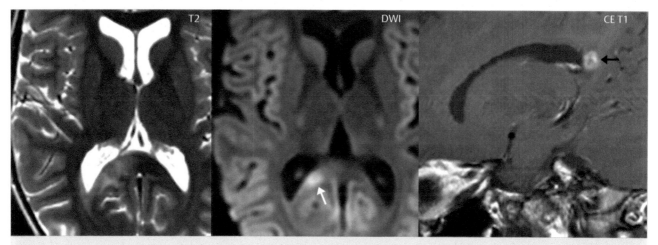

Fig. 1.174 Radiation necrosis. Abnormal high signal intensity is noted on the T2-weighted scan in the right splenium of the corpus callosum on axial imaging. Restricted diffusion (high signal intensity) is seen on the diffusion weighted axial image in the center of this abnormality (*white arrow*), which would favor recurrent tumor. The lesion (*black arrow*) enhances post-contrast, as visualized on a sagittal image. This pediatric patient received proton beam therapy for an anaplastic ependymoma, with biopsy of the lesion in question consistent with radiation necrosis, and follow-up MR showing persistent gliosis but without enhancement. On conventional MRI imaging, specifically without the acquisition of CBV perfusion studies, radiation necrosis and recurrent tumor have a similar imaging appearance—that of an enhancing lesion with surrounding vasogenic edema.

1.16.3 Normal Pressure Hydrocephalus

This entity is defined by ventriculomegaly with normal CSF pressure and altered CSF dynamics. The lateral and third ventricles will be enlarged, along with the sylvian fissures, disproportionate to enlargement of the cortical sulci (▶ Fig. 1.182). The hippocampi should be normal (not atrophic, as can be seen in generalized atrophy). Increased CSF velocity in the cerebral aqueduct is reported, with an accentuated CSF jet (signal void on T2-weighted scans) in the proximal fourth ventricle. The classic clinical triad is that of dementia, urinary incontinence, and gait disturbance. The pathogenesis is poorly understood. Findings on CT or MR are not specific, with the challenge clinically to identify patients that will be responsive to ventricular shunting. The major differential diagnosis is parenchymal atrophy.

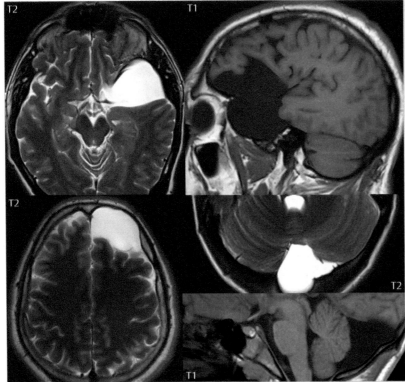

Fig. 1.175 Arachnoid cysts. Three common locations for an arachnoid cyst are illustrated. In the first patient, axial T2- and sagittal T1-weighted images depict a large CSF signal intensity fluid collection within the middle cranial fossa (by far the most common location for an intracranial arachnoid cyst), which extends superiorly. With an arachnoid cyst there may be simply displacement of adjacent brain, or, as in this instance, also loss of brain substance. In the second patient, a single axial T2-weighted image above the level of the ventricular system demonstrates a moderate in size convexity arachnoid cyst. Note the mass effect associated with this lesion, and in particular the remodeling (and thinning) of the adjacent calvarium. In the third patient, axial T2- and sagittal T1-weighted images depict a posterior fossa arachnoid cyst, with the remodeling of adjacent bone and the mild mass effect on the cerebellum (the latter best seen on the sagittal image) differentiating this lesion from a prominent cisterna magna.

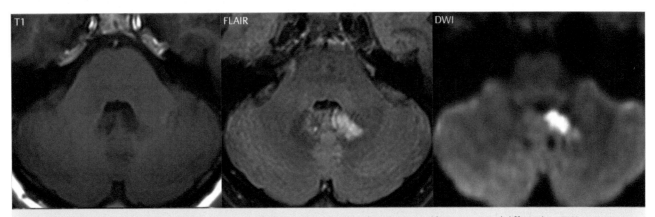

Fig. 1.176 Epidermoid cyst. A lesion with mild hyperintensity on FLAIR, and striking hyperintensity (due to restricted diffusion) on DWI is seen in one of the recesses of the fourth ventricle, a less common location than that classic for this lesion, the CPA cistern. Epidermoids are difficult to visualize on other pulse sequences (e.g., the T1-weighted scan illustrated), and contrast enhancement is not seen.

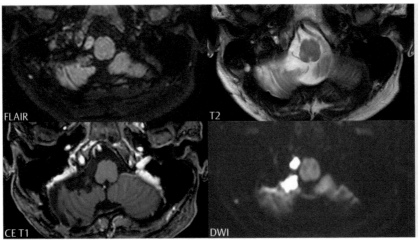

Fig. 1.177 Recurrent epidermoid. On the FLAIR scan there is a region of abnormal signal intensity, isointense to brain, to the right of the medulla. This could be related to abnormal soft tissue, or simply reflect artifact due to CSF pulsation. On the FSE T2-weighted scan, and the post-contrast T1-weighted scan, the question of subtle abnormal soft tissue in this region (nearly isointense with CSF) remains. The diffusion weighted scan is diagnostic in this instance, with several areas of marked hyperintensity seen within the subarachnoid space to the right of the medulla, consistent with an epidermoid.

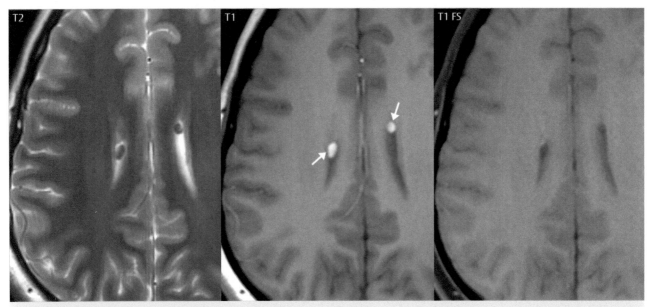

Fig. 1.178 Ruptured dermoid cyst. On the T2-weighted scan, two small round lesions are noted within the superior part of the lateral ventricles, each demonstrating a subtle chemical shift artifact (artifactual high signal intensity anterior rim). On the T1-weighted scan these are high signal intensity (*arrows*). With fat saturation, this is suppressed, confirming the lesions to be fat. Other scattered fat globules were noted in this patient in the ventricular system and subarachnoid space.

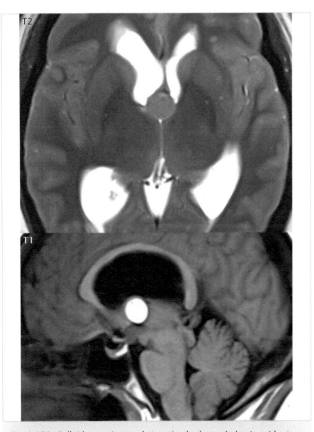

Fig. 1.179 Colloid cyst. Acute obstructive hydrocephalus is evident on the T2-weighted scan, with dilatation of the ventricles and periventricular high signal intensity (interstitial edema). A small round mass lesion is identified, in the anterior superiorthird ventricle, with intermediate signal intensity on axial T2- and high signal intensity on sagittal T1-weighted scans. Wedged into the foramina of Monro, this colloid cyst is acutely obstructing CSF outflow.

1.16.4 CSF Shunts and Complications

Of the long-term ventricular drainage catheters, the most common is a ventriculoperitoneal (VP) shunt. The presence of a shunt reservoir is an easily seen differentiating feature from a simple ventricular catheter. The reservoir can be used to acutely relieve pressure and to obtain CSF samples. In most patients with failure of a VP shunt, the lateral and third ventricles will enlarge. This can be visualized on CT or MR, with exams prior to shunt failure important for ventricular size comparison (▶ Fig. 1.183).

Exams performed following successful shunt revision will demonstrate a decrease in ventricular size. The tips of the temporal horns are a particularly sensitive area to assess for enlargement of the ventricular system, relative to a prior exam. In some patients with acute shunt obstruction interstitial edema will be visualized in the white matter surrounding the lateral ventricles. The variability in appearance on CT or MR of shunt malfunction is caused in part due to the compliance of the ventricular system. In a minority of patients there will be little to no change in ventricular size with shunt malfunction (presumably due to changes involving the ependymal lining of the ventricles). The integrity of a shunt is typically evaluated by a plain X-ray shunt series, examining the shunt along its entire course for integrity.

1.16.5 Idiopathic Intracranial Hypertension

In this entity, by definition, there is increased intracranial pressure without a known cause. Headache and papilledema are seen in almost all patients. Imaging findings (not all will be present in any individual patient) include dilatation of the sheath surrounding the optic nerves, tortuosity of the optic nerves, flattening of the posterior sclera, and protrusion of the optic papilla (disc) into the globe (▶ Fig. 1.184). The optic

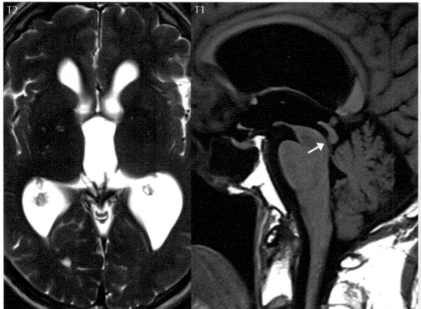

Fig. 1.180 Compensated obstructive hydrocephalus, due to a web or stenosis involving the distal cerebral aqueduct (*arrow*). There is prominent dilatation of the lateral and third ventricles. The proximal portion of the cerebral aqueduct is enlarged. Well illustrated on the sagittal image is thinning and upward bowing of the corpus callosum, with an enlarged rounded anterior recess of the third ventricle. There is mild enlargement of the opening of the sella, with the pituitary gland itself slightly compressed therein.

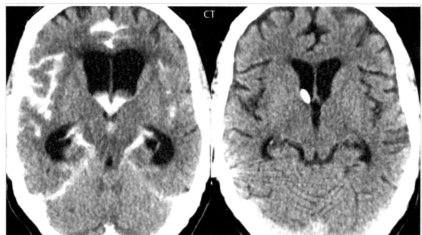

Fig. 1.181 Extraventricular obstructive hydrocephalus (communicating hydrocephalus). Axial CT scans are shown at clinical presentation, and on follow-up 4 months later. On the initial scan there is extensive acute subarachnoid hemorrhage, which is more prominent in the right sylvian fissure, a pattern consistent with the location of the ruptured aneurysm, which was at the right MCA trifurcation. Note that the frontal horns of the lateral ventricles are markedly dilated, as are the temporal horns, consistent with obstructive hydrocephalus in the setting of subarachnoid hemorrhage in this 54-year-old patient. On the follow-up CT, the ventricular system is normal in size (decompressed), and note is made of a ventriculoperitoneal shunt, with its tip in the right frontal horn of the lateral ventricle.

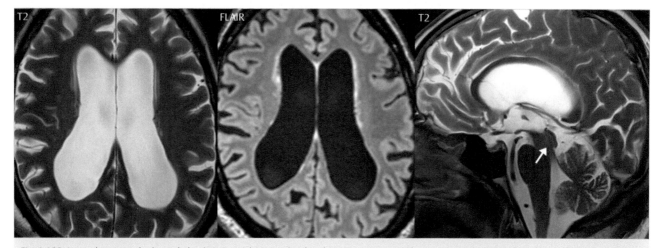

Fig. 1.182 Normal pressure hydrocephalus (NPH). Axial T2-weighted and FLAIR images reveal prominent dilatation of the lateral ventricles, without either substantial cortical atrophy (ventriculomegaly out of proportion to sulcal enlargement) or chronic small vessel white matter ischemic changes. The sagittal T2-weighted scan reveals a prominent flow void (*arrow*) in the cerebral aqueduct. These three findings are characteristic for NPH, but not definitive in terms of diagnosis, or more importantly for predicting those patients who will respond well clinically to placement of a ventriculoperitoneal shunt.

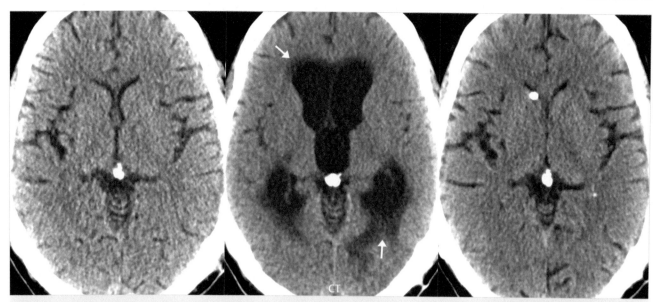

Fig. 1.183 Shunt malfunction. On the initial CT in this patient with a ventriculoperitoneal shunt (not present at the level illustrated), the ventricular system is normal in size. Several months later, there is gross enlargement of the ventricular system (middle image). Immediately periventricular, adjacent to the frontal horns and atria (*white arrows*) of the lateral ventricles, there is a thin zone of hypodensity, consistent with interstitial edema in obstructive hydrocephalus. Following shunt replacement (with the tip seen in the right frontal horn), the ventricular system is decompressed. Note also the compression of sulci and the sylvian fissures bilaterally in the middle image, due to increased intracranial pressure.

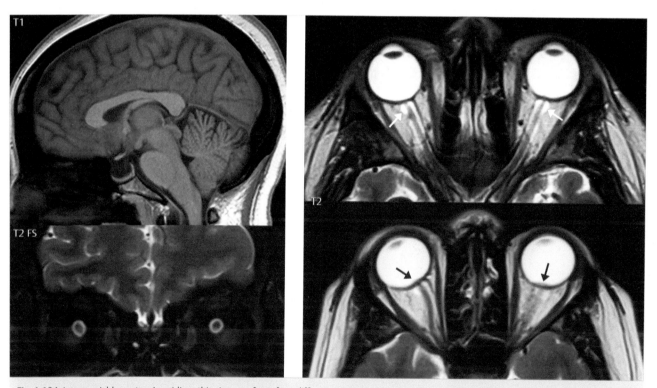

Fig. 1.184 Intracranial hypertension, idiopathic. Images from four different patients are presented. In **part 1**, the sagittal image depicts a partially empty sella, and the coronal image gross dilatation of the optic nerve sheaths. In **part 2**, the upper image displays in a different patient again the dilatation of the optic nerve sheaths, this time in the axial plane, with slight bulbous dilatation of the sheaths immediately posterior to the globes (*white arrows*). The lower image reveals tortuosity of the right optic nerve, flattening of the posterior sclera bilaterally, and intraocular protrusion of the optic nerves (papilledema, *black arrows*).

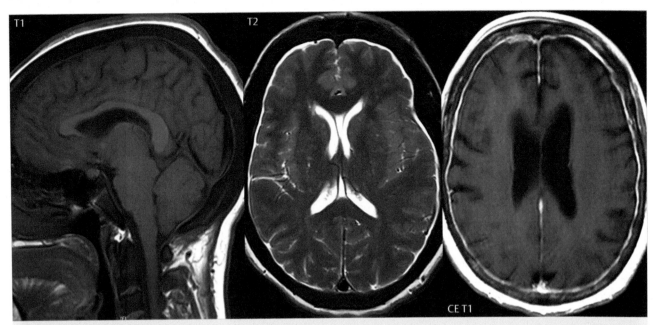

Fig. 1.185 Intracranial hypotension. Note on the sagittal T1-weighted image the generalized brain descent, with relative obliteration of CSF spaces adjacent to the midbrain, brainstem, and cerebellum. The pons is compressed against the clivus, and the optic chiasm and hypothalamus lie immediately adjacent to the sella. The axial T2-weighted scan in the same patient depicts small bilateral subdural fluid collections. In a second patient, on the post-contrast T1-weighted scan, there is diffuse intense dural enhancement, with all features presented characteristic for this entity.

nerves will both be involved. A secondary finding is a partially empty sella, with the increased intracranial pressure pushing against the diaphragma sellae with resultant flattening of the pituitary. It should be noted, however, that an empty sella is also a common incidental finding.

1.16.6 Intracranial Hypotension

Patients with this entity demonstrate classically on MR downward brain displacement, smooth, diffuse dural thickening (best seen post-contrast, with intense enhancement), and subdural fluid collections (usually hygromas) (▶ Fig. 1.185). The downward displacement of the midbrain ("sagging") is the most striking feature. There can be accompanying effacement of the CSF cisterns, with the pons flattened against the clivus. Venous engorgement is also described. Headache is a common presenting symptom. Intracranial hypotension can occur with a spontaneous spinal CSF leak or following intracranial shunt placement (overshunting).

2 Head and Neck

2.1 Skull Base

Addressing normal anatomy, the sphenoid bone forms the foundation of the central skull base. It forms the floor of the middle cranial fossa, provides structure for the cavernous sinus and a base for the pituitary gland. The shape of the sphenoid bone is bird-like with outstretched wings, being composed of the central body, two sets of wings (greater, lesser), and the medial and lateral pterygoid plates (inferiorly). Important foramina include the foramen rotundum, located medially in the anterior greater wing and containing the maxillary nerve (cranial nerve [CN] V2); the foramen ovale, located in the floor of the middle cranial fossa and containing the mandibular nerve (CN V3); and the foramen spinosum, located posterolateral to the foramen ovale and containing the middle meningeal artery and the meningeal branch of the mandibular nerve. The cavernous sinus borders the pituitary gland on each side, and contains medially the internal carotid artery (ICA), with the abducens nerve (CN VI) just inferior and lateral to the ICA.

Laterally, the cavernous sinus contains (from superior to inferior) the oculomotor nerve (CN III), the trochlear nerve (CN IV), and the ophthalmic (CN V1) and maxillary (CN V2) divisions of the trigeminal nerve. Blood flows into the cavernous sinus from the superior and inferior ophthalmic veins, superficial cortical veins, and the sphenoparietal sinus. The drainage of the cavernous sinus is via the superior and inferior petrosal sinuses. The clivus is not properly a separate bone, but rather the gradual sloping bony process that extends from the dorsum sellae to the foramen magnum. The clivus thus includes a portion of the body of the sphenoid bone (basisphenoid) and the basilar (anterior) portion of the occipital bone (basiocciput).

The most important (common) developmental abnormality affecting the middle cranial fossa (and thus by proximity the skull base) is an arachnoid cyst, a lesion that can also be traumatic in origin. By definition, an arachnoid cyst contains cerebrospinal fluid (CSF). It can expand with time. Of all locations,

for this entity, the middle cranial fossa is the most common. Bony changes may be present, including thinning and remodeling of the adjacent sphenoid wings.

Meningiomas are the most common benign skull base tumor. One-third of all meningiomas involve the skull base, with most of those involving the sphenoid wing. Bony hyperostosis is not uncommon. For lesions adjacent to the cavernous sinus, it should be kept in mind that sinus invasion is common. Other common locations for a meningioma include the olfactory groove and planum sphenoidale. Pituitary macroadenomas are discussed in depth in Chapter 1, but are relevant to the skull base and surrounding structures due to their propensity for cavernous sinus invasion and optic chiasm compression.

Chordomas and chondrosarcomas are the two malignant tumors of the skull base of note. Chordomas arise from remnants of embryonic notochord, with the second most common location being the clivus (after the sacrum). These are usually midline, destructive, infiltrative, slow-growing tumors and are often large on presentation with a poor prognosis. Areas of dystrophic calcification are common on computed tomography (CT). On magnetic resonance (MR), chordomas appear relatively well-defined and enhance postcontrast (▶ Fig. 2.1). A characteristic feature of this tumor is "thumb-printing" on the anterior brainstem, typically the pons.

Chondrosarcomas are found along synchondroses, with a propensity to occur in the skull base at the petrooccipital synchondrosis (▶ Fig. 2.2). Thus, these tumors are usually off midline (as opposed to chordomas). Tumor spread is usually by local invasion with destruction of adjacent bone. Calcification is characteristic, but the degree of calcification is widely variable. Resection is often incomplete, and recurrence is common. Increasingly, atypical presentations for lymphoma have been reported, and lymphoma needs to be included in the differential diagnosis of clivus lesions (▶ Fig. 2.3).

Metastases to the skull base are more common than primary bone tumors. Skull base invasion can also occur secondarily

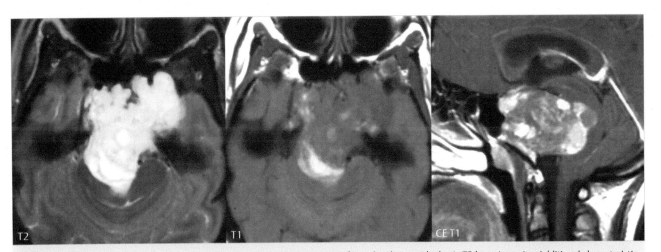

Fig. 2.1 Chordoma. A large destructive, expansile midline mass is seen, arising from the clivus, with classic T2 hyperintensity. Additional characteristic findings are seen on pre- and postcontrast T1-weighted scans. Foci of hyperintensity are present within the mass on the axial precontrast T1-weighted scan, consistent with hemorrhage and/or mucinous material. The sagittal postcontrast image reveals the thumb-like indentation of the lesion upon the pons, and the honeycomb-like enhancement due to large cystic/necrotic areas.

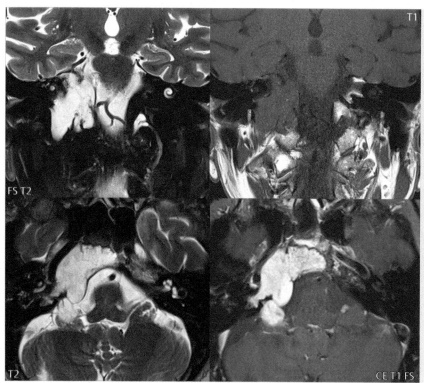

Fig. 2.2 Chondrosarcoma of the skull base. Chondroid tumors are most often located off midline, due to their propensity to occur (when located in the skull base) at the petroclival synchondrosis. High signal intensity on T2-weighted scans is common, as illustrated in this patient. Enhancement is reported to be often mild, in distinction to the case presented (with prominent enhancement). Most chondrosarcomas are well- or moderately differentiated and slow growing, with lobulated margins also characteristic.

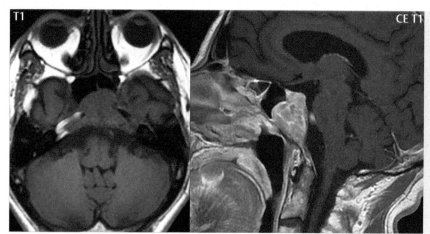

Fig. 2.3 Lymphoma, clivus. On the axial precontrast T1-weighted image, there is complete replacement of the normal high signal intensity fatty marrow of the clivus by an expansile mass lesion with intermediate signal intensity. The lesion was of intermediate to slight hyperintensity on T2-weighted images (not shown). The postcontrast sagittal image demonstrates prominent, slightly heterogeneous enhancement. The imaging appearance is nonspecific, other than being most consistent with a neoplastic process. Chordoma, metastasis, and lymphoma should all be considered in the differential diagnosis, with other entities less likely.

with adjacent malignant tumors—for example, nasopharyngeal carcinoma and, in children, rhabdomyosarcoma (▶ Fig. 2.4). Two other entities to keep in mind, due to some propensity for skull base involvement, are Paget disease and fibrous dysplasia (▶ Fig. 2.5).

Most fractures that involve the skull base are extensions of cranial vault fractures. Thin section CT with bone algorithm reconstruction is the method of choice for evaluation. Clinical presentations include CSF otorrhea/rhinorrhea, hemotympanum, and cranial nerve deficits.

2.2 Temporal Bone

The temporal bone is divided into five parts, which are subsequently described. The squamous portion (1) is anterolateral, forming the upper part of the temporal bone. It is thin and shell-like, and forms the lateral wall of the middle cranial fossa.

The temporalis muscle attaches to the squamous portion of the temporal bone. The zygomatic process arises from the lower portion and arches anteriorly, with the masseter muscle originating from its medial surface. The mastoid portion (2) contains the antrum (a large central mastoid air cell) which communicates posteriorly with the smaller mastoid air cells and anteriorly with the epitympanum (attic) via a small canal (the aditus ad antrum). The petrous portion (3) lies at the base of the skull between the sphenoid bone anteriorly and the occipital bone posteriorly. The petrous portion contains the internal auditory canal (IAC), with its opening (the porus acusticus), and the membranous and bony labyrinths of the inner ear. The IAC is divided into upper and lower compartments by a bony crest, the crista falciformis. The upper compartment contains the facial nerve (CN VII) anteriorly and the superior vestibular division of CN VIII posteriorly. The lower compartment contains the cochlear division of CN VIII anteriorly and the inferior vestibular

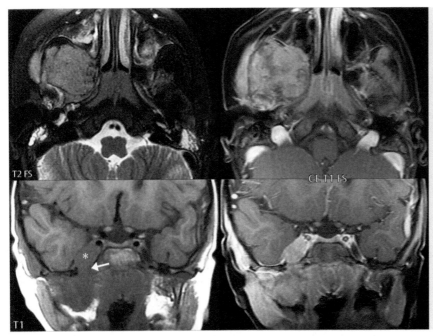

Fig. 2.4 Rhabdomyosarcoma. Axial images reveal a large, mildly heterogeneous, mass lesion in the right masticator space with local bone destruction and mild diffuse enhancement. The lesion is hyperintense to normal muscle on the T2-weighted scan and enhances postcontrast. Intracranial perineural tumor spread along CN V3 is evident extending through an enlarged foramen ovale (*arrow*) and into the Meckel cave (*asterisk*) and cavernous sinus, on coronal images. Clinical presentation is typically in the first two decades of life, with the patient in this instance a 3-year-old child.

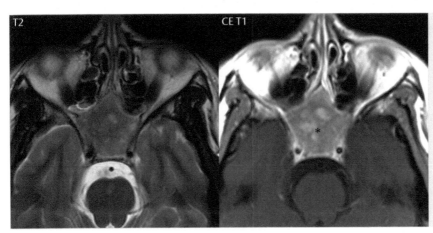

Fig. 2.5 Fibrous dysplasia, sphenoid sinus. There is a mildly expansile mass that fills the sphenoid sinus. The lesion is low to intermediate in signal intensity on the T2-weighted scan. There is moderate to prominent contrast enhancement (*asterisk*), the degree of enhancement being more apparent by comparison with the normal enhancing cavernous sinus.

division of CN VIII posteriorly. The jugular foramen is bordered by the petrous temporal bone anteriorly and the occipital bone posteriorly. The jugular foramen has two compartments, the smaller pars nervosa (anteromedial) which contains the inferior petrosal sinus and the glossopharyngeal nerve (CN IX), and the larger pars vascularis (posterolateral) which contains the internal jugular vein, the vagus nerve (CN X), and the spinal accessory nerve (CN XI). The tympanic part of the temporal bone (4) is a small curved plate surrounding the external auditory canal (EAC). The styloid process (5) projects down and anteriorly from the undersurface of the temporal bone, just anterior to the stylomastoid foramen.

The middle ear (tympanic cavity) is air-filled (via the eustachian tube from the nasopharynx) and traversed by the auditory ossicles (which connect the lateral and medial walls). The tympanic membrane (TM) separates the tympanic cavity from the EAC. There are three parts: the epitympanum, mesotympanum, and hypotympanum. The superior limit of the epitympanum (attic) is the tegmen tympani (which separates the epitympanum from the middle cranial fossa) and the inferior

margin is defined by a plane between the scutum (junction of lateral attic wall and roof of the EAC) and the tympanic segment of CN VII. Thus, it lies above the attachment of the TM. The lateral epitympanic recess, also known as Prussak space, is the classic location of acquired cholesteatomas. The head and body of the malleus and the short process of the incus lie in the epitympanum. The mesotympanum lies below the epitympanum, directly medial to the TM, separated from the hypotympanum below which lies inferior to the TM attachment. The mesotympanum contains the manubrium of the malleus, long process of the incus, the stapes, and the stapedius and tensor tympani muscles. The medial (labyrinthine) wall separates the middle and inner ears, and contains the oval and round windows, lateral semicircular canal, and tympanic segment of CN VII. The small hypotympanum is the inferior part of the tympanic cavity, below the cochlear promontory, and its floor separates the tympanic cavity from the jugular fossa.

The facial nerve (CN VII) enters the temporal bone via the porus acusticus/IAC. The labyrinthine segment extends from the fundus of the IAC to the geniculate ganglion (anterior genu).

The nerve then turns posteriorly in its tympanic segment and, subsequently, turns vertically (posterior genu) to become the mastoid (descending) segment, exiting the skull base at the stylomastoid foramen.

The vestibule, semicircular canals, and cochlea form the bony labyrinth (otic capsule) of the inner ear. The vestibule is a large ovoid perilymphatic space, which connects anteriorly to the cochlea and to the three semicircular canals: superior, lateral (horizontal), and posterior. The cochlea is shaped like a cone, with its apex pointing anteriorly, laterally, and slightly down, consisting of 2.5 to 2.75 turns. The cochlea is optimally visualized in its entirety on the Stenver reconstructed image (subsequently described). The membranous labyrinth is, by definition, the fluid-filled space within the bony labyrinth that is filled by endolymph (including the endolymphatic duct and sac) and perilymph (within the cochlear duct).

CT of the temporal bone is usually performed with very thin sections (≤ 1.5 mm) and reformatted in Poschl (vestibular oblique view), Stenvers (cochlear oblique view), and standard axial and coronal planes, focusing on images reconstructed to display fine bony detail. Screening MR exams are performed with thin section (≤ 3 mm) technique, utilizing both the axial and coronal planes, with the strength of MR being depiction of soft tissue and fluid structures. The MR exam is typically supplemented with intravenous contrast injection, which is essential for evaluation of neoplastic disease, infection, and inflammation. For detail involving the temporal bone (and specifically the membranous labyrinth) as well as the adjacent CSF cisterns on MR, high resolution three-dimensional (3D) sequences, employing either constructive interference in the steady state (CISS) or fast spin-echo (FSE) techniques, are routinely acquired. At 3 T images with a native isotropic resolution of ≤ 0.3 mm can be acquired in a clinically reasonable scan time.

Congenital anomalies can involve the outer, middle, or inner ear. There can be stenosis or atresia of the external auditory canal. Dysplasia or aplasia can involve the middle or inner ear structures. Some malformations are known to be associated with meningitis, due to CSF leaks. The most common vascular variant is the dehiscent jugular bulb (▶ Fig. 2.6). In this variant, which typically presents with pulsatile tinnitus, there is a dehiscent sigmoid (jugular) plate and the jugular bulb extends to lie within the inferior tympanic cavity. It will appear to clinicians as a "vascular" TM.

A large vestibular aqueduct, caused by enlargement of the endolymphatic sac and duct, is the most common anomaly associated with pediatric congenital sensorineural hearing loss (▶ Fig. 2.7). It is bilateral in 90% of patients and may be syndromic or nonsyndromic. The defining bony feature, as initially described, is enlargement of the vestibular aqueduct. There is a

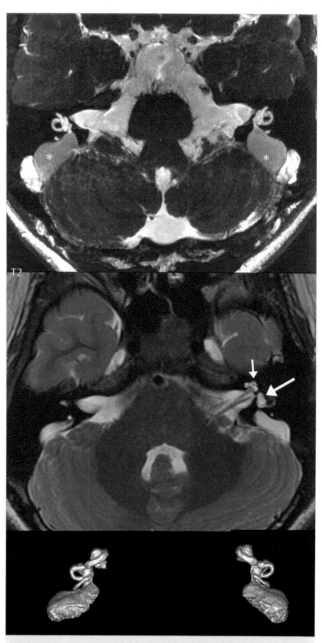

Fig. 2.7 Large endolymphatic sac anomaly. The images presented include a thick section MIP of a 0.6-mm axial FIESTA-C(CISS) acquisition, a 3-mm axial FSE T2-weighted section, and a volume rendered view of the cochlea, vestibule, semicircular canals, and the large endolymphatic sac. The abnormality is bilateral in this instance (which is seen in 90% of cases). As evident on both T2-weighted exams (better evaluated on the left given the images presented), the cochlea (*short arrow*) is dysplastic, the vestibule (*large arrow*) dilated, and the endolymphatic sac (*asterisk*) large. Although better seen on CT (not shown), the vestibular aqueduct (which extends from the vestibule to the posterior surface of the petrous bone) was also noted to be enlarged on the thick section MIP.

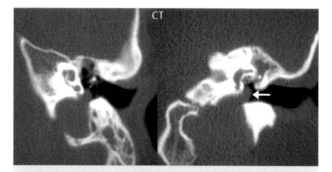

Fig. 2.6 Dehiscent jugular bulb. Thin section axial and coronal CT images of the temporal bone reveal focal dehiscence of the jugular plate with extension of a mass (part of the jugular bulb, *arrow*) into the hypotympanum.

spectrum of associated cochlear and/or vestibular anomalies, ranging from subtle to gross dysmorphism. The most common specific features include modiolar deficiency and cochlear abnormalities. High-resolution T2-weighted MR (CISS or 3D FSE) is the imaging approach of choice, both for characterization and detection of associated anomalies. Dehiscence of the superior semicircular canal (SCC) (and much less commonly the posterior SCC) is being increasingly encountered. It is likely a developmental anomaly and patients typically present with Tullio phenomenon (sound-induced vertigo with or without nystagmus). Thin section, bone algorithm, high resolution temporal bone CT is used for evaluation, with Poschl reformatted images best to demonstrate this entity.

Inflammation and infection of the temporal bone can take on many different appearances. A middle ear effusion in an adult is important to recognize on both CT and MR, since eustachian tube obstruction, secondary to a nasopharynx neoplasm, must be excluded (▶ Fig. 2.8). Mastoiditis on CT has a nonspecific appearance, with opacification of mastoid air cells. On MR, the air cells are opacified with debris that is of intermediate, not high, signal intensity on T2-weighted scans, with prominent contrast enhancement (▶ Fig. 2.9). Complications associated with mastoiditis include sigmoid sinus thrombosis (with or without venous infarction), (▶ Fig. 2.10) Bezold abscess (an abscess in the sternocleidomastoid muscle), and intraparenchymal/epidural abscesses (middle and/or posterior cranial fossae) (▶ Fig. 2.11 and ▶ Fig. 2.12). In chronic mastoiditis on CT, there will be demineralization of trabeculae, with eventual formation of one large cavity (coalescent mastoiditis). The specific subclassifications and procedures for mastoidectomy are complex and varied, with the term itself referring to resection of mastoid air cells (▶ Fig. 2.13). A mastoidectomy may be done to treat mastoiditis, chronic otitis media, or large cholesteatomas.

Labyrinthitis refers to inflammatory disease of the inner ear (specifically the membranous labyrinth), which can be secondary to a middle ear infection or meningitis. Of all infectious agents, a viral etiology is most common, resulting from upper respiratory infection. In this instance, the disease is usually self-limited and imaging is not performed. In acute and subacute labyrinthitis, CT is normal and the only imaging finding (which is still not seen in most patients) is faint enhancement of the fluid on MR within the labyrinth. Chronic labyrinthitis consists of a fibrous stage followed by an ossific stage. In the fibrous stage there is loss of the normal high signal intensity within the fluid-filled labyrinth on T2-weighted scans. In the ossific stage diffuse or focal ossification of the normally fluid-filled spaces is seen on CT, with hypointense signal therein on T2-weighted MR (▶ Fig. 2.14).

Patients with typical Bell palsy (herpetic peripheral CN VII paralysis) do not undergo imaging. Atypical cases are often evaluated with MR, not for imaging of the facial nerve, per se, but to exclude underlying pathology such as tumor. Paralysis of the facial nerve is thought to occur from latent herpes simplex infection of the geniculate ganglion, and is typically unilateral. On MR, the nerve in Bell palsy will be normal in diameter (occasionally slightly enlarged) and display uniform, linear enhancement, most common in the fundal and labyrinthine segments but, occasionally, throughout its entire course (▶ Fig. 2.15). Ramsey Hunt syndrome is caused by reactivation of a varicella zoster infection. As opposed to Bell palsy, however, it is typically

associated with external ear vesicles, involvement of the entire intratemporal facial nerve and the vestibulocochlear nerve, with involvement of the membranous labyrinth (▶ Fig. 2.16). Patients present with CN VII palsy and sensorineural hearing loss.

Petrous apex lesions are varied and can be confusing. A cholesterol granuloma is the most common primary lesion of the petrous apex (▶ Fig. 2.17). This expansile lesion causes adjacent cortical thinning, and has distinctive high signal intensity on

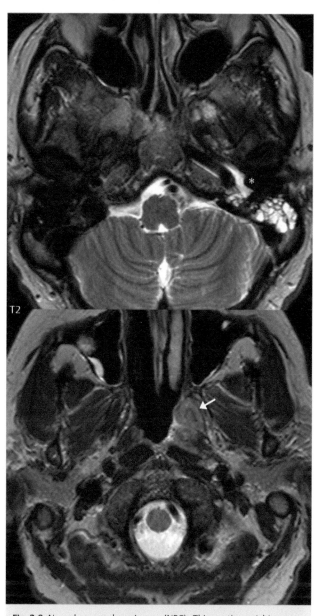

Fig. 2.8 Nasopharyngeal carcinoma (NPC). Thin section axial images are illustrated at two levels, from a screening brain exam performed in a 52-year-old man with chronic headaches (left occipital in location). The upper image reveals fluid within both the mastoid air cells and the middle ear (*asterisk*). The presence of the latter mandates a closer look at the exam for a possible cause. Although incidental mastoid air cell disease is common, fluid in the middle ear is not (and suggests obstruction and infection). Evaluation of the lower image reveals abnormal soft tissue (*arrow*) obliterating the opening of the eustachian tube (with mass effect upon the fossa of Rosenmüller), thus causing the effusions in the left middle ear and mastoid air cells. Biopsy revealed type III, undifferentiated, invasive NPC.

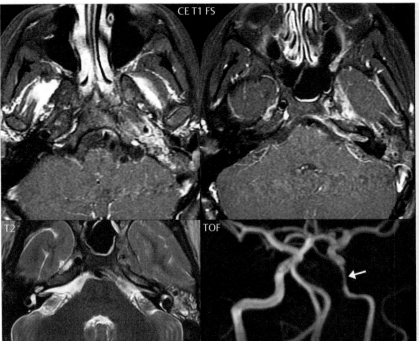

Fig. 2.9 Apical petrositis. There is opacification and abnormal enhancement of the petrous and mastoid air cells on the left. Note the intermediate signal intensity on the T2-weighted scan in the left mastoid air cells, consistent with infection (also reflected by the abnormal contrast enhancement). This should be distinguished from fluid signal intensity, seen commonly and not representing infection. There has been spread of infection to the adjacent meninges, with abnormal enhancement seen on the postcontrast scans within the left internal auditory canal and posterior to the clivus. There is also involvement of the left cavernous sinus and the Meckel cave, with abnormal enhancing soft tissue. Time-of-flight MRA reveals secondary narrowing of the cavernous carotid artery (*arrow*), confirmed on axial imaging. This 9-year-old patient presented with Gradenigo syndrome, specifically the triad of symptoms that include periorbital pain (due to trigeminal nerve involvement), diplopia (due to involvement of the abducens nerves), and otorrhea.

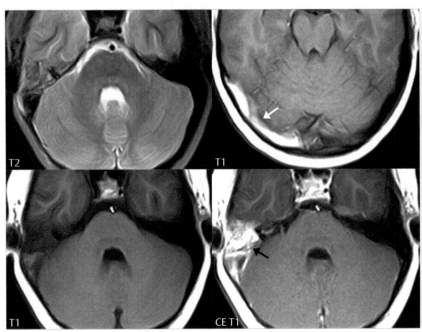

Fig. 2.10 Mastoiditis with secondary transverse sinus thrombosis. On the T2-weighted scan in this pediatric patient, there is complete opacification of the right mastoid air cells, seen as intermediate signal intensity that is more typical of infection as opposed to simple fluid. Postcontrast, there is intense enhancement (*black arrow*), also consistent with infection. A met-hemoglobin clot (with high signal intensity on the precontrast T1-weighted image, *white arrow*) is seen occluding the right transverse sinus, a known serious complication of acute otomastoiditis.

both T1- and T2-weighted images, the former due to the presence of hemorrhage and cholesterol. A cholesteatoma of the petrous apex (congenital or acquired) is less common but shares the characteristics of an expansile mass, with thinning and remodeling of adjacent bone. Its appearance on MR is, however, distinctive, consistent with its composition (an epidermoid), with low signal intensity on T1, high on T2, restricted diffusion, and no enhancement. Incidental lesions of the petrous apex that occasionally cause confusion include asymmetrical pneumatization and trapped fluid. The latter is common, and can be recognized by the presence of fluid with low T1 and high T2 signal intensity, without trabecular loss or any

expansile nature (▶ Fig. 2.18). Apical petrositis has a distinct appearance, consistent with infection, with prominent enhancement, including the adjacent meninges (▶ Fig. 2.19). In the middle ear, the lesion of importance is the cholesteatoma. This lesion represents an enlarging mass of stratified squamous epithelium containing exfoliated keratin. The vast majority are acquired pars flaccida cholesteatomas. The appearance on CT is that of a soft tissue mass originating in Prussak space with erosion of the scutum and often filling the epitympanum (▶ Fig. 2.19). Bony destruction is characteristic with larger lesions with erosion of the ossicles and Koerner's septum (a bony septum extending medially and inferiorly into the

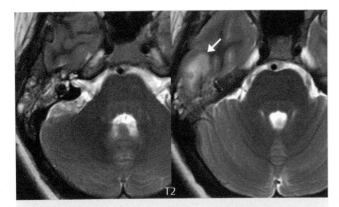

Fig. 2.11 Mastoiditis, with cerebritis, on T2-weighted imaging. There is complete opacification of the right mastoid air cells, of intermediate signal intensity (not as high as CSF), suggesting infection. There has been intracranial spread of infection, resulting in an area of edema/cerebritis in the adjacent temporal lobe (*arrow*).

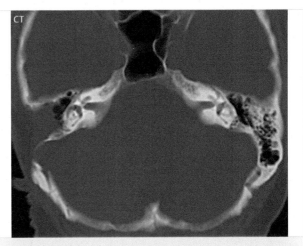

Fig. 2.13 Mastoidectomy. An extensive resection of mastoid air cells has been performed in the distant past on the right, with the inner ear cavity preserved.

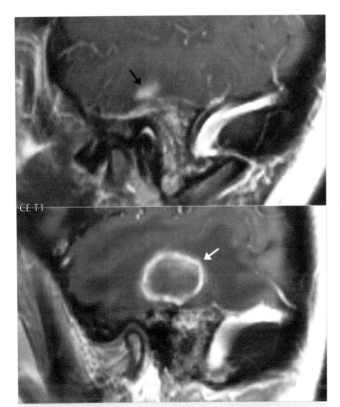

Fig. 2.12 Mastoiditis, with intracranial extension, the role of contrast enhancement. Sagittal postcontrast images from two different patients are presented, both demonstrating prominent enhancement of mastoid air cells consistent with infection. In the upper image, there is an ill-defined area of abnormal contrast enhancement (*black arrow*) in the adjacent temporal lobe, consistent with cerebritis. In the lower image, there is a mass lesion that exhibits a thin uniform enhancing rim (*white arrow*) and central necrosis, with extensive accompanying cerebral edema, in the adjacent temporal lobe, consistent with a brain abscess.

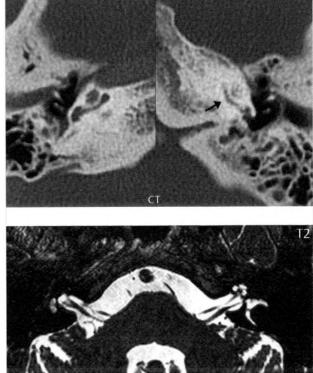

Fig. 2.14 Labyrinthitis ossificans. **Part 1:** Thin section axial CT images of the right and left temporal bones of a patient are presented, with the right inner ear normal. In chronic labyrinthitis, as illustrated on the patient's left side, there is ossification of the fluid-filled spaces of the inner ear, which can be diffuse and profound. In this patient, the result is near complete obliteration of the cochlea (*arrow*). **Part 2:** In a different patient, on axial thin section CISS images, there is diminished signal intensity within the cochlea, vestibule, and semicircular canals on the right, the MR presentation of chronic labyrinthitis ossificans (due to the normally fluid filled labyrinthine spaces becoming ossified).

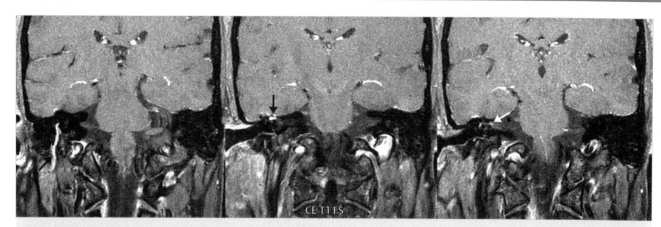

Fig. 2.15 Bell palsy. Enhancement of the facial nerve on the right is shown on coronal MR images, with the first image depicting enhancement of the entire mastoid (vertical) segment (*black arrow*). The subsequent two images depict enhancement in the region of the geniculate ganglion (*black arrow*) and in the distal internal auditory canal (*white arrow*), in this patient with acute facial nerve paralysis.

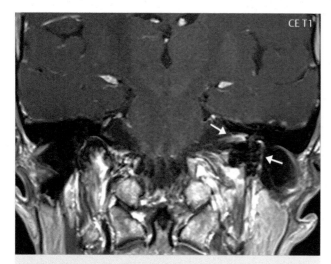

Fig. 2.16 Herpes zoster oticus (Ramsay Hunt syndrome). Abnormal enhancement is seen involving the intracanalicular and mastoid segments of the facial nerve on the left (*white arrows*). Enhancement of the entire course of the facial nerve was noted, including also the labyrinthine and tympanic segments (not shown).

antrum) being common. On MR, a cholesteatoma has low T1 and high T2 signal intensity and manifests restricted diffusion. MR is commonly performed in postoperative cases for differentiation, on the basis of diffusion-weighted images, of residual cholesteatoma from other lesions.

The term "otosclerosis" is actually a misnomer as the condition is actually "otospongiosis." There is resorption of the normal endochondral bony otic capsule (of unknown cause), with deposition of new spongy vascular bone. Clinically, these patients present with conductive hearing loss and bilateral disease in 80%. The majority of cases are fenestral in location, and can involve just the oval window or both the oval and round windows. Retrofenestral (cochlear) otospongiosis, which is less common, can be patchy or diffuse, and can occur with or without fenestral involvement. On CT, in the active phase of the disease, there is demineralization and, in the chronic phase, sclerosis. Treatment for the associated hearing loss includes hearing aids, early in the disease course, and, later, stapedectomy.

Cochlear implants are common today, with surgery performed for both congenital and acquired deafness, but require the presence of a functioning cochlear nerve. The electrode array is placed into the scala tympani (one of the two perilymph-filled cavities of the cochlear labyrinth) in the basal turn of the cochlea (▶ Fig. 2.20).

Although temporal bone fractures were traditionally categorized relative to their orientation to the long axis of the petrous bone, as longitudinal or transverse, the majority of fractures are actually complex or oblique. If the traditional categorization is used, the more common fracture is the longitudinal fracture which is parallel to the long axis of the petrous bone (▶ Fig. 2.21). Fractures can disrupt the ossicular chain, and transect either the cochlear nerve (with hearing loss) or facial nerve (with facial paralysis). CSF fistulas are not uncommon following a fracture involving the temporal bone.

2.2.1 Neoplasms

The most common neoplasm of the cerebellopontine angle is a vestibular schwannoma (arising from the vestibular division of CN VIII), which accounts for 10% of all intracranial tumors. Clinical symptoms consist of sensorineural hearing loss, tinnitus, and dysequilibrium. This benign, slow-growing, well delineated, encapsulated lesion typically arises within the internal auditory canal or (more commonly) is centered at the porus acusticus (▶ Fig. 2.22). Growth rates are variable. The typical presentation today, due to improved access to medical care and advanced imaging (MR), is that of a small lesion within the IAC. Presentation as a large mass lesion causing compression of the brainstem is uncommon (▶ Fig. 2.23). Although larger lesions can be seen on modern CT scanners, this modality does not play a clinical role in screening or diagnosis.

Vestibular schwannomas on MR are intensely enhancing lesions, identified by their location and focal nature. The majority have both an intra- and an extra-canalicular component, with mild enlargement of the porus acusticus and with the extra-canalicular portion rounded in appearance. Very large lesions can have a cystic component. Up to one-third of vestibular schwannomas are purely intracanalicular, and, thus, are very small lesions (▶ Fig. 2.24). For small to intermediate size lesions,

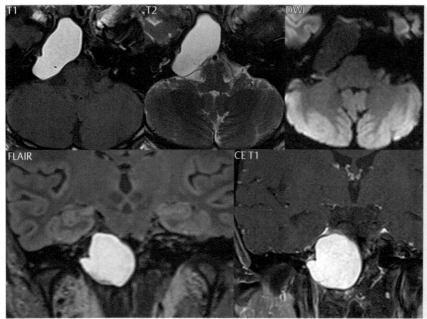

Fig. 2.17 Cholesterol granuloma. A large expansile lesion is noted in the right petrous apex, hyperintense on both T1- and T2-weighted scans, without diffusion restriction or internal contrast enhancement. The imaging findings are characteristic, with one exception—that a peripheral hemosiderin rim is not present. The lesion was resected through a transnasal, trans-clival approach.

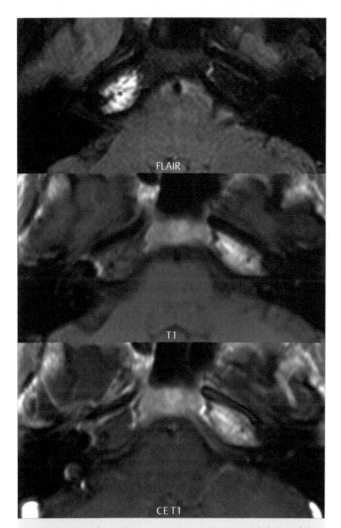

Fig. 2.18 Retained secretions, petrous apex. A nonexpansile lesion of the right petrous apex is identified, with fluid signal intensity precontrast (note the high signal intensity on FLAIR, *asterisk*), and no abnormal enhancement. The lack of bone expansion differentiates this entity from other much less common lesions such as an epidermoid cyst or mucocele.

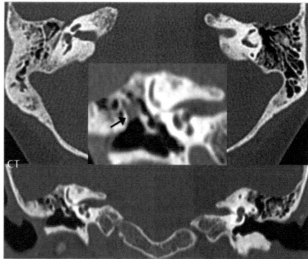

Fig. 2.19 Cholesteatoma. On axial and coronal high resolution, thin section CT, abnormal soft tissue (*black arrow*, magnified view of the coronal section) is noted within Prussak space extending into the attic (epitympanum) on the right. There is also erosion of the scutum, seen on the coronal image.

stereotactic radiation is increasingly being recommended as the treatment of choice (▸ Fig. 2.25). Although much less common, schwannomas of the cochlear and facial nerves do occur (▸ Fig. 2.26). The latter can be, depending on extent, indistinguishable in appearance from a vestibular schwannoma.

The differential diagnosis for a mass lesion at the cerebellopontine angle includes, in decreasing order of incidence, a (vestibular) schwannoma, meningioma, arachnoid cyst, and epidermoid.

Meningiomas can occur in the cerebellopontine angle; however, as opposed to vestibular schwannomas, they are usually located eccentric to the porus acusticus. A meningioma should not enlarge the porus acusticus, and will only, uncommonly, extend into the internal auditory canal (▸ Fig. 2.27). A broad-based lesion along a dural surface and calcification are common

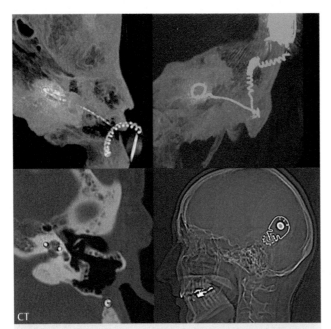

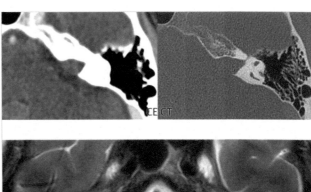

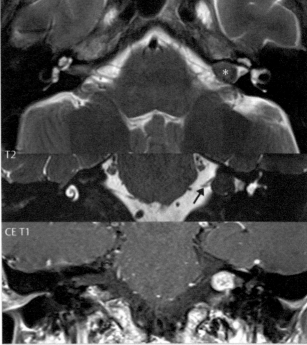

Fig. 2.20 Cochlear implant. Thick section axial and coronal MIP, thin section axial, and lateral scout images from a CT exam reconstructed using a bone algorithm are presented. Both the electrode array, lying within the basal turn of the cochlea, and the receiver and stimulator, lying within the post-auricular soft tissues, are illustrated.

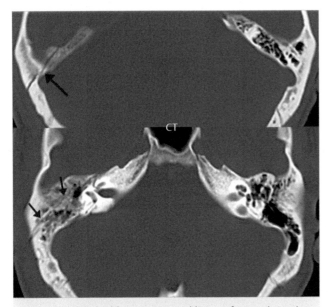

Fig. 2.21 Longitudinal fracture, temporal bone. A fracture (arrows), parallel to the long axis of the petrous bone on the right, is seen on two axial sections. On the lower image, the mastoid air cells are noted to be opacified (compare with the normal left side), a clue in the setting of acute trauma to an underlying fracture. The fracture (small black arrows) traverses the mastoid air cells, with involvement of the facial nerve common in these fractures.

Fig. 2.22 Vestibular schwannoma, CT and MR. Part 1: Axial CT, reconstructed with a soft tissue algorithm and a bone algorithm, suggests the presence of a soft tissue mass within the internal auditory canal. There is widening of both the opening (the porus acusticus internus) and the proximal canal. Part 2: Axial and coronal T2-weighted scans, and a coronal postcontrast T1-weighted scan, depict a moderate sized vestibular schwannoma (asterisk), which expands the porus acusticus, and displays typical prominent enhancement. Note the displacement superiorly of nerves (small black arrow, specifically two of the four divisions that lie within the internal auditory canal) by the mass on the thin section (1 mm) high-resolution coronal T2-weighted scan.

findings. Although a dural "tail" is a characteristic sign for a meningioma, this can also be seen with a vestibular schwannoma and is not a differentiating feature.

Epidermoids are very slow growing lesions, and can reach substantial size prior to clinical presentation (usually as an adult). An epidermoid tends to insinuate itself into the cisterns, incorporating cranial nerves and vessels, and causing mild (and sometimes massive) irregular compression of adjacent brain. On CT epidermoid tumors will manifest as "dirty" CSF. On MR these lesions are near isointensity with CSF, being only slightly hyperintense on FLAIR, but with distinctive hyperintensity on diffusion-weighted imaging (DWI). A little appreciated caveat is that the high signal intensity (SI) of an epidermoid on DWI is not due to restricted diffusion, but, rather, to T2 shine-through (thus the apparent diffusion coefficient [ADC] map will not show the lesion to have lower diffusion as compared to adjacent brain).

A trigeminal (CN V) schwannoma can arise anywhere along the course of the nerve, and, thus, can also occur at the cerebellopontine angle (CPA). A minority of trigeminal schwannomas in

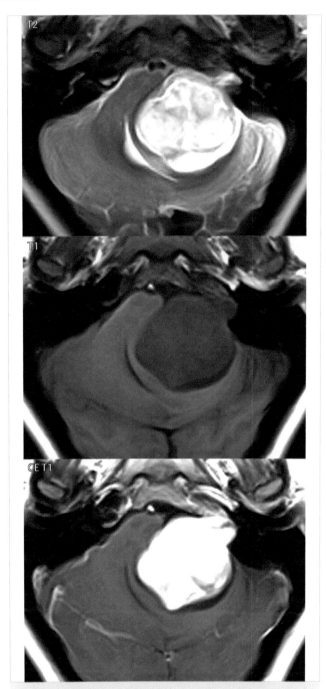

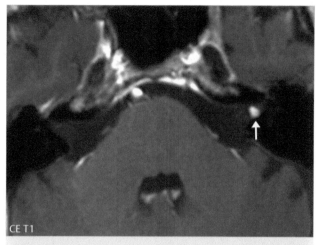

Fig. 2.24 Intracanalicular vestibular schwannoma. On thin section axial MR imaging, a very small soft tissue mass (*arrow*) is identified within the left internal auditory canal, with prominent contrast enhancement.

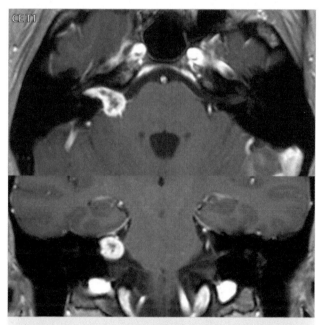

Fig. 2.25 Stereotactic radiation therapy, vestibular schwannoma. One option for treatment of vestibular schwannomas is stereotactic radiation therapy. In the early months following radiation, central necrosis is observed, reflected on axial and coronal postcontrast scans by a central region of nonenhancement With time, the lesion dimensions, overall, will regress.

Fig. 2.23 Large vestibular schwannoma. A very large mass lesion widens and extends into the left internal auditory canal, with the bulk of the lesion extracanalicular in location. There is prominent deformity and displacement of the brainstem and fourth ventricle. There is little if any vasogenic edema. Vestibular schwannomas are, in general, very slow growing, and, if undetected, may result in large mass lesions such as that illustrated, with few symptoms (other than the loss of hearing) due to the ability to of the CNS to adapt well to slow chronic changes. Such lesions, common in the past, are rarely seen today due to more intensive screening and readily available medical care.

this location extend into both the middle and posterior fossae, having a dumbbell shape. The three major branches (ophthalmic, maxillary, and mandibular) of the trigeminal nerve exit the trigeminal ganglion (also known as the gasserian ganglion) which is located in the Meckel cave, with trigeminal schwannomas also rising in this location (▶ Fig. 2.28). Trigeminal schwannomas are much less common than vestibular schwannomas, with the latter accounting for 95% of intracranial schwannomas. Facial nerve and cochlear schwannomas (▶ Fig. 2.29) also occur, but are uncommon. The vast majority of CPA tumors are vestibular schwannomas (between 60 and 90%, in literature series), with other nonvestibular schwannomas much less common (4%).

Head and neck paragangliomas occur in four common locations: in the tympanic cavity (glomus tympanicum paragangliomas [most common tumor of the middle ear]), at the skull base

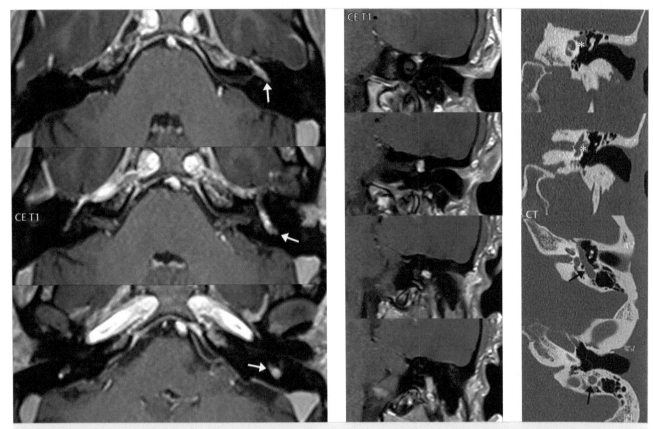

Fig. 2.26 Facial nerve schwannoma. On axial thin section post-contrast T1-weighted scans (**part 1**) the facial nerve on the left is noted to be enlarged in diameter and enhancing, with involvement of the ganglionic, horizontal and vertical, segments (*arrows*). These findings are also well visualized on thin section postcontrast T1-weighted coronal scans (**part 2**). On thin section temporal bone CT, with both coronal and axial reformatted images (**part 3**), the facial nerve canal is noted to be enlarged (*white asterisk* on coronal and *black arrow* on axial images) and to contain soft tissue.

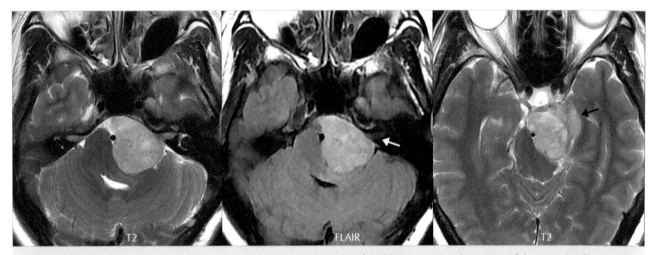

Fig. 2.27 Cerebellopontine angle meningioma. A large mass lesion is seen on the left with its epicenter at the opening of the internal auditory meatus (the porus acusticus). There is marked compression of the pons, with displacement and compression of the fourth ventricle, but no edema. These findings, taken together, suggest that the mass is long-standing in nature (thus slow growing and benign). The basilar artery (with a black flow void, medial to the mass) is partially encased. There is no evidence of extension of the lesion into the internal auditory canal (the signal intensity within the IAC is that of CSF on both the T2-weighted sequence and FLAIR, *white arrow*). These findings are consistent with a meningioma, which was proven on resection. An additional finding on imaging, consistent with the diagnosis of a meningioma (as opposed to a vestibular schwannoma), is extension of the lesion into the cavernous sinus on the left (*black arrow*), seen on the T2-weighted image at a higher level.

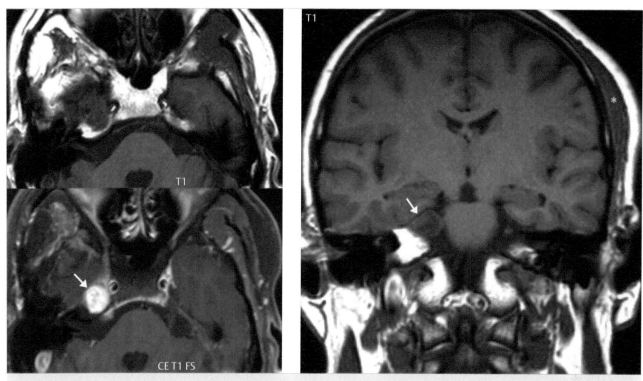

Fig. 2.28 Trigeminal schwannoma. **Part 1:** A small, extraaxial, round, enhancing lesion (*arrow*) is seen on axial scans in the region of the Meckel cave. Note the chronic denervation fatty atrophy of the temporalis muscle on the right. Trigeminal schwannomas can involve multiple compartments—for example, both intracranial and the masticator space—and thus can be dumbbell in shape with a "waist" where it traverses the foramen ovale. **Part 2:** The portion of the tumor (*arrow*) involving the cisternal segment of the nerve is seen on a coronal image, with the contralateral normal trigeminal nerve serving as a reference. Note also the atrophy of the right temporalis muscle, which is difficult to even visualize, in comparison to the normal left temporalis muscle (*asterisk*).

in the region of the jugular bulb (glomus jugulare paragangliomas [most common tumor of the jugular foramen]) (▶ Fig. 2.30), in the high retrostyloid parapharyngeal (carotid) space (glomus vagale paragangliomas), and at the common carotid artery bifurcation (carotid body paragangliomas). The latter tumor classically splays the ICA and ECA and completely "fills" the carotid bifurcation (▶ Fig. 2.31). Within the carotid sheath, glomus vagale paragangliomas displace the ICA anteriorly (as the vagus nerve is located posterior to the artery within the sheath) (▶ Fig. 2.32). However, some large glomus vagale paragangliomas extend caudally and can also splay the internal and external carotid arteries, much like a carotid body paraganglioma. The classic, more specific, location of a glomus tympanicum paraganglioma is on the cochlear promontory (▶ Fig. 2.33). This is the tumor known for its appearance as a red retrotympanic mass on otoscopic exam. One must be *very* careful to assess for presence of an aberrant internal carotid artery, which also presents with pulsatile tinnitus and a red retrotympanic mass. Look for integrity of the carotid canal wall. Large glomus tympanicum paragangliomas can fill the middle ear cavity (▶ Fig. 2.34).

Paragangliomas, other than the glomus tympanicum paragangliomas, are typically smoothly contoured and ovoid in shape. Large tumors may be inhomogeneous, with areas of necrosis. On both T1- and T2-weighted images, the classic appearance is that of "salt and pepper," with tiny areas of high

signal intensity (salt) due to slow flow (or hemorrhage), and low signal intensity (pepper) due to fast flow (flow voids). Paragangliomas are hypervascular tumors, with early prominent enhancement. Digital subtraction angiography (DSA) reveals enlarged feeding arteries, and rapid venous drainage. Contrast enhancement on MR, in addition to providing lesion characterization (for all paragangliomas), assists in detection of small glomus tympanicum paragangliomas. However, this is typically not required as a noncontrast temporal bone CT is usually diagnostic (soft tissue mass on the cochlear promontory) and best to exclude a potential aberrant ICA. Bone destruction is common with glomus jugulare paragangliomas and is classically permeative-destructive. Glomus jugulare paragangliomas may also extend into the internal jugular vein. Although much less common, a schwannoma or meningioma can occur in the region of the jugular foramen, and should be kept in mind in terms of differential diagnosis.

2.3 Orbit

Addressing normal anatomy, the optic foramen (the opening of the optic canal) lies at the orbital apex and contains the optic nerve and the ophthalmic artery. The superior orbital fissure lies inferolateral to the optic canal and contains the oculomotor (CN III), trochlear (CN IV), and abducens (CN VI) nerves,

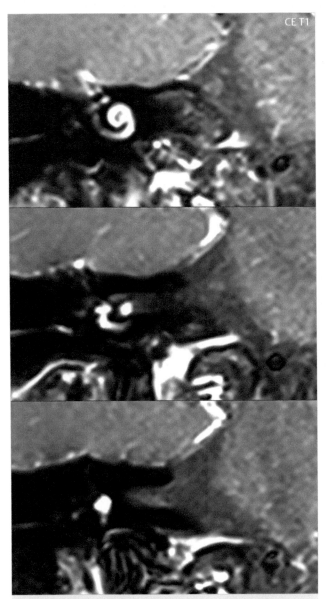

Fig. 2.29 Cochlear schwannoma. Three adjacent coronal thin section postcontrast T1-weighted scans are presented (from anterior to posterior). Abnormal enhancement is seen in the cochlea, the adjacent section of the internal auditory canal, and the vestibule.

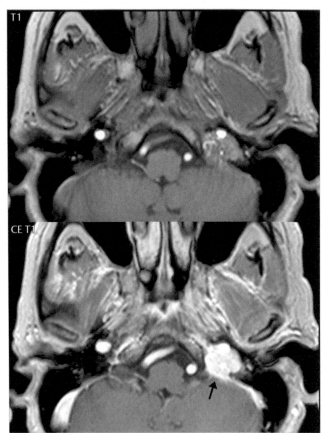

Fig. 2.30 Glomus jugulare paraganglioma. A mass involves the jugular bulb on the left, with intense enhancement postcontrast (*arrow*). Paragangliomas are hypervascular (thus their enhancement), with larger lesions also displaying a salt and pepper appearance on T1- and T2-weighted images.

together with the ophthalmic nerve (CN V1) (and branches therein) and the ophthalmic veins. The inferior orbital fissure lies more inferiorly, and slightly laterally, and contains the maxillary nerve (CN V2). The medial wall of the orbit is referred to as the lamina papyracea (paper thin). The extraocular muscles include the superior, inferior, medial, and lateral recti, together with the superior and inferior obliques and the levator palpebrae superioris. The superior oblique muscle is the longest and thinnest, passing anteriorly and medially through the trochlea and then turning posterolaterally and downward to insert on the lateral sclera. The inferior oblique, the only muscle not to originate from the orbital apex, originates from the maxilla. The levator palpebrae superioris muscle lies between the superior rectus muscle and the roof of the orbit, and may be difficult to separate from the superior rectus. The rectus muscles separate the intraconal space from the extraconal space. The lacrimal gland is located superolaterally in the orbit, with its vascular supply being the lacrimal artery. Tears produced by the lacrimal gland pass across the cornea and are absorbed through the lacrimal canaliculi of the upper and lower lids. In regard to innervation, CN III supplies the superior, inferior, and medial recti; the inferior oblique; and the levator palpebrae superioris muscles. CN IV supplies the superior oblique muscle and CN VI the lateral rectus muscle.

Evaluation of the orbit by CT includes reformatted thin sections in all three primary planes, with intravenous contrast necessary for soft tissue evaluation and assessment of lesion vascularity. MR scans are also typically obtained in all three planes, with fat suppression essential for evaluation of orbital contents and the optic nerve. Intravenous contrast is routinely employed, in particular, for evaluation of mass lesions and the optic nerve.

A few basic definitions are in order, in regard to orbital anomalies. In hypertelorism, the eyes (orbits) are farther apart than normal and, in hypotelorism, the eyes are abnormally too close. Exophthalmos (proptosis) is abnormal anterior protrusion of the globe.

2.3.1 Inflammation/Infection

Orbital inflammation includes a number of diverse entities. Orbital cellulitis is divided into pre-septal and post-septal (orbital) types. In pre-septal cellulitis, infection is limited to the skin and subcutaneous tissues (▶ Fig. 2.35). In post-septal cellulitis inflammation involves the orbital contents. In the textbooks, it is stated that most orbital cellulitis is secondary to paranasal sinus infection (most commonly from the adjacent ethmoid sinuses). Spread from sinus infection can result in a subperiosteal or orbital abscess (▶ Fig. 2.36). This is usually treated as a surgical emergency. Cystic fibrosis is a predisposing condition. In severe cases of an orbital abscess there can be thrombosis of the ophthalmic veins and cavernous sinus. The term orbital pseudotumor refers to idiopathic orbital inflammation and is a diagnosis of exclusion. This entity is divided into subtypes, spe-

cifically anterior orbital inflammation, diffuse orbital pseudotumor, and orbital myositis (▶ Fig. 2.37).

In the anterior subtype, inflammation predominately involves the anterior orbit and globe. In the myositis subtype, one or more of the extraocular muscles is primarily infiltrated and the tendons are typically involved. The differential diagnosis for the myositis subtype is thyroid orbitopathy. In thyroid associated orbitopathy, involvement of extraocular muscles is usually bilateral and symmetric (with accompanying exophthalmos). The most commonly involved muscles (in order of decreasing frequency) are the inferior, medial, superior, lateral, and oblique muscles (I'M SLO mnemonic). The enlargement of the muscles involves principally the bellies, sparing the tendons (▶ Fig. 2.38). On CT there may be heterogeneous areas of lower density within the muscles. On MR typical findings include muscle edema in the acute phase and prominent enhancement of the involved muscles.

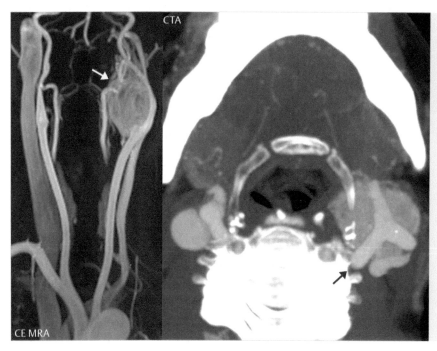

Fig. 2.31 Carotid body paraganglioma. At the bifurcation of the left common carotid artery, a large prominently enhancing mass (*white arrow*) is noted. The external and internal carotid artery branches are splayed by the mass, best seen on the axial thick MIP of the CTA (*black arrow*, common carotid artery).

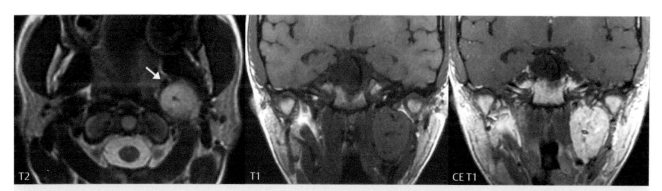

Fig. 2.32 Glomus vagale paraganglioma. In the retrostyloid parapharyngeal (carotid) space, vagal paragangliomas are less common than schwannomas. An ovoid mass is noted on the left, with several small flow voids, the latter finding being characteristic for this diagnosis (**part 1**). On the axial T2-weighted scan, the internal carotid artery (*arrow*) is noted to be displaced anteromedially. There is prominent contrast enhancement.

(*Continued*)

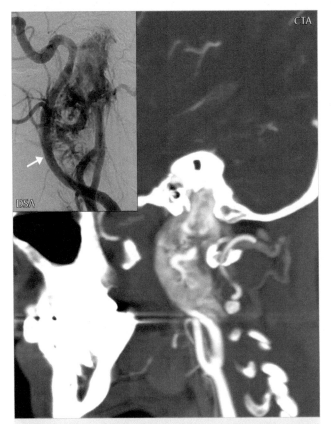

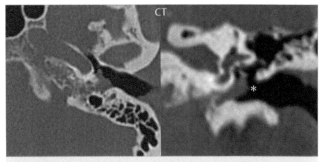

Fig. 2.33 Glomus tympanicum paraganglioma, CT. On axial and coronal reformatted images, a soft tissue mass (*asterisk*) is noted along the medial wall of the left middle ear, abutting the cochlear promontory. Osteolytic areas are also noted in the temporal bone, posterior to the carotid artery, on the axial image.

Fig. 2.32 (*Continued*) CTA and DSA (**part 2**) reveal additional characteristic findings (with the anterior displacement of the internal carotid artery well seen on DSA, *arrow*), including the intense vascular blush and dilated feeding vessels.

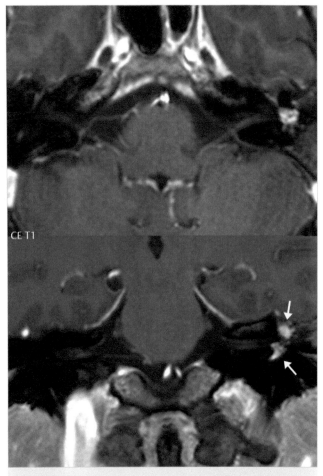

Fig. 2.34 Glomus tympanicum paraganglioma, MR. The axial postcontrast image depicts an enhancing lesion involving the middle ear cavity. As opposed to a small tumor, which would lie only on the cochlear promontory, this more extensive lesion occupies much of the middle ear (*small arrows*), as depicted on the coronal postcontrast image.

2.3.2 Neoplasms

Optic nerve gliomas histologically are low grade (i.e., pilocytic and fibrillary astrocytomas). Involvement can be limited to the nerve within the orbit, or can involve any portion of the visual pathway. Extension posteriorly from the orbit to involve the chiasm and optic tracts is not uncommon. Most optic nerve gliomas present in the first decade of life. There is fusiform enlargement of the optic nerve, often with proptosis (▶ Fig. 2.39). Homogeneous enhancement is seen in some lesions, with no enhancement in others (▶ Fig. 2.40). Optic nerve gliomas are associated with neurofibromatosis type 1 and, in this disease, can be bilateral.

Intraorbital meningiomas can occur at the orbital apex, along the optic nerve (perioptic meningiomas), or unrelated to the nerve in the extraconal space. Meningiomas in the orbit are much more common in females and occur principally in middle-aged adults with painless, progressive visual loss and proptosis. When these occur in juvenile patients, they are usually associated with neurofibromatosis type 2. Linear ("tram-track") or stippled calcifications are seen on CT in half of cases (▶ Fig. 2.41). The term "tram-track" is also used to reference circumferential uniform enhancement along/around the nerve. As opposed to nerve enlargement in optic nerve gliomas, the optic nerve is normal in size with perioptic meningiomas (▶ Fig. 2.42).

Common benign tumors of the orbit further include hemangiomas and lymphatic malformations, with schwannomas much less common. Capillary hemangiomas are seen in infants in the first year of life, most commonly located in the superior nasal quadrant. They typically grow rapidly for 1 to 2 years, regress over 3 to 5 years, and completely regress by late childhood (with proliferative, involuting, and involuted phases). A cavernous hemangioma, the most common intraconal vascular orbital tumor in adults, is seen most often in the second to fourth decades and appears as a well-defined, smoothly marginated,

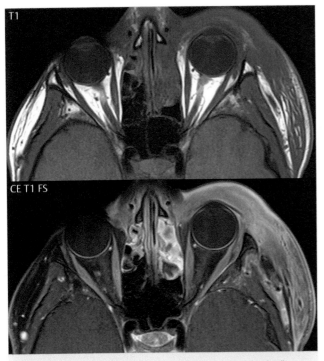

Fig. 2.35 Pre-septal cellulitis. There is extensive left periorbital inflammation, pre-septal in location, without involvement of the contents of the orbit itself. This is to be differentiated from post-septal cellulitis, which is more commonly referred to as orbital cellulitis. There is increased thickness of the periorbital soft tissues on the left, with obliteration of normal fat planes, reflecting extensive soft tissue inflammation and edema. Although sinus infection can lead to pre-septal cellulitis, as in this patient, other etiologies including trauma are also common.

homogenous mass. It has a strong female predominance. Hemangiomas typically manifest patchy, central enhancement early and "fill-in" on delayed scanning (▶ Fig. 2.43). A lymphatic malformation is an unencapsulated mass seen in children and young adults which is poorly circumscribed, multicystic, typically heterogeneous and may demonstrate characteristic fluid-fluid levels. Not infrequently, venous vascular elements are often present (venolymphatic malformation) (▶ Fig. 2.44).

A carotid cavernous fistula deserves mention in this section because it can present with proptosis. CT and MR typically demonstrate engorgement of the superior ophthalmic vein, which can be accompanied by enlargement of the extraocular muscles. Schwannomas of the orbit are rare, most common in the intraconal space and, on imaging, are sharply marginated and oval or fusiform in shape. Imaging features are those of other schwannomas in the head and neck. Most tumors of the lacrimal gland are benign, with benign mixed tumor (previously termed pleomorphic adenoma) most common. It is a well-encapsulated round lesion often producing scalloped remodeling of the lacrimal fossa. The most common malignant lacrimal gland tumor is adenoid cystic carcinoma. Lymphoma of the lacrimal gland may also be encountered, unilateral or bilateral, typically B-cell lymphoma.

Dermoid and epidermoid inclusion cysts of the orbit are among the most common childhood orbital tumors. Clinical presentation can be delayed to early adulthood. The most common location is the superior temporal quadrant of the orbit, adjacent to the frontozygomatic suture (with their origin being sequestration of ectoderm along suture lines of orbital bones). On CT, these are well-circumscribed, smoothly marginated, and low density. On MR, the imaging appearance of epidermoid lesions (absent dermal adnexa) is predominately that of fluid (low on T1 and high on T2). Fat-containing dermoid tumors will manifest high signal intensity on T1-weighted images, with the signal suppressed on fat-saturated, postcontrast scans.

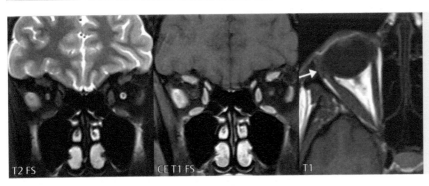

Fig. 2.36 Subperiosteal abscess, orbit. An axial unenhanced CT, reconstructed with a soft tissue algorithm, demonstrates confluent density in the medial left orbit, extraconal in location. The ethmoid air cells are opacified bilaterally, of relevance to the diagnosis specifically on the left. A coronal reformatted image, from the same exam but reconstructed with a bone algorithm, demonstrates dehiscence (*asterisk*) involving the lamina papyracea on the left. Sinusitis is the most common cause of a subperiosteal abscess involving the orbit.

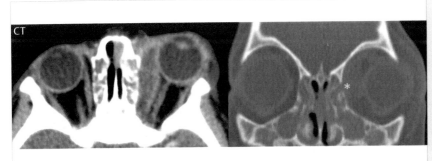

Fig. 2.37 Orbital pseudotumor, MR. Coronal and axial images are presented. There are several forms of orbital pseudotumor, one being the myositis form illustrated. The lateral rectus muscle on the right is affected in this instance, with enlargement that extends to involve the tendon insertion anteriorly (*arrow*). The latter differentiates orbital pseudotumor from thyroid orbitopathy. The lateral rectus is also noted to be mildly hyperintense on the T2-weighted scan, with moderate enhancement postcontrast.

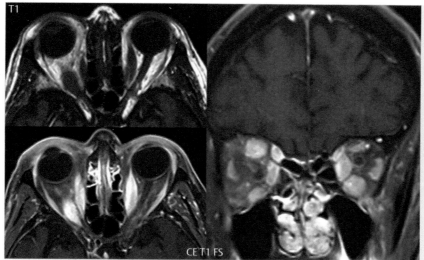

Fig. 2.38 Thyroid orbitopathy (Graves disease). Precontrast axial T1 and postcontrast T1 fat-saturated axial and coronal images are presented. All of the extraocular muscles are enlarged to some degree, and somewhat asymmetrically when comparing the left and right orbits. The enlargement predominantly involves the bellies of the respective muscles with sparing of the tendinous insertions. The lateral rectus muscles appear least involved.

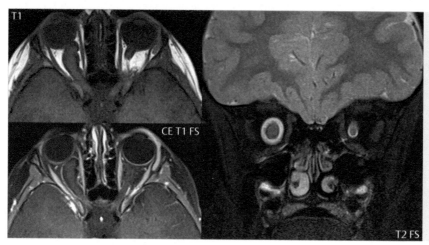

Fig. 2.39 Optic nerve glioma, neurofibromatosis type 1 (NF1). In this 4-year-old child, there is fusiform enlargement of the right optic nerve, with characteristic kinking. As is common, in childhood NF1 cases, there is no abnormal enhancement. There is accompanying prominent dilatation of the optic nerve sheath (with increased fluid circumferential to the lesion).

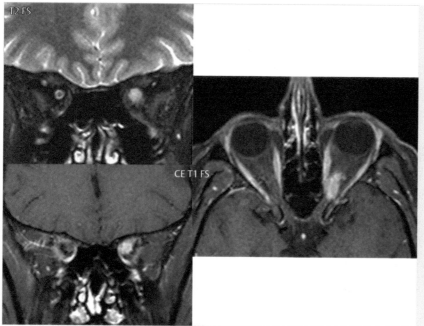

Fig. 2.40 Optic nerve glioma (enhancing). There is fusiform enlargement of a segment of the left optic nerve, within the orbit, seen on coronal and axial MR images. The lesion itself is hyperintense on the coronal T2-weighted scan, and displays intense homogeneous enhancement postcontrast.

2.4 Globe

Aqueous humor is secreted by the epithelium of the ciliary body, and is present in both the smaller anterior chamber and the larger posterior (vitreous) chamber of the globe. The globe is comprised of three concentric layers: the sclera, uvea, and retina. The sclera is the outermost layer and is composed of collagen-elastic tissue. The uvea is the middle layer, is vascular in nature (providing the vascular supply to the eye), and contains the iris, ciliary body, and choroid. The retina is the innermost layer, separated from the vitreous by the hyaloid membrane. The retina has two layers, the inner being the complex sensory layer and the outer being the retinal pigment epithelium.

There are three potential spaces and, thus, three types of retinal detachment: that between hyaloid and sensory retina (the posterior hyaloid space), that between the sensory retina and retinal pigment epithelium (the sub-retinal space), and that between the choroid and the sclera (the suprachoroidal space). Posterior hyaloid detachment is seen in adults > 50 years of age, with macular degeneration. Separation of the sensory retina from retinal pigment epithelium produces the classic V-shape imaging appearance (of a retinal detachment), with convergence at the optic disc (▶ Fig. 2.45). Etiologies include masses (e.g., malignant melanoma), diabetes, inflammatory disease, trauma, and senile macular degeneration. Choroidal detachment can be due to surgery, trauma, or inflammatory disease, with the fluid either serous or hemorrhagic in nature. Retinal detachments are well-visualized on MR. Because of the high incidence of retinal detachments in older adults, a scleral buckle (placed to repair a retinal detachment) (▶ Fig. 2.46) is a common finding on screening CT (or MR) performed for other reasons.

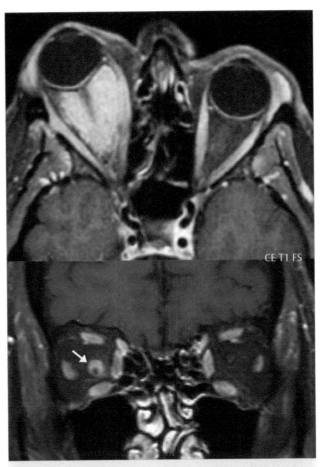

Fig. 2.42 Optic nerve meningioma, MR. Two patients are illustrated. In the first, on an axial scan, a large intraconal enhancing mass is noted circumferential to the optic nerve, with prominent proptosis. In the second, a small meningioma is visualized on a coronal image, with abnormal enhancing soft tissue (*arrow*) surrounding the optic nerve within the posterior orbit.

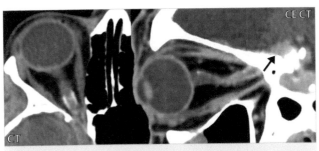

Fig. 2.41 Optic nerve meningioma, CT. Axial and sagittal reformatted CT images from two different patients are presented. In the first patient, the posterior portion of the optic nerve within the orbit is slightly prominent, with distinctive "tram track" calcification. In the second patient, linear calcification and abnormal enhancement are demonstrated along the optic nerve sheath within the orbit, with extension of this meningioma along the nerve through the optic canal to involve the dura intracranially (*arrow*).

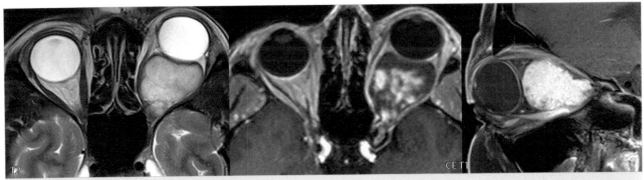

Fig. 2.43 Cavernous hemangioma of the orbit. A well-defined, smoothly marginated mass is identified in the intraconal space, the most common location for this tumor. The tumor is hyperintense on the T2-weighted scan. Note also the patchy enhancement on the axial postcontrast scan, that "fills-in" on the delayed sagittal scan. These features are all very characteristic for this tumor.

Retinoblastoma is the most common childhood intraocular tumor (98% of cases present before 6 months of age), often presenting with leukocoria. It is bilateral in 25 to 30%. Histologically these are primitive neuroectodermal tumors. The entity trilateral/quadrilateral retinoblastoma refers to a patient with bilateral retinoblastomas and an additional tumor in either the

suprasellar and/or pineal region (▶ Fig. 2.47). Imaging is performed to look for retrobulbar spread, optic nerve invasion, and intracranial metastases. Both on ophthalmologic exam and imaging, a variety of benign mass lesions can mimic retinoblastoma. *CT* shows calcification (punctate or speckled) in more than 90% of retinoblastomas, in marked distinction to other intraocular lesions. On MR, retinoblastoma is visualized as a mass with short T1 and T2 (mildly hyperintense on T1 and hypointense on T2). Enhancement is typically moderate to

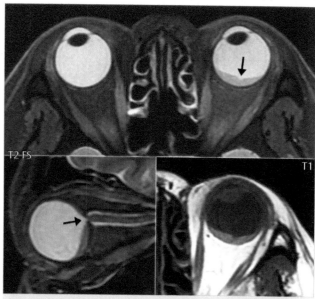

Fig. 2.45 Retinal detachment. A lentiform fluid collection is noted posteriorly in the left globe, on axial and sagittal T2-weighted scans obtained with fat saturation, and on the axial T1-weighted scan. There is a characteristic V-shaped indentation (*arrow*), representing infolding of the retinal leaves, pointing toward the optic disc.

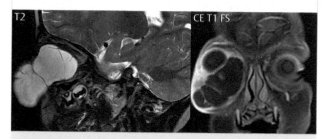

Fig. 2.44 Lymphatic malformation, orbit. Axial T2-weighted (**part 1**) together with sagittal T2- and coronal postcontrast fat sat T1-weighted (**part 2**) scans are presented in this 2-year-old child. A large, lobulated, multilocular, trans-spatial orbital mass is noted, which is T2 hyperintense consistent with fluid. The globe is compressed and deformed, and the orbit expanded. Although there is a small solid component, the lesion is predominantly cystic with prominent enhancement postcontrast of the cyst margins.

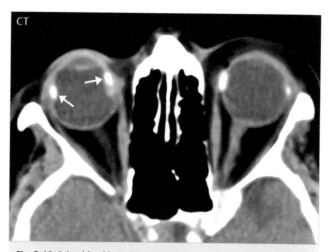

Fig. 2.46 Scleral buckle. Scleral banding or buckling is performed for retinal detachment. The band is placed around the equator of the globe, with compression promoting apposition of the choroid and sclera to the retina. These bands are typically dense on CT and low signal intensity on MR. Bilateral scleral buckles (*arrows*, right globe) are visualized in this patient.

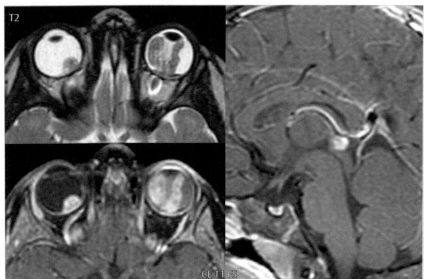

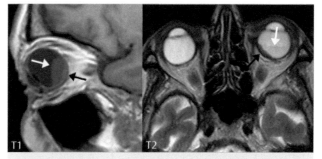

Fig. 2.47 Trilateral retinoblastoma. Enhancing soft tissue masses involve both globes in this 16-month-old child. Also noted is an 8-mm enhancing pineal region mass. Presence or development of an intracranial lesion defines a trilateral retinoblastoma, with the majority of such lesions noted in the pineal region. These patients carry a poorer prognosis, with lower survival and a propensity to leptomeningeal tumor spread.

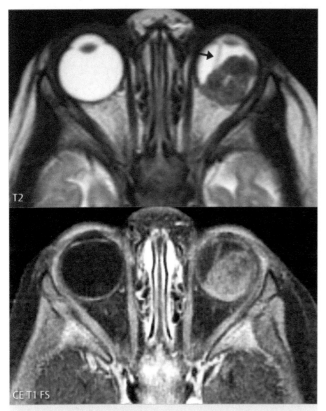

Fig. 2.49 Ocular metastasis. This 70-year-old patient presented to her ophthalmologist with painless loss of vision in the left eye. Her history was pertinent for a prior gastrectomy (adenocarcinoma). Sagittal and axial images reveal both a retinal detachment (*white arrow*), and a small, posteromedial choroidal mass (*black arrow*) on the left. The latter, a metastasis, also demonstrated contrast enhancement (image not shown). Incidentally noted is prior bilateral cataract surgery (with removal of the lenses).

Fig. 2.48 Retinoblastoma. Retinoblastomas can have similar signal intensity characteristics to melanoma due to hemorrhage, necrotic elements, or calcification therein. Detection of calcification—limited on MR—on CT distinguishes retinoblastoma from melanoma, as does patient age since retinoblastomas are found almost exclusively in children. On the T2-weighted axial image, this large retinoblastoma demonstrates characteristic low signal intensity. Although not shown, it also was slightly hyperintense on the T1-weighted image. Enhancement is present on the postcontrast image. Fat saturation is routinely used for postcontrast imaging in the orbits, suppressing the signal intensity from retrobulbar fat that might otherwise obscure findings. For retinoblastoma, specifically, evaluation for possible optic nerve enhancement is important, with the latter indicative of contiguous tumor spread. Lesions may also cause retinal detachment, present in this patient (*small black arrow*).

marked (▸ Fig. 2.48). There are many uncommon, benign diseases that occur in the globe, some of which can mimic retinoblastoma, which are beyond the scope of this textbook. These include persistent hyperplastic primary vitreous, Norrie disease, Warburg syndrome, retinopathy of prematurity, Coats disease, and ocular toxocariasis.

Ocular choroidal melanoma and choroidal metastases (▸ Fig. 2.49) are usually diagnosed by ophthalmoscopy, which is true of all ocular tumors. Ocular melanoma is the most common primary intraocular neoplasm in adults, typically unilateral, with retinal detachment frequent. MR plays a limited role for characterization and definition of extent. Lesions that present for MR are usually small and mound-shaped with a broad choroidal base (▸ Fig. 2.50). Although choroidal melanomas are described as having a classic MR appearance, due to melanin, with marked hyperintensity on T1 and hypointensity on T2, this is observed in just slightly more than half of these tumors. Thus, differentiation on MR between choroidal metastases and melanomas is limited.

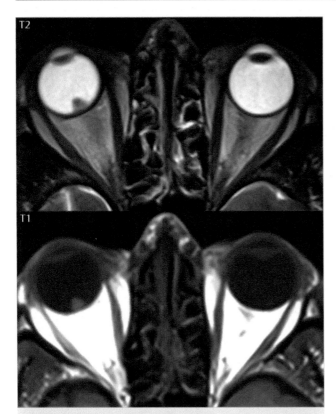

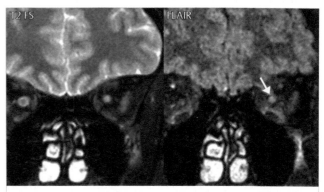

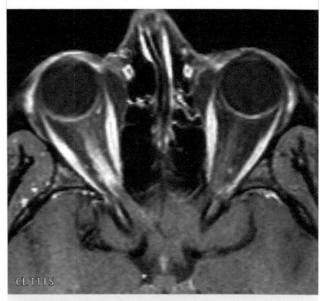

Fig. 2.50 Choroidal melanoma. A small soft tissue lesion lies along the posterior wall of the right globe of this 52-year-old patient, with slight hyperintensity on the T1-weighted image. Binding of paramagnetic metals by melanin is responsible for this appearance, which is characteristic and somewhat unique. Thus a choroidal melanoma in most instances is relatively hyperintense on T1- and hypointense on T2-weighted images, as in this patient. There was moderate contrast enhancement (image not shown), also characteristic.

Fig. 2.51 Optic neuritis. **Part 1:** On coronal T2-weighted scans obtained with fat saturation, the left optic nerve is hyperintense, consistent with edema (*arrow*). This is best demonstrated on the FLAIR scan. **Part 2:** In a second patient, on an axial postcontrast scan, there is abnormal enhancement of a long segment of the right optic nerve.

2.5 Visual Pathway

At the optic chiasm, the axons from the nasal half of the retina cross to the contralateral optic tract. The axons from the temporal half of the retina, however, do not cross. Thus, in terms of visual fields, the right side (present on the nasal half of the right retina and the temporal half of the left retina) projects to the left hemisphere (optic tract, lateral geniculate ganglion [located in the thalamus], optic radiations, and visual cortex), and vice versa. An optic nerve lesion leads to monocular blindness. An optic chiasm lesion leads to bitemporal hemianopsia (vision loss in the outer halves of both eyes), and an optic tract lesion leads to contralateral homonymous hemianopsia (vision loss on the same side in both eyes).

Any portion of the visual pathway can be involved by an optic glioma, as previously noted. Involvement of the optic chiasm and tract are common. Contrast enhancement of these lesions is variable (from little to prominent). Involvement of the visual pathway is well-identified in these tumors by MR especially on FLAIR scans. As discussed in the brain section, pituitary macroadenomas can extend superiorly, splaying and compressing the optic chiasm, leading to bitemporal hemianopsia.

An ophthalmic artery aneurysm is the most common aneurysm to cause visual symptoms, due to impingement on the visual pathway. Ischemia—for example, due to retinal or ophthalmic artery emboli—can lead to transient loss of vision in one eye (monocular blindness). Ischemia involving the visual cortex (occipital lobe) will lead to contralateral homonymous hemianopsia. Optic neuritis can cause either complete or partial loss of vision in one eye, with the most common etiology being multiple sclerosis. Thin-section axial and coronal FLAIR and postcontrast T1-weighted scans (both obtained with fat suppression) are critical for identification of inflammation involving the optic nerve, with edema seen on the former and abnormal contrast enhancement on the latter (typically extending along a relatively long section of the nerve) (▶ Fig. 2.51).

2.6 Paranasal Sinuses, Nasal Cavity, and Face

The roof of the nasal cavity is formed by the cribriform plate and the floor by the hard palate. The olfactory mucosa is found in the upper portion of the nasal cavity, above the superior turbinates. The nasal septum is formed by the ethmoid bone posteriorly, cartilage anteriorly, and the vomer posteroinferiorly. The turbinates (nasal concha), of which there are three (inferior,

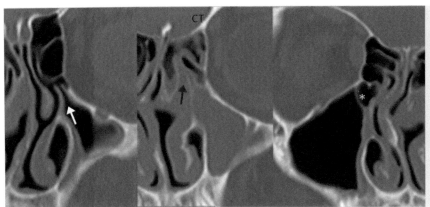

Fig. 2.52 Ostiomeatal unit, normal and opacified. Coronal CT studies in three different patients are illustrated. In the first, a normal, aerated, ostiomeatal unit (extending from the maxillary sinus ostium [*white arrow*], up over the uncinate process, and down to the middle meatus) is illustrated. In the second, the entire ostiomeatal unit is opacified (*black arrow*), together with the associated left maxillary sinus. In the third patient, a Haller cell (a low ethmoid air cell) is present (*asterisk*).

middle, and superior), lie along the lateral walls of the nasal cavity, with a space (meatus) beneath each turbine, named according to the turbinate immediately above. The nasolacrimal duct opens into the inferior meatus. The semilunar hiatus is a crescent-shaped groove in the middle meatus, with the ostium for the maxillary sinus located posteriorly therein. The ostium lies high on the medial sinus wall. Therefore, gravity cannot drain the maxillary sinus. There is a normal nasal cycle, with alternating partial congestion and decongestion of the nasal turbinates with time, from the left side to the right side, which can be commonly observed on imaging, either with the appearance of unilateral congestion or with alternation between different exams of the side of congestion.

The frontal sinus is typically divided by a septum along the midline, with the two resulting sinuses usually asymmetric in size, but each a single cavity. The ethmoid sinuses, which are composed of multiple individual small air cells, are today typically divided into anterior and posterior groups. In regard to the sphenoid sinus, pneumatization varies widely. There is typically a septum which is midline anteriorly, but can deviate to one side posteriorly. Two major air cells are common for the sphenoid sinus, with one often substantially larger than the other. Extension of the sphenoid sinus, specifically the lateral recesses, into the greater wing of the sphenoid, is common. The maxillary sinuses are usually symmetric. Asymmetry in size should immediately raise the question of chronic sinus disease (with chronic sinusitis leading to a small sinus with thickened walls.). Plain film exam grossly underestimates the extent of soft tissue disease and bone erosion/destruction versus cross-sectional imaging. CT of the paranasal sinuses is often reformatted in a tilted coronal plane, which well displays the ostiomeatal unit (▶ Fig. 2.52). This term refers to the collecting channel that drains the anterior ethmoid air cells and frontal and maxillary sinuses into the middle meatus. The posterior ethmoid air cells and the sphenoid sinus drain via the sphenoethmoidal recess into the superior meatus. Viewing of images reconstructed with both soft tissue and bone algorithms on CT is recommended. MR, as always, offers superior soft tissue visualization/differentiation, but inferior depiction of fine bony change.

2.6.1 Inflammation/Infection

Acute bacterial sinusitis can occur following viral infection (the "common cold"), with mucosal inflammation and swelling of the turbinates causing obstruction of the sinus ostia, which then leads to bacterial infection. Dental infection or tooth

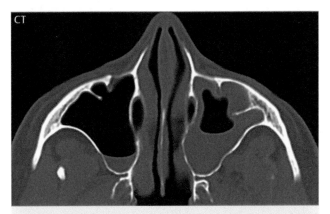

Fig. 2.53 Acute sinusitis, CT. An air-fluid level is present on this axial scan in the right maxillary sinus. This finding alone has several possible etiologies. On the left, there is both mucosal thickening and an air-fluid level, a combination of findings that is more specific for acute sinusitis.

extraction can also lead to acute bacterial sinusitis. The clinical presentation is one of pain over the affected sinus, with mucopurulent discharge. Disease is often limited to a single sinus. With repeated or persistent infection (chronic sinusitis), the bony walls of the sinus become thickened and sclerotic. With persistent maxillary obstruction, hypoventilation and negative pressure occur leading to retraction of the sinus walls and craniocaudad orbital enlargement and enophthalmos (silent sinus syndrome). Allergic sinusitis is characterized by symmetrical involvement and nasal polyposis (a differentiating point from bacterial sinusitis). However, profuse secretions in this disease process, with resultant obstruction, can lead to bacterial sinusitis.

The most reliable sign of acute bacterial sinusitis on imaging is the combination of mucosal thickening with an air-fluid level (▶ Fig. 2.53 and ▶ Fig. 2.54). Another presentation is that of complete sinus opacification by fluid (typically easily identified, and differentiated from soft tissue, on T2-weighted images), with DWI an important additional MR sequence (for identification of infection). Of all the paranasal sinuses, the maxillary sinus is the most commonly involved (▶ Fig. 2.55). Other causes of an air-fluid level include trauma (with hemorrhage), placement of a nasal tube, and sinus lavage. Complications from paranasal sinusitis include orbital involvement (most often due to ethmoid sinus infection), meningitis, intracranial abscess formation, subgaleal abscess (Pott puffy tumor, most often from frontal sinus involvement), and osteomyelitis (in patients with

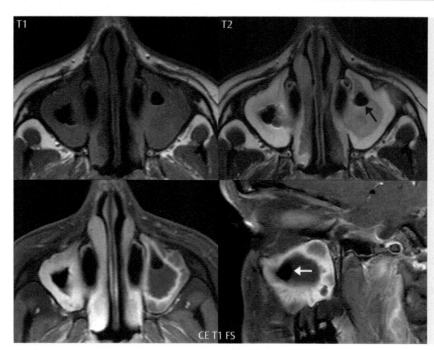

Fig. 2.54 Acute and chronic sinusitis. There is prominent mucosal thickening bilaterally, reflecting acute inflammatory disease, with enhancement postcontrast. An air-fluid level (*arrows*) is demonstrated in the left maxillary sinus, consistent with infection involving this sinus. Note the improved differentiation of the fluid from the mucosal thickening on the postcontrast scan. The walls of the maxillary sinuses bilaterally (visualized as a thin, low signal intensity line) are also thickened, consistent with chronic inflammatory disease.

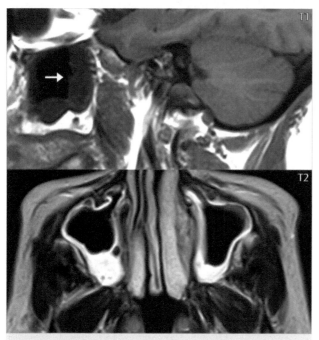

Fig. 2.55 Acute sinusitis, MR. The question is often raised whether fluid signal intensity within a sinus on a T2-weighted scan reflects a retention cyst or an air-fluid level. Although this differentiation should be simple on axial scans, posteriorly located retention cysts may cause confusion. Thus a sagittal scan, such as the T1-weighted image illustrated, can be of great use, clearly defining an air-fluid level (*arrow*) in this patient with acute sinusitis (with the scans demonstrating both an air-fluid level and mucosal thickening in the affected sinus).

chronic disease) (▶ Fig. 2.56). Intracranial spread of infection (cerebritis, epidural abscess, etc.), involving the anterior cranial fossa, can occur within 48 hours following development of frontal sinusitis (due to the rich venous network).

Cysts and polyps are a common local complication of inflammation. A very large cyst can resemble an air-fluid level on imaging, with close inspection of images mandated, in particular considering the direction of gravity and inspection of the cyst/fluid border, which should be slightly convex with a cyst. A mucous retention cyst is the most common of the different cysts and polyps, with the floor of the maxillary sinus the most frequent location (▶ Fig. 2.57). A mucous retention cyst is generally considered an incidental finding. A polyp is due to a local upheaval of mucosa, with the two common etiologies being inflammation and allergy (with allergic polyps being multiple). Polyps can be expansile in nature, cause bony destruction, and most often involve the maxillary sinus. As the polyp expands in size, it may prolapse through the sinus ostium, forming an antrochoanal polyp (in the literature 5% of all polyps, thus not uncommon) (▶ Fig. 2.58).

The most common causes of invasive fungal sinusitis include aspergillosis, mucormycosis, and candidiasis. Mucormycosis especially occurs in poorly controlled diabetes and other chronic disease states. Candidiasis occurs in immunocompromised patients. Fungal sinusitis often involves multiple sinuses, with additional clues being increased attenuation (calcification) within the opacified sinus on CT and hypointense signal intensity on T2-weighted scan centrally (▶ Fig. 2.59). Orbital and intracranial complications are not uncommon, including cavernous sinus thrombosis.

Two additional entities that involve the paranasal sinuses are of note. Granulomatosis with polyangiitis (previously termed Wegener granulomatosis) is a necrotizing vasculitis, which can affect the nose and paranasal sinuses. The common presentation, when there is nasal involvement, is that of a soft tissue mass involving the nasal cavity with bone destruction (septal perforation). On MR, the mass will be low signal intensity on T2-weighted images, with homogeneous enhancement postcontrast. Cocaine abuse also causes a necrotizing vasculitis, with inflammatory changes and septal erosion/perforation (▶ Fig. 2.60).

Mucoceles are the most common expansile lesion involving a paranasal sinus (▶ Fig. 2.61). A mucocele is caused by obstruction of a sinus ostium (or of a compartment in a septated sinus). The incidence, by sinus, is frontal > ethmoid > maxillary > sphenoid.

The sinus will be devoid of air and expanded, with remodeling of the walls. The most common appearance on MR is low on T1 and high on T2. If present for a long time the signal intensity on T1 may be high, due to protein content and resorption of water.

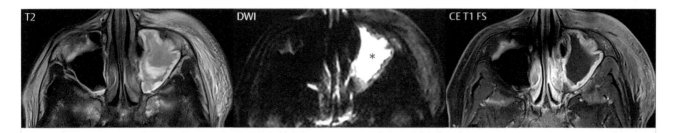
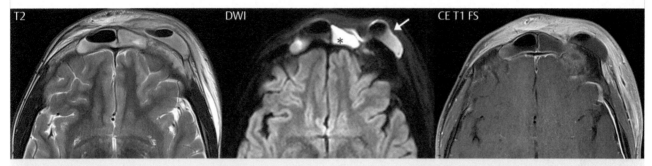

Fig. 2.56 Acute sinusitis, diffusion-weighted imaging (DWI). Axial images of both the maxillary **(part 1)** and frontal **(part 2)** sinuses are presented in a 15-year-old patient. The left maxillary and frontal sinuses are completely opacified, with mild mucosal thickening in the former. An air-fluid level is noted in the right frontal sinus. Diffusion-weighted imaging in this instance offers a key to diagnosis, suggesting infection (confirmed clinically), due to high signal intensity on DWI (*asterisk*) in the sinuses in question. This was confirmed on ADC maps to represent restricted diffusion (images not shown). Infection in this instance has spread from the frontal sinus to the supraorbital extracranial soft tissues, with a subperiosteal abscess (*arrow*, also hyperintense on DWI) and extensive inflammatory soft tissue reaction identified. These findings are consistent with a Pott's puffy tumor, a rare entity seen primarily in adolescents, with a subperiosteal abscess and osteomyelitis, as a complication of frontal sinusitis (in the case presented) or trauma.

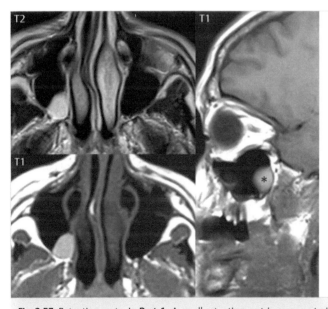
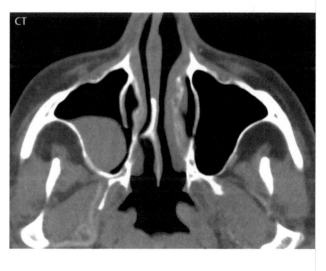

Fig. 2.57 Retention cysts. In **Part 1:** A small retention cyst is seen posteriorly in the right maxillary sinus on axial T2- and T1-weighted scans, as well as on the sagittal T1-weighted scan (*asterisk*). Retention cysts have rounded margins, a base along a sinus wall, occur in all sizes and typically demonstrate fluid signal intensity, low on T1-, high on T2-weighted scans. This small retention cyst is unusual for its signal intensity on the T1-weighted scan, being slightly hyperintense, due to either proteinaceous content or hemorrhage. **Part 2:** Illustrates a large right maxillary retention cyst on CT, with these lesions typically incidental (asymptomatic) regardless of size. Note the rounded margins and flat base along the sinus wall.

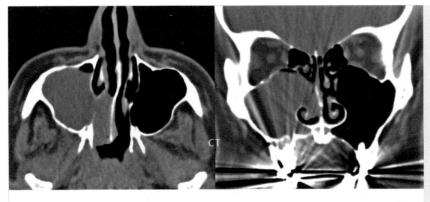

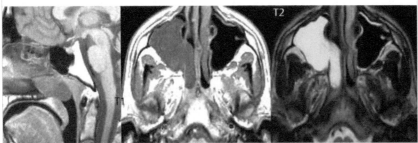

Fig. 2.58 Antrochoanal polyp (sinonasal polyp). **Part 1:** Axial and coronal reformatted CT images reconstructed with a soft tissue algorithm depict abnormal soft tissue, on the right, filling the maxillary antrum with extension through an enlarged maxillary ostium into the middle meatus. Mild thickening of the walls of the right maxillary sinus is also noted (best seen on the axial image), consistent with chronic sinus disease. **Part 2:** Sagittal and axial MR scans depict a mass with fluid signal intensity (the polyp) occupying the right maxillary sinus and extending into both the nasal cavity and, best seen on the sagittal image, the proximal nasopharynx. (Courtesy of Lindell R. Gentry, MD.)

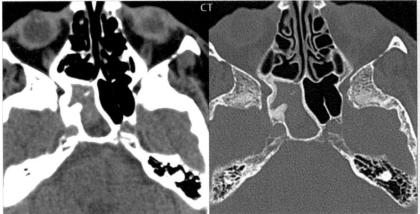

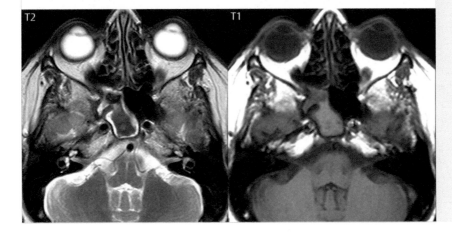

Fig. 2.59 Fungal sinusitis. **Part 1:** On the axial CT images (reconstructed with soft tissue and bone algorithms), the right sphenoid sinus is opacified with hyperdense material and its walls thickened and sclerotic. A small calcification is also noted anteriorly within this air cell. Fungal disease, for example aspergillosis, is known for such intrasinus calcifications (together with high density sinus contents). **Part 2:** On MR, the low signal intensity on the T2-weighted scan is characteristic for fungal infection, which typically also has low signal intensity on the scan (not seen in this patient).

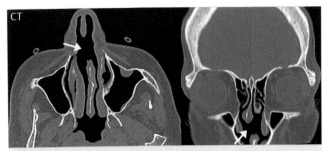

Fig. 2.60 Nasal septal perforation, cocaine. Axial and coronal CT scans reconstructed with a bone algorithm reveal destruction of a portion of the anterior nasal septum, involving predominately cartilage (*arrow*), in a patient with chronic cocaine abuse.

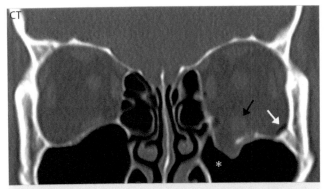

Fig. 2.62 Blowout (orbital floor) fracture. A coronal CT of the orbits in an assault victim demonstrates herniation of orbital fat (*asterisk*) through a comminuted fracture involving the floor of the left orbit. Indicative of acute trauma is the orbital emphysema (*white arrow*). The inferior rectus muscle (*black arrow*) is displaced interiorly, adjacent to the fracture fragments of the orbital floor, but without definite entrapment.

2.6.2 Fractures

Blowout fractures of the orbit (▶ Fig. 2.62) occur due to a blow by an object too large to enter the orbit. With inferior blowout fractures, the orbital contents rupture into the maxillary sinus, often with associated antral hemorrhage. The globe is usually not damaged. Diplopia can occur due to edema and hemorrhage, or muscle entrapment. This injury is often accompanied by a fracture of the medial wall of the orbit, which can be difficult to visualize. Small amounts of orbital emphysema adjacent to one of the walls of the orbit can be key to recognition of a fracture involving the orbit. A medial blowout fracture can lead, long term, to dehiscence of the lamina papyracea. Hemorrhage or fluid is seen acutely in the adjacent ethmoid air cells, but otherwise the etiology of a long-standing dehiscence is difficult to establish, and may be posttraumatic, postsurgical, or congenital (▶ Fig. 2.63).

Nasal bone fractures are the most common fracture of the face (▶ Fig. 2.64) and most often involve the distal third of the nasal bone. The majority of frontal sinus fractures are limited to

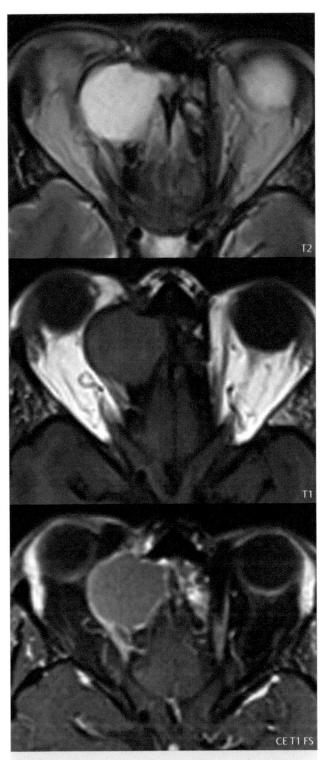

Fig. 2.61 Ethmoid mucocele. There is opacification and expansion of a right ethmoid air cell. The imaging characteristics are consistent with fluid, with high signal intensity on the T2-weighted scan, intermediate to low signal intensity on the T1-weighted scan, and only minimal peripheral enhancement (the mucosal lining of the air cell).

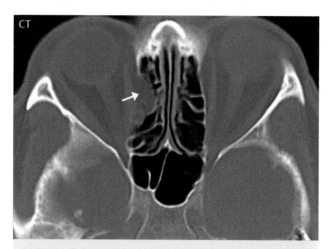

Fig. 2.63 Dehiscence (*arrow*) of the lamina papyracea. There is medial deviation of the lamina papyracea on the right, with the absence of opacification of adjacent ethmoid air cells indicating that this finding is chronic. This can be due either to congenital dehiscence or remote trauma, with the latter the more likely etiology. The finding is relatively common in the adult population.

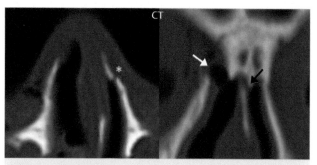

Fig. 2.64 Nasal bone fractures. On an axial scan, a fracture (*asterisk*) of the left nasal bone is identified. There is subcutaneous emphysema adjacent to a fracture of the right nasal bone, with assessment of the overlying soft tissues helpful in identifying fractures and also assessing their time frame. The coronal reformatted image identifies the fracture of the right nasal bone (*white arrow*) and nasal septum (*black arrow*), together with lateral displacement of the nasal bone.

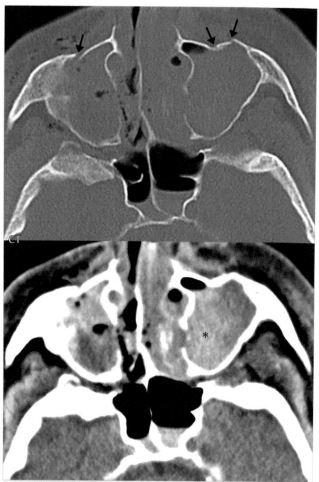

Fig. 2.65 Maxillary sinus fractures. On the image reconstructed with a bone algorithm (top), a comminuted fracture of the anterior wall of the left maxillary sinus is noted, together with an isolated fracture of the anterior wall of the right maxillary sinus (*black arrows*). There is near complete opacification of the two sinuses. Subcutaneous emphysema is also noted on the right. Air-fluid levels are present in the sphenoid sinus. On the image reconstructed with a soft tissue algorithm (bottom), much of the contents of the maxillary sinuses display high density, consistent with hemorrhage (*asterisk*), together with the fluid in the sphenoid sinus.

the anterior wall. Maxillary sinus fractures are extremely common both with local trauma and high speed injuries (▶ Fig. 2.65). Sphenoid sinus fractures are associated with severe trauma and basal skull fractures. The zygomaticomaxillary complex (ZMC) fracture (previously termed a tripod fracture) includes a fracture separating the zygoma and maxilla, through the zygomatic arch, and through the lateral orbital wall and floor (▶ Fig. 2.66).

Le Fort fractures, as originally described, are similar to low velocity impact fractures seen today. High velocity impact forces are common in modern injury, although the same fracture lines are still observed but often in different combinations than originally described. Thus it is important to describe, in detail, each fracture line visualized, with a summary using a Le Fort classification if pertinent. In a Le Fort I fracture, the tooth-bearing portion of the maxilla is separated from the lower maxillary sinus and nasal septum (▶ Fig. 2.67). The fracture also extends through the lower pterygoid plates. A Le Fort II fracture is caused by a blow over the central face, as opposed to a blow over the upper lip, which is responsible for a Le Fort I fracture. A Le Fort II fracture runs through the nose root, lacrimal bones, medial orbital walls, orbital floor, zygomaticomaxillary suture, anterior wall of the maxilla, and lower pterygoid plates. In a Le Fort III fracture, the facial skeleton is separated from the skull base. This fracture is most easily conceptualized as a Le Fort II fracture with extension to involve the zygomatic arches and lateral orbital walls.

2.6.3 Sinus Surgery

Sinus surgery is most frequently performed for infection. Often observed on imaging is the end result of one of several common surgeries. The objective of surgery is to improve

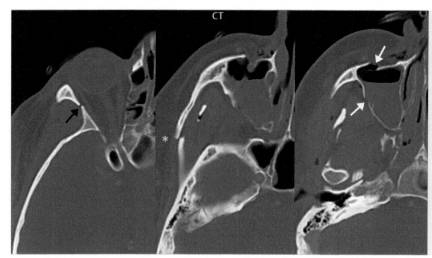

Fig. 2.66 Zygomaticomaxillary complex fracture. Fractures are noted of the lateral wall of the orbit (*black arrow*), zygomatic arch (*asterisk*), and involving the anterior and posterior walls of the right maxillary sinus (*white arrows*). The sinus fracture separates the zygoma from the maxilla. There is slight displacement involving the latter two parts of this fracture. An air-fluid level with hemorrhage is noted in the maxillary sinus, together with some subcutaneous emphysema.

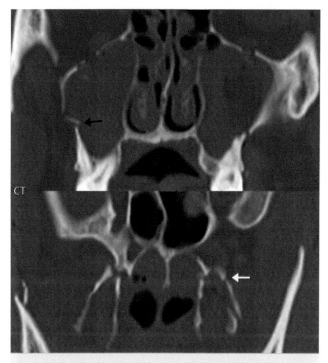

Fig. 2.67 Le Fort I fracture. On coronal reformatted CT, reconstructed with a bone algorithm, there are fractures of the lateral walls (*black arrow*) of the maxillary sinuses bilaterally. There were accompanying fractures of the medial walls, not well depicted on the images presented. Also noted are minimally displaced fractures (*white arrow*) of the medial and lateral pterygoid plates bilaterally.

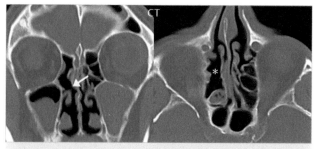

Fig. 2.68 Partial ethmoidectomy. There has been surgery in the past involving the right ethmoid air cells, visualized on both coronal and axial images. Note the absence of septa therein (*asterisk*) with the exception of the most posterior portion of the ethmoid sinus. On the coronal image, a bony defect (*arrow*) is noted between the nasal cavity and the ethmoid sinus, surgical in origin, created for functional endoscopic sinus surgery and to promote drainage. Additional sinus inflammatory disease illustrated includes a large retention cyst in the right maxillary sinus and complete opacification of the left maxillary sinus.

drainage. Ethmoid sinus surgery often involves removal of all or a large portion of the ethmoid septae (▶ Fig. 2.68). Maxillary sinus surgery often involves the (endoscopic) creation of a large antrostomy (opening) in the medial wall, generally in the middle meatus, communicating with the nasal cavity (▶ Fig. 2.69). Individual or multiple turbinates may be resected. In the Caldwell-Luc procedure, the maxillary sinus is entered surgically under the lip above the canine teeth. A medial antrostomy is also part of this procedure. On imaging, prior Caldwell-Luc surgery can be recognized by the presence of a lower anterior sinus wall defect (▶ Fig. 2.70). Sphenoid sinus surgery involves enlargement (variable in extent) of the sphenoid sinus ostium (sphenoethmoidal recess), along the anterior wall. In the transethmoidal approach, this involves simply extension of the ethmoidectomy posteriorly.

2.6.4 Neoplasms

Tumors of the sinonasal cavity frequently present at an advanced stage (▶ Fig. 2.71), often accompanied by chronic inflammatory disease (and thus overlooked). On CT, intravenous contrast administration is important for lesion visualization and differentiation from inflammatory disease. MR is much more valuable in this regard, with most inflammatory change seen as high signal intensity on T2 as distinguished from most sinonasal tumors, which are highly cellular and have intermediate T2 signal intensity. For MR evaluation intravenous contrast administration is also mandated. Treatment is altered by extension into anterior/middle cranial fossae, pterygopalatine fossa, orbit, or palate, and, thus, careful image evaluation is critical (▶ Fig. 2.72).

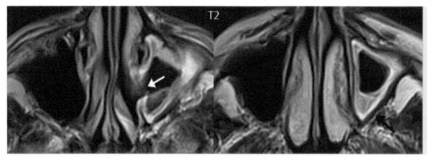

Fig. 2.69 Maxillary antrostomy. The first axial image demonstrates a surgically created defect/communication between the left maxillary sinus and the nasal cavity, an antrostomy. The second axial image (inferior to the first) demonstrates a small left maxillary sinus with thickening of the posterior wall (*black arrow*), seen as a linear low signal intensity structure (cortical bone), and moderate mucosal thickening, all indicative of chronic sinus disease.

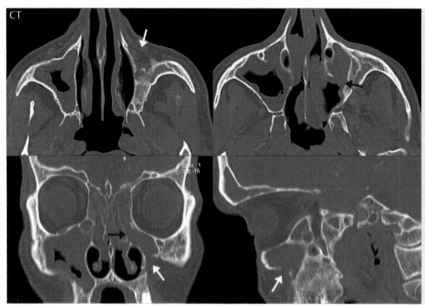

Fig. 2.70 Caldwell Luc antrostomy. In this surgery, which is still performed (although most antral and ostiomeatal complex procedures today are endoscopic), the maxillary sinus is entered via the canine fossa under the lip (thus avoiding a facial scar), and a medial antrostomy performed. CT images reconstructed using a bone algorithm demonstrate characteristic findings of a Caldwell Luc procedure performed many years prior to the imaging exam. Both the anterior bony wall defect (*white arrow*) and the medial antrostomy (*black arrow*) are visualized on axial, coronal, and sagittal reformatted images. The left maxillary sinus is small, with thickening of its walls, due to chronic sinus disease.

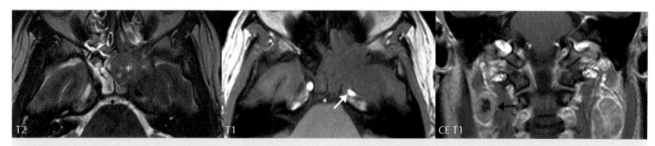

Fig. 2.71 Squamous cell carcinoma, sphenoid sinus, MR. On axial scans, a soft tissue mass (*asterisk*) is noted to involve the left sphenoid sinus, with extension into the nasal cavity and middle cranial fossa. The left internal carotid artery (*white arrow*) is compressed and displaced posteriorly. The coronal postcontrast T1-weighted scan demonstrates bilateral grossly enlarged lymph nodes with central necrosis (nonenhancement) seen in the node on the right (*black arrow*), consistent with metastatic involvement. The lesion, histologically, was confirmed to represent moderately to poorly differentiated squamous cell carcinoma.

With aggressive bone destruction, squamous cell carcinoma or sinonasal undifferentiated carcinoma (SNUC) are the most likely diagnoses (▶ Fig. 2.73). Adenoid cystic carcinoma is the most common of the malignant minor salivary gland tumors in the sinonasal cavity. Another less common tumor in the sinonasal cavity is adenocarcinoma (▶ Fig. 2.74). On MR, fibrous dysplasia may mimic a tumor within the sinuses, although often the appearance on CT is characteristic (with mixed sclerotic and lytic disease, or a ground-glass appearance).

An osteoma is a benign proliferation of bone which most commonly occurs in the frontal sinus (although an osteoma can occur in any sinus), and is typically an incidental finding.

Multiple osteomas, including involvement of the skull and mandible, raises the question of Gardner syndrome.

Osteogenic sarcoma, chondrosarcoma, and lymphoma can all occur in the sinonasal cavity, but are rare. The same is true for benign neurogenic tumors (which typically remodel bone), specifically schwannoma and neurofibroma.

An inverted papilloma is a benign lesion that arises from the lateral nasal wall, near the middle turbinate, extending secondarily into the sinuses (maxillary or ethmoid) (▶ Fig. 2.75). Symptoms include prominently nasal obstruction. There is a high recurrence rate following resection. When visualized, a convoluted cerebriform appearance is characteristic (▶ Fig. 2.76).

A juvenile angiofibroma is a highly vascular, nonencapsulated, polypoid, histologically benign, locally aggressive tumor with intense enhancement on CT and MR (▸ Fig. 2.77). Flow voids may be seen on MR. Enlarged feeding vessels from the external carotid artery, together with an intense capillary blush, are seen on angiography. Clinical presentation is in adolescent males with nasal obstruction and epistaxis. This tumor occurs in the nasopharynx, classically arising adjacent to the sphenopalatine foramen. The lesion epicenter will thus be in the posterior nasal cavity off the midline. The majority extend through the sphenopalatine foramen into the pterygopalatine fossa. Tumor extension into adjacent paranasal sinuses, in particular the sphenoid sinus, is common. Intracranial tumor extension, into the middle cranial fossa, and involvement of the cavernous sinus can also occur.

Esthesioneuroblastoma (olfactory neuroblastoma) is a malignant tumor that arises from the olfactory neuroepithelium lining the roof of the nasal vault (▸ Fig. 2.78). Large tumors can

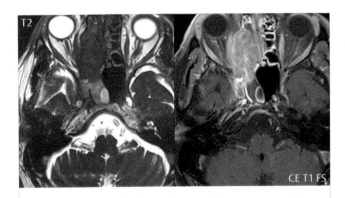

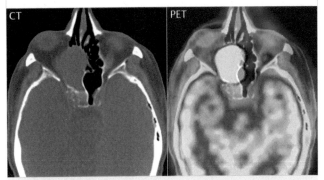

Fig. 2.72 Squamous cell carcinoma of the ethmoid sinus. An expansile, destructive mass with moderate contrast enhancement is noted on axial MR scans (part 1) with its epicenter in the right ethmoid sinus. The lesion is of intermediate to low signal intensity on the T2-weighted scan. There is extension laterally to involve the right orbit and posteriorly to involve the sphenoid sinus and orbital apex. Bony destruction is present on CT, with avid tumor 18F-fluorodeoxyglucose uptake on PET (part 2).

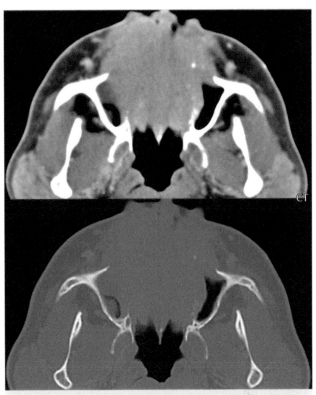

Fig. 2.73 Squamous cell carcinoma, with extensive bone destruction, CT. There is a large soft tissue mass with its epicenter in the lower nasal cavity anteriorly. The mass extends to involve the maxillary sinuses bilaterally, with destruction of portions of the medial and anterior walls. There is destruction of much of the nasal septum, with abnormal soft tissue encompassing the inferior nasal turbinates anteriorly.

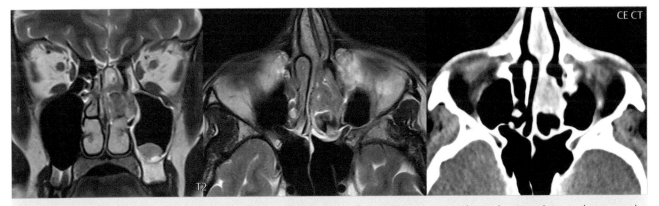

Fig. 2.74 Adenocarcinoma of the nasal cavity. Like squamous cell carcinomas, adenocarcinomas occur in the nasal cavity and sinuses, but are much less common. The imaging characteristics are, however, indistinguishable. In the case presented, a small expansile lesion is noted in the left nasal cavity, with destruction of the middle turbinate. The tumor is slightly hypointense to the turbinates on the coronal and axial T2-weighted scans, and displayed moderate enhancement on both MR (not shown) and CT.

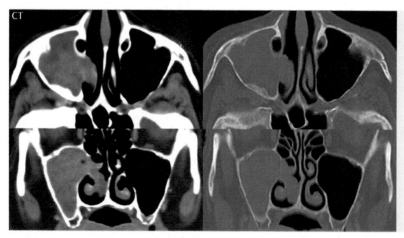

Fig. 2.75 Inverted papilloma (CT). Abnormal soft tissue is noted along the right lateral nasal wall, centered on an enlarged middle meatus. The mass extends into the maxillary sinus, with complete opacification.

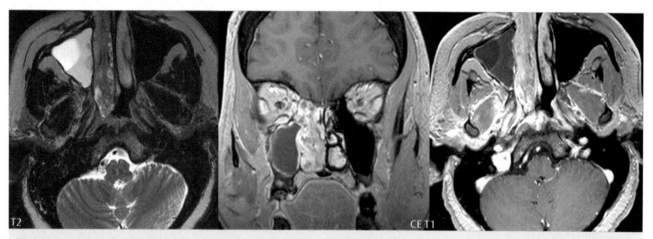

Fig. 2.76 Inverted papilloma (MR). A soft tissue mass is noted within the right nasal cavity (middle meatus), with extension into the nasopharynx posteriorly and ethmoid sinus superiorly, causing obstruction of the right maxillary sinus—all classical imaging findings for this diagnosis.

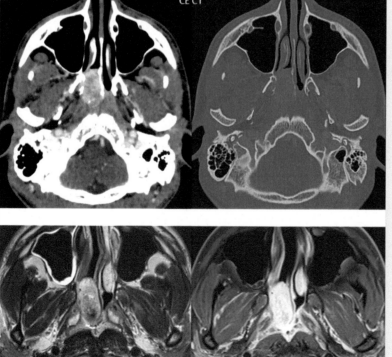

Fig. 2.77 Juvenile nasopharyngeal angiofibroma. On contrast-enhanced CT **(part 1)**, an oval, well-delineated enhancing mass is noted, on the right, in the posterior nasal cavity/nasopharynx near the sphenopalatine foramen (the latter is not well seen at the anatomic level depicted). There is mild bone remodeling/destruction involving the medial pterygoid plate on the right. Intense enhancement is seen on MR **(part 2)**.

(Continued)

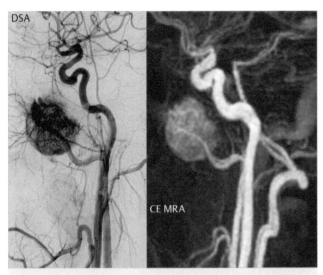

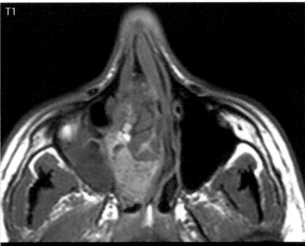

Fig. 2.77 (*Continued*) The arterial supply is delineated by both DSA and CE MRA (**part 3**) to be primarily from the external carotid artery, with an intense capillary blush demonstrated.

extend into the anterior cranial fossa and ipsilateral ethmoid and maxillary sinuses. Esthesioneuroblastomas occur over a broad age range, and present with mild epistaxis and unilateral nasal obstruction. Treatment is by surgical excision, combined with radiation therapy. On CT, an esthesioneuroblastoma appears as a homogeneous, enhancing lesion which can both remodel and destroy bone. Avid tumor enhancement is seen on MR. In the presence of intracranial extension, identification of peripheral tumor cysts is highly suggestive of these tumors.

2.7 Mandible

The mandible is divided into the body anteriorly and the ramus posteriorly, with the angle of the mandible interposed between. The ramus ascends dividing into the coronoid process anteriorly and the condyle with its neck and head posteriorly. The masseter muscle inserts on the outer surface of the ramus and the medial pterygoid on the inner surface. The temporalis muscle inserts anteriorly on the coronoid process. The lateral pterygoid muscle inserts anteriorly on the neck of the condyle. There are 20 deciduous teeth: 2 incisors, 1 canine, and 2 molars in each quadrant. There are 32 permanent teeth: 2 incisors, 1 canine, 2 premolars, and 3 molars in each quadrant.

A Panorex is the standard plain film exam, for screening, of the mandible. It provides a survey (panoramic view) of the entire mandible and maxilla on a single image. CT provides excellent bony detail regarding the mandible, and a Panorex-like image can also be reconstructed. Dental caries are commonly incidentally visualized on CT, whether performed for trauma involving the face or inflammatory disease involving the paranasal sinuses (▶ Fig. 2.79). In regard to neoplastic disease, MR provides excellent assessment of extraosseous lesion extent, and is very sensitive to tumor invasion (of the mandible). Abnormalities involving the marrow of the mandible can be assessed on MR by the use of fat suppressed T2-weighted scans, T1-weighted scans (with obliteration of the normal high signal intensity fatty marrow implying tumor

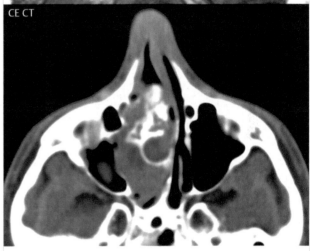

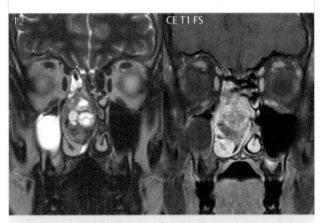

Fig. 2.78 Esthesioneuroblastoma. An expansile mass is noted in the right nasal cavity (**part 1**), with bone remodeling and marked tumoral calcifications. On coronal imaging (**part 2**), extension to involve the inferior right ethmoid air cells is seen. The lesion in this instance is heterogeneous in signal intensity (although they are more often homogeneous), with prominent enhancement postcontrast. Presentation with epistaxis and the location/imaging appearance are important keys to the diagnosis.

invasion), and fat suppressed T1-weighted postcontrast imaging.

Osteonecrosis of the jaw (with that of the mandible most common) may be associated with osteomyelitis (due to dental infections), osteoradionecrosis in patients with prior radiation, metastatic disease, or with bisphosphonate use (bisphosphonate-related osteonecrosis of the jaw [BPONJ]). Patients with BPONJ typically present with tooth loosening and nonhealing extraction sockets. Bisphosphonates inhibit osteoclast-mediated bone resorption and are standard treatment for skeletal-related manifestations of multiple myeloma, breast carcinoma, and other solid cancers. *CT* demonstrates mixed sclerotic and lytic changes and occasionally pathologic fractures (▶ Fig. 2.80). MR typically manifests low T1 and high T2 signal intensity, with lesion enhancement. BPONJ is fluorodeoxyglucose (FDG) avid.

Dental cysts can be either odontogenic (associated with tooth development) or nonodontogenic. Radicular cysts (a.k.a. periodontal cysts) are the most common odontogenic cysts (▶ Fig. 2.81) and occur with untreated dental caries. Dentigerous (follicular) cysts are the next most common odontogenic

cyst. They are unilocular and surround the crown of an unerupted tooth (▶ Fig. 2.82).

Fissural cysts are the most frequently encountered nonodontogenic cysts, the most common being the nasopalatine duct cyst (incisive canal cyst), with some cysts attaining sizes of 2 to 3 cm. The normal canal should measure approximately 6 mm and canals larger than this should be regarded with suspicion. Fissural cysts are most commonly encountered in the fourth to sixth decades with surgical enucleation the treatment of choice. Keratocystic odontogenic tumors are characterized by local aggressiveness and infiltration into surrounding tissues with a high rate of recurrence. They appear as an expansile multi- or unilocular cyst (not associated with a crown or unerupted tooth) with undulating borders, cortical thinning, and root resorption often occurring near the third molar tooth. They can be associated with Marfan and Noonan syndromes. When multiple, 50% are associated with nevoid basal cell carcinoma (Gorlin) syndrome.

An ameloblastoma is a benign, locally invasive neoplasm of odontogenic origin. Although it can involve either the mandible or maxilla, most are mandibular (80%). They occur in the third and fourth decades of life, and are slow growing and painless. On imaging ameloblastomas are usually bubbly multiloculated lesions (80%) often with extensive bony destruction (▶ Fig. 2.83). Ameloblastomas have a tendency to break through the cortex with formation of a soft tissue mass.

The mandible is commonly injured in trauma, due to its prominent position and ring-like configuration. Motor vehicle accidents and assaults are the primary causes of injury, and

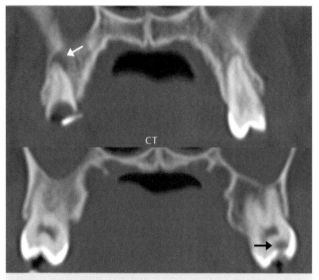

Fig. 2.79 Periodontal disease and dental caries. These two common diseases are often seen incidentally on CTs obtained for other purposes. In periodontal disease, there is loss of bone and widening of the space between bone and the tooth root (*white arrow*). In dental caries, there is formation of a cavity most commonly at the tooth occlusal surface, as a result of mineral dissolution of part of the dense enamel crown (*black arrow*).

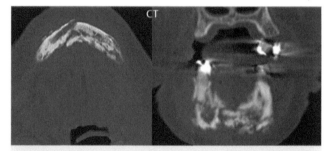

Fig. 2.80 Osteonecrosis of the mandible. Axial and coronal CT scans reconstructed with a bone algorithm reveal areas of osteolysis with thickening and fragmentation of the cortex. The patient was a woman with breast cancer, treated with Zometa, a bisphosphonate given intravenously to slow bone resorption.

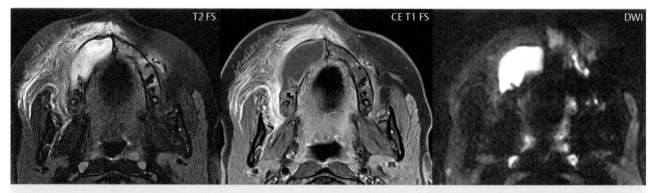

Fig. 2.81 Infected radicular cyst. A large, expansile unilocular cyst (of the right maxilla) is seen on axial scans, which was associated with a tooth root (image not shown). There is extensive edema and enhancement in the adjacent soft tissues. On DWI, the cyst is hyperintense, consistent with restricted diffusion (confirmed on the ADC map) and thus infection.

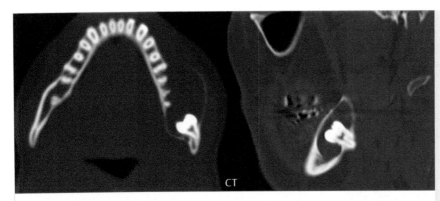

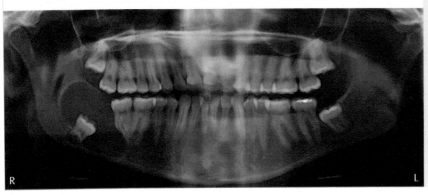

Fig. 2.82 Dentigerous (follicular) cyst. **Part 1:** CT scans (an axial image, and a reformatted sagittal image) from two different patients are illustrated. In each instance, a large cyst in noted involving the mandible, consistent with a dentigerous cyst as defined by its association with the crown of an unerupted tooth. **Part 2:** In a third patient, a Panorex (dental panoramic radiograph) identifies a cyst of the right mandible associated with the crown of the third molar, the most common location for a dentigerous cyst.

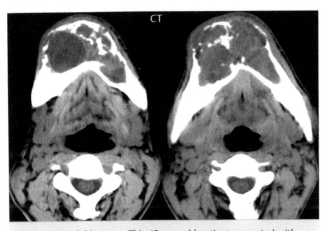

Fig. 2.83 Ameloblastoma. This 43-year-old patient presented with swelling and discomfort involving the mandible for more than 20 years. Two axial CT images are presented, depicting a large, expansile, destructive lytic mandibular lesion. The mass is at least, in part, multiloculated, a feature best seen on the more caudal of the two images. Although matrix calcification is not typical of an ameloblastoma, fragmented bone can be present, as in this case, due to the destructive nature of the lesion.

specifically fracture. A Panorex exam can miss subtle nondisplaced fractures, with CT advocated for optimal evaluation (▶ Fig. 2.84). Fractures involving the body may traverse the inferior alveolar canal, which runs from the mandibular foramen to the mental foramen, and can impair function of the inferior alveolar nerve (a branch of the mandibular [CN V3] nerve) resulting in lip/chin numbness. Due to its ring-like configuration, 50% of mandibular fractures are multiple (usually two breaks) (▶ Fig. 2.85) such as a parasymphyseal fracture and associated contralateral subcondylar fracture.

2.8 Temporomandibular Joint

The osseous components of the temporomandibular joint (TMJ) include the mandibular condyle, glenoid (mandibular) fossa, and, anteriorly, the articular tubercle (the bony eminence of the temporal bone). The TMJ disk is a biconcave structure, with a thick periphery and a thin center. In the sagittal plane the disk appears biconcave, in the coronal plane crescent-shaped. The anterior and posterior parts of the disk are referred to as the anterior and posterior bands. In the normal closed position, the posterior band is located at 12:00 over the condyle. In a normal joint, regardless of position (open or closed), the central thin portion of the disk remains interposed between the condyle and the articular tubercle.

The most common internal derangement of the TMJ is disk displacement, which is usually anterior or anteromedial. Displacement (dislocation) can occur with or without reduction (the disk reverting to its normal position) on opening (▶ Fig. 2.86). A "click" heard on opening can occur due to reduction of an anterior disk displacement. In a disk displacement without reduction, the disk remains displaced anteriorly regardless of jaw position. Jaw opening may be limited, in this instance, on the affected side. Disk deformity occurs late in the disease stage, with associated degenerative bony changes including flattening of the condyle and small osteophytes. The upper and lower compartments (joint spaces, above and below the disk) normally do not communicate. TMJ arthrography is routinely performed in specialty centers, either of the lower joint space alone or of both joint spaces. CT of the TMJ is the best means of examining the osseous joint structures. On MR today, at 3 T using bilateral dedicated multichannel surface coil arrays, true dynamic imaging of the TMJ can be accomplished, with a temporal resolution of one-

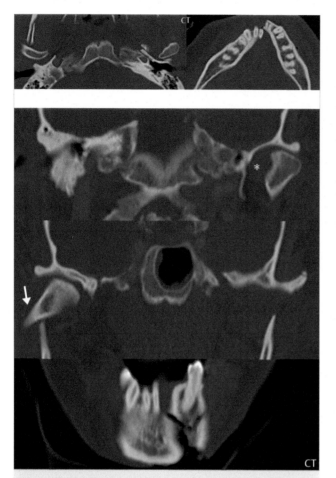

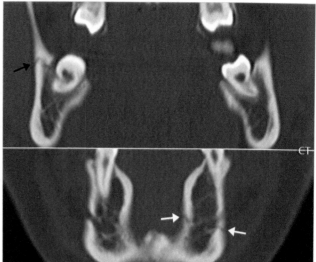

Fig. 2.85 Mandibular fracture. Because it is, in essence, a ring (when considered with the skull base), fractures of the mandible are often—but not always—multiple. Coronal reformatted images display two fractures, one at the angle of the mandible on the right (*black arrow*) and one through the body on the left (*white arrows*), parasymphyseal in location. For a single fracture that involves the mandible, the angle of the mandible is the most common location. The fracture on the right did traverse the inferior alveolar canal (images not shown), with thus the potential for damage to the inferior alveolar nerve.

Fig. 2.84 Mandibular fracture with condylar displacement. Axial images (**part 1**) display a subcondylar fracture on the right, and a parasymphyseal fracture on the left. Coronal reformatted images (**part 2**) display well both fractures, with the subcondylar fracture grossly angulated (*arrow*) and, in addition, dislocation or subluxation of the left mandibular condyle (*asterisk*). Close inspection of the condyles, evaluating for displacement/subluxation, is advised in all facial trauma.

fourth of a second. This should be supplemented by high resolution static images in both the open and closed position in the sagittal and coronal planes. Regardless of pulse sequence, the disk will have low signal intensity. T2-weighted images can also be acquired to identify abnormal joint fluid or edema in the adjacent tissues.

2.9 Nasopharynx

The roof of the nasopharynx is formed by the sphenoid sinus and upper clivus. The posterior margin is formed by the lower clivus and upper cervical spine. Anteriorly lies the nasal cavity. The lateral walls are formed by the pterygoid plates (anteriorly) and the fascia and muscles of the airway (posteriorly). The nasopharynx is separated from the oropharynx below by the soft palate. The levator and tensor veli palatini muscles arise from the skull base, attach to the soft palate, and function to elevate and tense the palate. The pharyngobasilar fascia holds the airway patent. It surrounds the mucosa, superior constrictor, and levator veli palatini muscles, and separates the nasopharyngeal mucosal space from surrounding fascial spaces.

The nasopharyngeal mucosal space contains mucosa, adenoidal tissue, the superior constrictor muscle, the torus tubarius, levator veli palatini muscles, and many minor salivary glands. The mucosa and normal adenoidal tissue are high signal intensity on T2-weighted MR images. The eustachian tubes end in the torus tubarius (a lateral cartilaginous enlargement). The lateral pharyngeal recess (fossa of Rosenmüller) is formed by mucosal reflection over the longus colli and capitis muscles (flexors of the cervical spine), and is the site of origin for the vast majority of nasopharyngeal carcinomas (NPC). The levator veli palatini muscle is intrapharyngeal, just lateral to the torus tubarius. The tensor veli palatini muscle is lateral to the pharyngobasilar fascia and surrounded by fat. The retropharyngeal space is a potential space between the pharyngeal constrictor muscles anteriorly and the prevertebral muscles posteriorly. The prevertebral (perivertebral) space is bounded by the prevertebral fascia anteriorly and the vertebral bodies posteriorly, contains the prevertebral muscles, and extends from the skull base to the coccyx.

Infection involving the nasopharynx is usually secondary to either dental or tonsillar infection. Dental infection can spread to the masticator and prestyloid parapharyngeal spaces, in

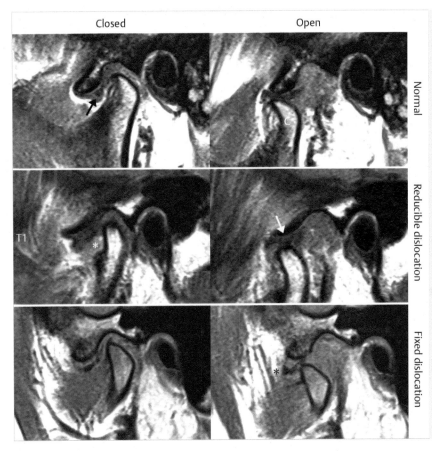

Closed	Open

Normal

Reducible dislocation

Fixed dislocation

T1

Fig. 2.86 Temporomandibular joint, disk displacement The normal appearance of the TMJ is demonstrated in closed and open mouth views (first row). The mandibular condyle is located anterior to the external auditory meatus with its head articulating with the glenoid fossa and articular eminence of the temporal bone. When the mouth is closed (first column), the mandibular condyle lies centered in the glenoid fossa with the meniscus (*black arrow*) lying along its anterosuperior aspect. With mouth opening, the condyle (*C*) translocates anteriorly with the meniscus moving into the one o'clock position. The most common cause of TMJ dysfunction is an anterior reducible dislocation of the meniscus (second row). In the closed mouth view, the low SI meniscus (*white asterisk*) is located anterior to the mandibular condyle with the condyle resting on retrodiskal tissue. In the open mouth view, second column, the condyle translocates anteriorly underneath the posterior band of the meniscus, with the meniscus (*white arrow*) now assuming a normal position (reduction of the dislocation). In a fixed-type of dislocation (third row), the meniscus is seen anterior to the mandibular condyle in the closed-mouth view, and remains dislocated (*black asterisk*) anteriorly to the condyle in the open mouth view. Often a fixed, chronically dislocated meniscus will appear deformed or compressed due to repetitive trauma during opening and closing of the mouth.

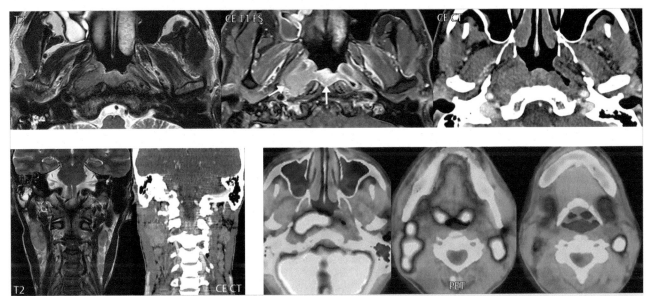

Fig. 2.87 Nasopharyngeal carcinoma, undifferentiated, with extensive cervical nodal metastases. Abnormal enhancing soft tissue is present on the right in the posterior nasopharynx at the level of the ostium of the eustachian tube, centered on (and obliterating) the fossa of Rosenmüller (pharyngeal recess), as well as extending slightly across the midline (**part 1**, *arrow*). Tumor margins are relatively well delineated on MR, as compared to CT, with the latter modality demonstrating only soft tissue prominence. Coronal imaging, both MR and CT (**part 2**), reveals extensive bilateral lymphadenopathy, consistent with metastatic spread. Also note the middle ear and mastoid fluid due to eustachian tube obstruction. Positron emission tomography (PET) CT (**part 3**) identifies the primary lesion in the right nasopharynx with slight extension across the midline, together with involved level II lymph nodes bilaterally.

addition to causing osteomyelitis. Tonsillar infection can result in an abscess that can extend to the retropharyngeal space or the prestyloid parapharyngeal space.

Benign, incidental soft tissue masses in the nasopharynx include adenoidal hypertrophy (seen in children and young adults), and the Tornwaldt cyst. The latter is very common, seen in 4% of patients, and is a small midline cyst that lies along the posterior nasopharyngeal wall. A Tornwaldt cyst will have high signal intensity on T2, reflecting fluid, and intermediate to high signal intensity on T1-weighted images, dependent on the protein concentration.

Nasopharyngeal carcinoma is by far the most common malignant tumor of the nasopharynx, strongly associated with Epstein-Barr virus infection. The lateral pharyngeal recess is the most common site of origin. These tumors often cause eustachian tube obstruction, due to involvement of the levator veli palatine muscle, resulting in a middle ear effusion (▶ Fig. 2.8). A tumor in this location can grow in any direction, with lateral extension most common. Eighty to 90% of patients have nodal involvement on presentation (retropharyngeal, level II and level V) (▶ Fig. 2.87). Involvement of lymph nodes can be suggested on many different bases—by size criteria, with visualization of necrosis, and by restricted diffusion, with FDG PET extremely valuable for identification of tumor involvement (above a certain size). It is important to note that radiation therapy causes a substantial change in appearance of tissues in this region on both CT and MR, with fibrosis having low signal intensity on both T1- and T2-weighted images.

Rhabdomyosarcoma is the most common sarcoma in pediatrics and young adults. Forty percent of these lesions occur in the head and neck, with the most common locations being the orbit and nasopharynx. This tumor is locally invasive, often with bone destruction and perineural tumor extension.

2.10 Oral Cavity, Oropharynx

The oral cavity includes the anterior two-thirds of the tongue, the lingual and buccal mucosa, the sublingual space (which houses the sublingual gland, and the neurovascular pedicle of the tongue), the deep lobe of the submandibular gland, and the mylohyoid muscle (the sling that forms the floor of the mouth). Extrinsic muscles of the tongue include the genioglossus, hyoglossus, styloglossus, and palatoglossus muscles while intrinsic muscles include vertical, horizontal, and oblique fibers. All muscles are innervated by CN XII. The anterior digastric muscles lie outside of the oral cavity proper, below the mylohyoid muscle and above the platysma muscle. The anterior digastric and mylohyoid muscles are innervated by the mylohyoid nerve, a distal branch of CN V3. The oropharynx includes the posterior one-third of tongue (the tongue base), the palatine tonsils, lymphoid tissue at base of tongue (lingual tonsils), the soft palate, and the oropharyngeal mucosa, held in place by the constrictor muscles.

Infections in this area usually involve the mandible (due to dental caries), salivary glands (with an obstructive calculus), or tonsils (▶ Fig. 2.88). Extensive infection involving the sublingual and submandibular spaces, typically bilateral (Ludwig angina), is a serious, potentially life-threatening infection, usually occurring in adults (▶ Fig. 2.89). It is the result of dental caries and, if untreated, can lead to airway obstruction.

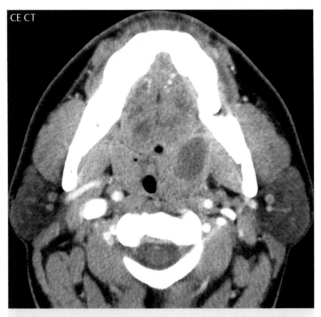

Fig. 2.88 Peritonsillar abscess, CT. There is a 2.4 × 1.6 cm oval low-density lesion within the region of the left palatine tonsil. There is subtle peripheral enhancement. Mild mass effect upon, and displacement of, the oropharynx is noted. These findings are consistent with a peritonsillar abscess. Prominent reactive upper cervical lymphadenopathy (not shown) was also present on the left.

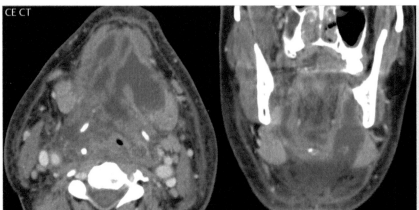

Fig. 2.89 Ludwig angina. This polymicrobial infection, which involves the soft tissues of the floor of the mouth, can spread rapidly in the absence of adequate antimicrobial treatment, dissecting into the mediastinum and causing chest pain (thus the name "angina"). In this patient, a 49-year-old substance abuser, the lesion was of odontogenic origin. On axial and coronal images there is an extensive phlegmon involving the floor of the mouth, with contiguous spread along connective tissue, fascia, and muscle planes. There is associated stranding of soft tissue and subcutaneous fat. Airway compromise, present in this case, is the dreaded complication.

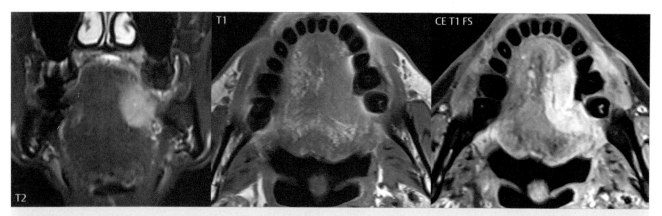

Fig. 2.90 Squamous cell carcinoma, tongue. There is a mass within the tongue on the left, hyperintense on the coronal T2-weighted scan, intermediate signal intensity on the T1-weighted axial scan precontrast, and enhancing on the postcontrast scan with fat suppression. The lesion approaches, but does not cross the midline. Note that the tumor can be distinguished from normal adjacent tongue, even on the precontrast T1-weighted scan, with the latter demonstrating mild fatty changes.

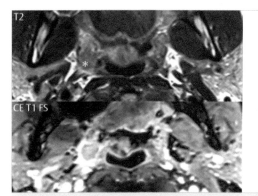
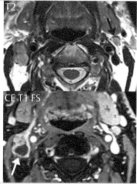
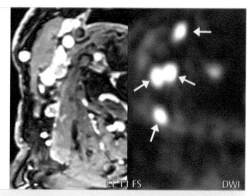

Fig. 2.91 Tonsil carcinoma (poorly differentiated squamous cell carcinoma). A small soft tissue lesion (*asterisk*) is noted on the right, with intermediate signal intensity on the T2-weighted scan (slightly hyperintense to muscle) and mild contrast enhancement (**part 1**). An enlarged, necrotic level IIa lymph node is noted on the right (*white arrow*), which compresses the internal jugular vein medially (**part 2**). The jugulodigastric node on the left (*black arrow*) is normal by size criteria, but was partially necrotic on the adjacent section (not shown) and had restricted diffusion (also not illustrated). On axial images, cropped to the right neck (**part 3**), at a level just below the hyoid bone, four small necrotic level III lymph nodes are noted, with improved detection of tumor involvement (*arrows*) on the basis of DWI.

More than 90% of malignant tumors involving the oral cavity and oropharynx are squamous cell carcinomas. These are associated with alcohol and tobacco use, and some are associated with the human papilloma virus (HPV). Other much less common malignant lesions include non-Hodgkin lymphoma and minor salivary gland tumors. Half of all minor salivary gland tumors in this region are malignant. In regard to the tongue, squamous cell carcinoma easily spreads along the intrinsic muscles. In image interpretation, it is important to assess spread in relation to the midline. Without midline extension, hemiglossectomy is a surgical option (▶ Fig. 2.90). The most common oral cavity tumor is squamous carcinoma of the lower lip. Other common sites include the tongue, floor of the mouth, retromolar trigone, and hard palate.

Within the oropharynx, tonsil carcinoma is the most common squamous cell carcinoma, with a strong HPV association (▶ Fig. 2.91). In this location in particular, there is a very high incidence of nodal metastases at presentation (60–75%, usually level II). Regardless of specific location, bilateral lymph node involvement at presentation is common. Squamous cell carcinoma is well visualized on MR in the oral cavity and oropharynx, with slight high signal intensity on T2-weighted scans and enhancement on postcontrast scans, which should be both performed using fat saturation.

2.11 Salivary Glands

The major salivary glands include the parotid, submandibular, and sublingual glands. The parotid gland is artificially divided into deep and superficial lobes by the facial nerve. The main duct of the parotid gland is Stensen duct, which runs anteriorly to pierce the buccinator muscle and open into the vestibule opposite the second maxillary molar. The main duct of the submandibular gland is Wharton duct, which opens at the top of a small papilla in the sublingual space.

With inflammation and infection, a salivary gland will be enlarged and, on CT, demonstrate increased attenuation. Eighty percent of salivary glands stones occur in Wharton duct (▶ Fig. 2.92) with only 15% in Stenson duct (▶ Fig. 2.93). The majority of salivary gland stones are radiopaque. Sialolithiasis (salivary stones) presents clinically with pain and swelling and,

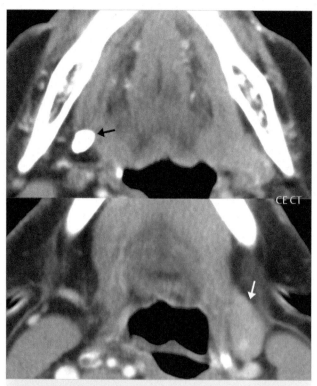

Fig. 2.92 Submandibular sialolithiasis. The right submandibular gland is not visualized (due to atrophy). A normal left submandibular gland is present (*white arrow*). A dense calcification (ductal stone, *black arrow*), the etiology for the gland atrophy, is noted lying along the course of Wharton duct.

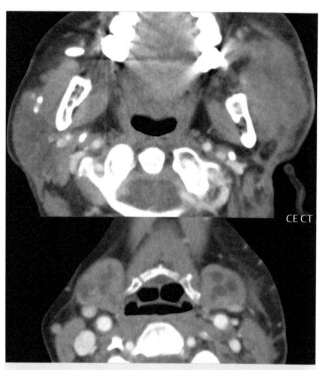

Fig. 2.93 Acute parotitis. Multiple ill-defined cysts are seen within the right parotid gland and numerous well-defined cysts within enlarged submandibular glands bilaterally, in this patient with chronic sialadenitis and an acute exacerbation. Multiple calcifications are present on the right, all likely in Stensen duct. The left parotid is surgically absent, with accessory parotid tissue overlying the masseter muscle anteriorly and stranding of the adjacent subcutaneous fat, consistent with inflammation.

when untreated, can lead to infection of the involved gland. Sjögren syndrome is a chronic systemic autoimmune disease, with bilateral enlargement of the parotids due to multiple cystic and solid lesions, occasionally associated with calcifications. Five percent of patients with HIV develop benign lymphoepithelial lesions, specifically multiple cystic and solid masses within and enlarging the parotid glands. This is often accompanied by tonsillar hyperplasia and benign, reactive cervical adenopathy.

A ranula is a mucous retention cyst (mucocele) of the sublingual gland, which occurs due to rupture of the salivary gland duct (usually caused by trauma). A "simple" ranula is most common and is confined to the sublingual space (▶ Fig. 2.94). These may be difficult to differentiate from epidermoid cysts, which are common in this location, but fat-containing dermoid cysts are easily distinguished. A "diving" or "plunging" ranula forms following rupture of a simple ranula and presents in the submandibular space, often with a residual tail in the sublingual space.

A good general rule is that the smaller the salivary gland, the greater the likelihood of malignancy, when a mass is detected. A benign mixed tumor (pleomorphic adenoma) is the most common salivary gland tumor. The majority occur in the parotid gland, with most in the superficial lobe. On imaging they are solitary, ovoid, and well-demarcated (▶ Fig. 2.95).

On CT, these will be higher in attenuation than the adjacent parotid tissue. On MR, the most common appearance is a lesion with low signal intensity on T1, intermediate to high signal intensity on T2, with moderate contrast enhancement. Warthin tumors are the second most common type of benign parotid

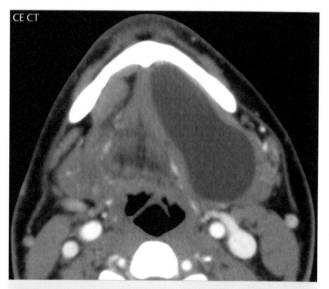

Fig. 2.94 Simple ranula. A well-defined, thin-walled, unilocular, non-enhancing, cystic low-attenuation lesion is seen, within the sublingual space. A pertinent negative is the lack of adjacent soft tissue swelling or abnormal enhancement.

lesions. These lesions arise from intraparotid lymph nodes and are isolated to the parotid gland as other salivary glands do not contain lymph nodes (▶ Fig. 2.96). A classic presentation is that of a well-marginated, heterogeneous, parotid tail mass (although

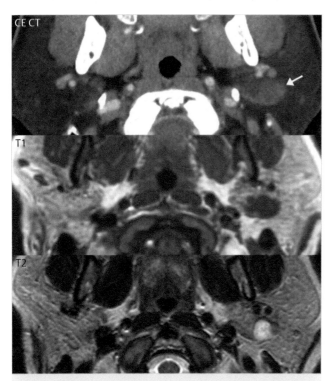

Fig. 2.95 Benign mixed tumor (pleomorphic adenoma). There is a small, smoothly marginated, round mass lesion (*arrow*) in the deep lobe of the left parotid gland. The mass displays characteristic low signal intensity on T1- and high signal intensity on T2-weighted images, and demonstrates prominent enhancement (image not shown). The diagnosis was confirmed by fine needle aspiration and at subsequent resection.

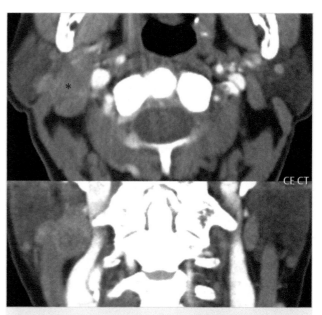

Fig. 2.96 Warthin tumor. On axial and coronal reformatted CT images obtained during bolus intravenous contrast administration, a mass lesion (*asterisk*) is seen continuous with and medial to the right parotid gland, with slightly higher density. A portion of the lesion is lower in density, raising the question of a cystic component (common with this diagnosis). As with most Warthin tumors, the lesion is located more posteriorly near the parotid tail. The lesion is ovoid and smoothly marginated. Tissue diagnosis was confirmed by fine needle aspiration.

these can be located anywhere within the parotid, or adjacent to the parotid). Overall, they appear more complex than benign mixed tumors. Multiple lesions, unilateral or bilateral, occur in 20% to 30% of cases. Two malignant salivary gland tumors are of note, although much less common than benign tumors, mucoepidermoid and adenoid cystic carcinomas (▶ Fig. 2.97).

Perineural spread is particularly common with adenoid cystic carcinoma (▶ Fig. 2.98). Although lesion heterogeneity and ill-defined lesion margins favor more aggressive lesions in the salivary glands, low-grade malignant salivary gland tumors may have an imaging appearance indistinguishable from benign masses, being well-circumscribed, homogeneous, and enhancing. Metastases to intraparotid lymph nodes may occur as they represent first order drainage from malignancies of the face, auricle, and scalp.

2.12 Parapharyngeal Space

The parapharyngeal space is a triangular fat-filled space that extends from the skull base superiorly to the level of the hyoid bone, and is subdivided into the prestyloid (parapharyngeal [PPS]) space and the post-styloid (carotid space [CS]). In addition to fat, the major contents of interest in the PPS are minor salivary glands. Medially is the pharynx, posteromedially the retropharyngeal space, posterolaterally the CS, and laterally the masticator space. PPS displacement medially occurs by masses in the masticator space, the PPS may be displaced anteriorly by

deep lobe parotid masses or masses in the CS and lateral displacement is caused by pharyngeal mucosal space lesions, particularly tonsil pathology.

Salivary gland tumors (arising from the minor salivary glands) are the most common primary lesions in the PPS, with most being benign mixed tumors. Neurogenic tumors (usually vagal schwannomas) (▶ Fig. 2.99) and glomus vagale paragangliomas are the most common lesions to arise in the CS. Second branchial cleft cysts typically produce medial displacement of the CS, as well as lateral or posterior displacement of the sternocleidomastoid muscle and anterior displacement of the submandibular gland. One must be careful making this diagnosis in an adult as a level II necrotic node may mimic a branchial cleft cyst.

2.13 Larynx

The mucosal surface of the larynx is well evaluated by laryngoscopy, with the role of imaging to determine deep tumor extent and tumor margins. The epiglottis has an upper free margin and is attached inferiorly to the thyroid cartilage. The hyoid bone is the ceiling from which the larynx is suspended. The largest of the laryngeal cartilages is the thyroid cartilage consisting of an anterior body, two small superior horns (cornua), and two large posterior horns. The thyrohyoid membrane extends from the hyoid bone superiorly to the superior cornua inferiorly. Inferior to the thyroid cartilage is the cricoid cartilage, which resembles a "signet" ring that faces posteriorly. The inferior margin of the cricoid cartilage is the junction between the larynx and trachea. The cricothyroid membrane closes the gap between the cricoid and the thyroid cartilages. The arytenoid cartilages articulate superolaterally with the cricoid

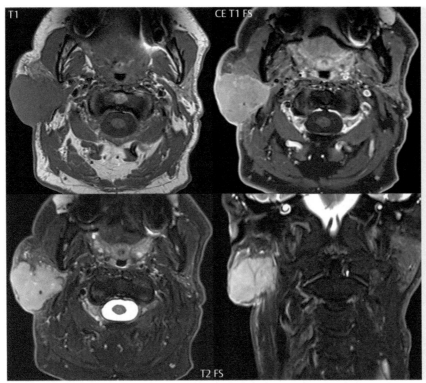

Fig. 2.97 Epithelial carcinoma. A large mass lesion is identified involving the right parotid gland. The mass is homogeneous, well defined, and slightly lobulated. Although malignant lesions can have irregular borders and heterogeneity suggesting their diagnosis, benign and malignant salivary gland tumors cannot be differentiated on imaging alone, with malignant lesions often having what otherwise might be considered benign features, as in this case. Malignant epithelial tumors represent up to 20% of all salivary gland tumors, and include adenoid cystic and mucoepidermoid carcinomas.

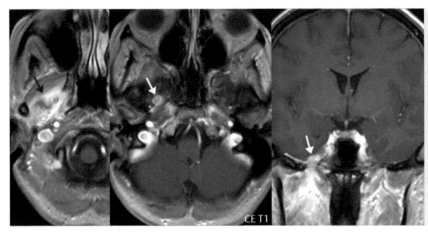

Fig. 2.98 Perineural tumor spread. This patient is status post resection of a mucoepidermoid carcinoma in the parotid. The first image depicts tumor recurrence (*black arrow*) in the lateral pterygoid muscle. The subsequent axial and coronal images depict enhancing tumor extending along the third division (CN V3) of the trigeminal nerve through the foramen ovale (*white arrows*), which is enlarged, with extension to the Meckel cave.

posteriorly. The thyroarytenoid (vocalis) muscles attaches to the lower anterior surface of the arytenoid, forming the bulk of the true vocal cord. The true cord is inferior to the false cord, with the glottis defined as the horizontal space between the true and false vocal cords.

The valleculae are the small bilateral recesses between the tongue base and free margin of the epiglottis. The aryepiglottic folds lie above the false vocal cords and form the lateral margins of the vestibule (the supraglottic airspace), extending from the arytenoid cartilages to the free margin of the epiglottis. The pyriform sinuses are lateral to the aryepiglottic folds, being mucosal recesses between the thyroid cartilage and the aryepiglottic folds. The ventricles are the lateral recesses between the true and false cords. The anterior commissure lies in the midline between the true vocal cords anteriorly, and, on thin section CT at this level, air should directly abut the thyroid cartilage. In a Valsalva maneuver, the patient attempts to exhale against a closed glottis, with the true cords adducted. In quiet respiration, the true cords will be slightly abducted but not completely effaced.

Innervation of the larynx is by the recurrent laryngeal nerve (RLN). These paired nerves emerge from the vagus nerve with different courses. The right RLN arises at the level of, and loops under, the subclavian artery while the left arises at the level of the aortopulmonary window and loops under the aorta. The nerves then ascend in the tracheoesophageal grooves. Supraglottic lymphatics drain to upper jugular nodes and subglottic lymphatics drain to paratracheal and pretracheal nodes and then, eventually, to lower jugular nodes.

A Zenker diverticulum is a posterior outpouching of the pharyngeal wall just above the cricopharyngeus muscle (thus just above the esophagus). The cricopharyngeus muscle is often prominent, with the diagnosis of a Zenker diverticulum typically made on the basis of a barium swallow.

A laryngocele is a dilatation of the laryngeal ventricle. They are typically air-filled but may be fluid-filled in which case

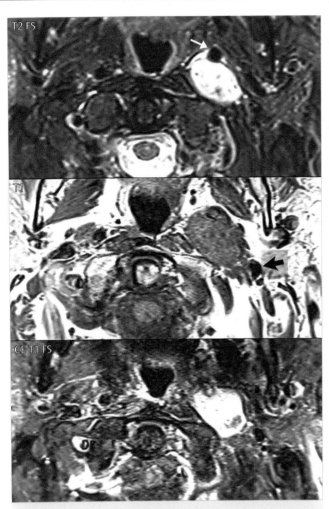

Fig. 2.99 Vagal schwannoma. Neurogenic lesions account for up to 25% of tumors of the retrostyloid parapharyngeal (carotid) space, with most being schwannomas of the vagus nerve. As the nerve lies behind the internal carotid artery (ICA), most tumors displace the ICA (*white arrow*) anteriorly and medially, and the internal jugular vein (*black arrow*) posteriorly and laterally, as do glomus vagale paragangliomas. Most schwannomas are fairly homogeneous in composition; however, there can be areas of hemorrhage or necrosis, leading to a heterogeneous appearance. Schwannomas are typically well-defined, ovoid masses, with hyperintensity on T2-weighted scans and prominent enhancement. However, as opposed to glomus vagale paragangliomas, schwannomas do not exhibit flow voids or a "salt and pepper" appearance.

they are termed saccular cysts. The classic acquired laryngocele was seen in glassblowers and trumpet players, due to constant increased pressure in the larynx with forced expiration. They may also be caused by an obstructing tumor. A laryngocele may be internal (confined within the larynx) (▶ Fig. 2.100) or external (extending through the thyrohyoid membrane).

Foreign bodies can result from ingestion or aspiration. A foreign body may initially lodge in the pyriform sinus, from which point it can migrate into the larynx (▶ Fig. 2.101).

Ninety-five percent of all malignancies of the larynx are squamous cell carcinoma. These tumors arise on the mucosal surface, with deep lesion extent relative to precise landmarks not possible to be assessed by endoscopy, thus the role of imaging.

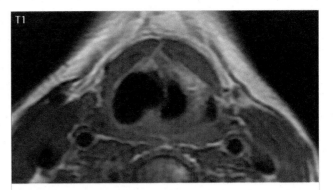

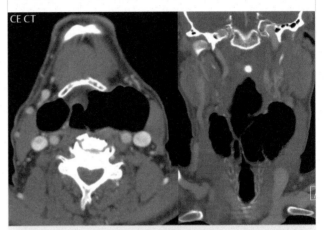

Fig. 2.100 Laryngocele. **Part 1:** On an axial MR image, a thin walled air-filled lesion is visualized lateral to the false vocal cord on the right, consistent with an internal (simple) laryngocele. There is mild airway compression. **Part 2:** In a second patient (a 56-year-old trumpet player), huge bilateral laryngoceles are seen on axial and coronal CT images. There is extension bilaterally through the thyrohyoid membrane, with these lesions thus representing mixed (internal/external) laryngoceles.

Smoking and heavy consumption of alcohol are important risk factors. Treatment options include several voice sparing operations, typically coupled with radiation therapy (▶ Fig. 2.102). The supraglottic region includes the false vocal cords, aryepiglottic folds, preepiglottic and paraglottic spaces, and epiglottis. In a supraglottic laryngectomy (which is voice sparing), the larynx above the ventricle is removed, with the resection line made through the ventricle. The key to feasibility is inferior tumor extension (▶ Fig. 2.103) and tumor must be clearly separated from the anterior commissure. Part of one arytenoid can be removed, but the thyroid cartilage cannot be involved by tumor. Lymph node involvement with supraglottic tumor is common. Tumors of the true vocal cord (glottic carcinomas) present early, due to a change in voice (early vocal cord paralysis), with lymph node involvement uncommon. Contraindications to surgery, specifically hemilaryngectomy (unilateral removal of the true and false cords, and thyroid ala—an operation which is also voice sparing), include extension across the anterior commissure, subglottic extension, involvement of the cricoarytenoid joint, and thyroid cartilage invasion. Cartilage involvement is best identified on MR by the demonstration of cartilage enhancement. Tumors of the subglottic larynx (inferior surface of true vocal cords to cricoid cartilage) are least common, often presenting as T4 lesions (defined by invasion of

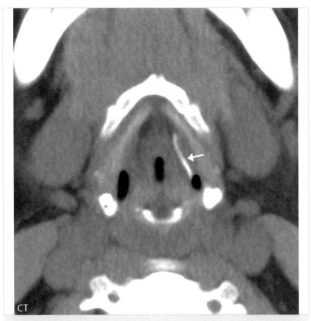

Fig. 2.101 Foreign body. There is a linear radiopaque density (a wire, *arrow*), approximately 2 cm in length, which lies in the vicinity of the left false vocal cord parallel to the thyroid cartilage. The anterior extent of the foreign body appears to lie within the left false cord anteriorly. The posterior tip of the foreign body abuts the left pyriform sinus. There is mild surrounding soft tissue swelling likely related to inflammatory changes.

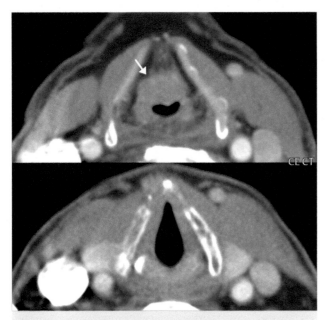

Fig. 2.103 Supraglottic squamous cell carcinoma. A mass lesion (*arrow*) involves the laryngeal surface of the epiglottis, with some involvement of the pre-epiglottic fat. On the lower axial image, there is no evidence of extension to the level of the true cord.

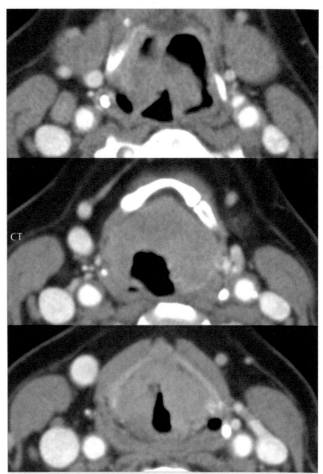

Fig. 2.102 Extensive supraglottic squamous cell carcinoma. A bulky soft tissue mass involves the epiglottis, aryepiglottic folds, preepiglottic space, and supraglottic region. The lesion did not, however, extend to the level of the false vocal cords (image not shown).

include malignancy involving the vagus or recurrent laryngeal nerves, and iatrogenic injury (prior surgery, especially thyroid).

2.14 Soft Tissues of the Neck

For descriptive purposes on MR and CT, particularly on axial imaging, the neck is divided into spaces. The masticator space contains the muscles of mastication (lateral and medial pterygoid, temporalis, and masseter muscles-all innervated by CN V3), the ramus and posterior body of mandible, and the pterygoid venous plexus. Infection and tumor can spread from the masticator space to the PPS and skull base. The submandibular space is directly continuous with the sublingual space at the posterior free margin of the mylohyoid muscle. The CS extends from the skull base to the aortic arch and is enclosed by the carotid sheath. It contains the internal carotid artery, internal jugular vein (with the right greater in size than the left in 80% of patients), cranial nerves IX to XII, and the sympathetic plexus. The PPS was previously described, and lies anteromedial to the CS. The prevertebral space is that between the prevertebral fascia and the vertebrae. The posterior cervical space lies posterolateral to the CS, deep to the sternocleidomastoid and trapezius

the thyroid cartilage and/or extension beyond the larynx). Cricoid invasion is common. Large lesions require total laryngectomy and radiation therapy.

In unilateral vocal cord paralysis, the affected vocal cord rests in a paramedian position. Etiologies outside of the larynx

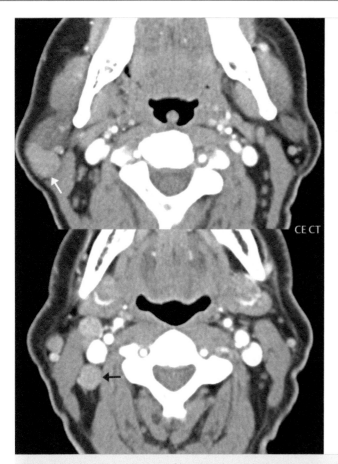

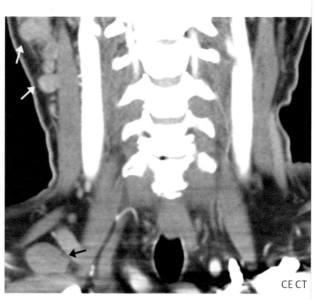

Fig. 2.104 Metastatic involvement of lymph nodes. Multiple prominent and grossly enlarged (by size criteria) lymph nodes are seen in the right neck on axial images (**part 1**). There is a mass (*white arrow*) immediately adjacent and posterior to the right parotid gland (and thus, by definition, a parotid mass). A right jugular digastric lymph node is prominent, but not enlarged by size criteria. There is an 11-mm level IIA lymph node on the right (*black arrow*). Multiple additional level IIA and IIB lymph nodes on the right are prominent, but not enlarged by size criteria. There were no comparable enlarged lymph nodes on the left. Also noted (**part 2**) on a coronal reformatted image is an enlarged, 14-mm right supraclavicular lymph node (*black arrow*). Other prominent and grossly enlarged nodes are also seen (*white arrows*). Fine needle biopsy of the parotid lesion revealed metastatic melanoma, with the clinical history pertinent for a small melanoma resected 7 years prior to the current exam.

muscles. The retropharyngeal space (RPS) lies posterior to the pharynx and anterior to the prevertebral muscles extending from the skull base to the mediastinum. In addition to its main fat component, the suprahyoid RPS contains important medial and lateral RPS nodes.

2.14.1 Lymph Nodes

Lymph nodes lie throughout the soft tissues of the neck. A common radiologic classification of lymph nodes in the neck, which is used predominately for squamous cell carcinoma, defines seven levels. Level I is subdivided into Ia, the submental nodes, and Ib, the submandibular nodes. Level II encompasses the internal jugular chain of lymph nodes, and extends from the base of the skull to the hyoid bone. It is subdivided into level IIa, those anterior, lateral, or medial to the vein and those immediately posterior but inseparable from the internal jugular vein, and level IIb, those posterior to the vein but with a fat plane interposed. Level III is composed of the internal jugular chain of lymph nodes from the hyoid level to the cricoid, with level IV nodes being those from the cricoid to the clavicle. Level V nodes are those within the posterior cervical space (posterior to the

sternocleidomastoid muscle), level VI nodes are anterior triangle nodes (anterior to the sternocleidomastoid muscle), and level VII are superior mediastinal nodes. Nodes of importance that are not contained in this nodal classification include the intraparotid nodes and the retropharyngeal nodes (not amenable to physical examination).

On CT, size is an important criterion for identification of abnormal lymph nodes. Nodes larger than 10 mm in the short axis are considered abnormal, with the exception of level I nodes and the jugulodigastric node, where 15 mm is used as the cutoff (▶ Fig. 2.104). By size criteria alone, up to 20% of lymph nodes are incorrectly classified (in regard to involvement by neoplastic disease). It should also be kept in mind that there are many benign causes of lymph node enlargement. These include infectious mononucleosis (▶ Fig. 2.105) and cat-scratch disease.

Size independent criteria include loss of the fatty hilum and necrosis (the latter reinforcing the importance of contrast enhancement, whether imaging with *CT* or MR). DWI has added a new dimension to MRI in the head and neck (with recent technologic advances making possible diagnostic quality DWI in this region), providing improved sensitivity and specificity,

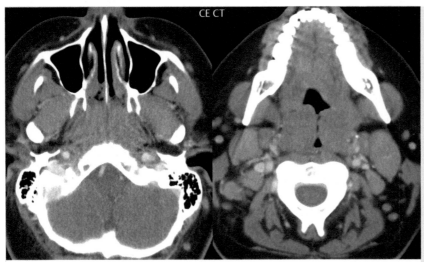

CE CT

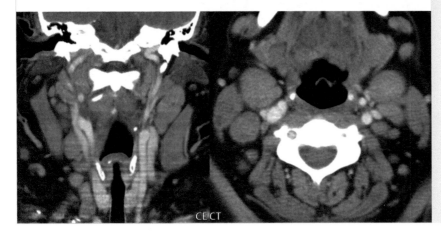

CE CT

Fig. 2.105 Infectious mononucleosis. This 21-year-old patient presented with a sore throat, tonsillar swelling, enlarged lymph nodes in her neck, and difficulty eating and drinking fluids. On axial CT, with images presented from two levels (**part 1**), there is prominent adenoidal soft tissue in the posterior nasopharynx, and grossly prominent tonsillar tissue. On coronal and axial reformatted CT images (**part 2**), grossly enlarged lymph nodes are seen throughout the soft tissues of the neck, bilaterally. In this instance, the etiology was benign, being infectious mononucleosis.

with increased utility for evaluation of treatment response and detection of local recurrence. Although restricted diffusion is a marker of lymph node involvement by neoplastic disease, experience in this area is still limited with evolution of standards and diagnostic criteria.

2.14.2 Congenital Anomalies

Congenital anomalies in the neck include branchial cleft anomalies, thyroglossal duct cysts, and lymphatic/venolymphatic malformations. The vast majority of branchial cleft cysts (95%) arise from the second branchial cleft. Only 5% are first branchial cleft cysts. Third and fourth branchial cleft cysts are quite rare. Sinus tracts, communicating with the skin (or gut), occur but are rare. Most second branchial cleft cysts are located at the angle of the mandible (▸ Fig. 2.106). Most first branchial cleft cysts are either periauricular in location or close to the parotid (▸ Fig. 2.107). Clinically, branchial cleft cysts present classically in a child or young adult as a painless mass.

A thyroglossal duct cyst (TGDC) is the most common congenital neck lesion, and usually presents in children. During embryogenesis, the thyroid develops at the base of the tongue (foramen cecum), and subsequently descends (along the thyroglossal duct), looping behind the hyoid bone, to reach the thyroid bed. The duct then normally involutes. Migration of the thyroid can be arrested at any point—for example, a lingual thyroid being total failure of migration. Thyroid tissue may lie along any portion of the tract. A TGDC can be midline (suprahyoid) or paramedian (infrahyoid, typically lying deep to, or embedded within, the strap muscles) (▸ Fig. 2.108). Approximately 50% of cysts lie at the level of the hyoid, 25% in the suprahyoid neck and 25% infrahyoid in location.

Seventy-five percent of lymphatic malformations occur in the neck, mainly in early childhood, presenting as a painless mass. Many of these lesions harbor components of venous malformations and are termed venolymphatic malformations. The imaging appearance is that of a nonenhancing cystic mass, typically multiloculated, with an imperceptible wall (▸ Fig. 2.109). Hemorrhage can occur within these malformations, and there can be fluid-fluid levels which are virtually pathognomonic. The most common location of these lesions is in the posterior cervical space.

Infantile hemangiomas are classified as benign vascular neoplasms (not a congenital anomaly); however, 90% involute over time without treatment. One-third are seen at birth, with the median age of presentation being 2 weeks. Visually they appear

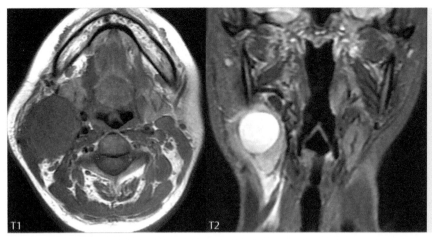

Fig. 2.106 Second branchial cleft cyst. Axial T1- and coronal T2-weighted images, in this young woman, reveal a moderate size, ovoid cyst on the right (with low SI on T1, and high SI on T2), in a classic location for this congenital lesion: posterolateral to the submandibular gland, anteromedial to the sternocleidomastoid muscle, and lateral to the carotid space. Also characteristic is the location just caudal to the angle of the mandible, well displayed on the coronal image. The wall of the cyst is thin and not clearly discernible.

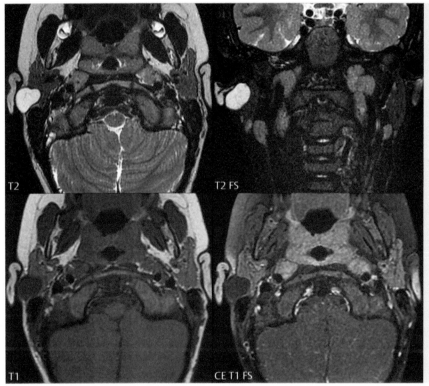

Fig. 2.107 First branchial cleft cyst. A small, ovoid, cystic lesion is noted in this 4 year old, just below and posterior to the pinna. There is no abnormal contrast enhancement. The cyst is well-circumscribed and unilocular, with low SI on T1- and high SI on T2-weighted scans.

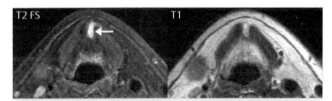

Fig. 2.108 Thyroglossal duct cyst. On axial imaging, at a level just inferior to the hyoid bone, a small midline cyst is identified (*arrow*), with hyperintensity on both T2- and T1-weighted images. Thyroglossal duct cysts are usually hypointense on T1-weighted scans, with hyperintensity reflecting increased proteinaceous content, a less common appearance. These can be found in the midline anywhere between the tongue base to the thyroid bed.

as cutaneous red, purple, or blue, plaque, or berry-like lesions. On MR, these demonstrate intense, uniform enhancement, with vascular flow voids common (▶ Fig. 2.110). Infantile hemangiomas are hyperintense on T2-weighted scans. Most occur in the head and neck region, often parotid or buccal in location. Enlarged feeding arteries can be visualized on contrast enhanced MR angiography. Twenty percent are multifocal (▶ Fig. 2.111).

2.14.3 Inflammation/Infection

Both CT and MR well detect and characterize infection in the soft tissues of the neck (▶ Fig. 2.112). An abscess is differentiated from cellulitis by the presence of a fluid collection. It is

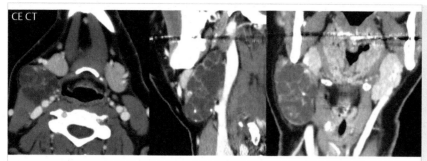

Fig. 2.109 Lymphatic malformation, neck. Axial, sagittal, and coronal reformatted images from a contrast-enhanced CT exam of the neck are presented. A multiloculated cystic neck mass is present on the right, posterior to the submandibular gland, lateral to the carotid space, and anterior to the sternocleidomastoid muscle. This location is classic for a second branchial cleft cyst. However, the multicystic nature of this lesion would be inconsistent with the typical unilocular second branchial cleft cyst.

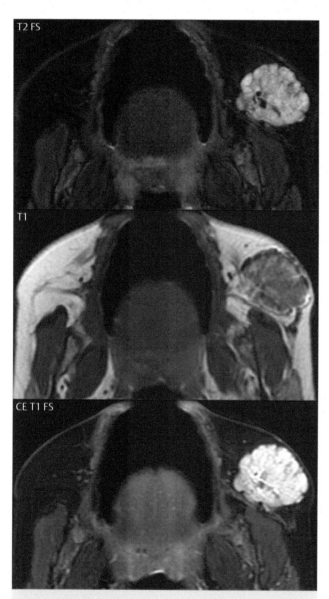

Fig. 2.110 Proliferating infantile hemangioma, buccal space. In this 3-year-old child, a well-defined, somewhat lobulated, buccal space mass is seen on the left, hyperintense on the T2-weighted scan and with intense, uniform enhancement postcontrast. Note the characteristic, prominent vascular flow voids within the mass best seen on the T2-weighted scan.

important to describe any associated complications, for example, venous thrombosis and airway compression. An abscess can be uni- or multiloculated, and will demonstrate an enhancing rim, with thickening of the overlying skin and inflammation within the adjacent fat. There can be accompanying myositis. Spread of infection is limited by fascial planes. However, it should be noted that both the visceral and prevertebral spaces communicate with the mediastinum and, thus, infection in these compartments can spread to the mediastinum (which can be life threatening) (▶ Fig. 2.113).

2.14.4 Neoplasms

Soft tissue masses within the neck in children are mainly benign, including inflammatory lymphadenopathy and congenital lesions. Of malignant pediatric lesions, lymphoma is most common (▶ Fig. 2.114) and rhabdomyosarcoma next most common. After the age of 40, most neck masses represent metastatic disease, with squamous cell carcinoma the most common primary. Nodal metastases in the neck with an occult primary tumor are usually attributable to head and neck SCCa, with common sites of primary tumor including the nasopharynx, pyriform sinus, tongue base, and tonsil. As previously discussed, paragangliomas also occur in the neck, including specifically glomus vagale paragangliomas and carotid body tumors. These benign tumors are painless and slow growing.

Muscle denervation results from many causes, with neoplasia and trauma the leading etiologies in the head and neck. In the early time period following denervation, edema (on T2-weighted scans) and abnormal contrast enhancement can be seen in the affected muscle, with visualization of both improved by the use of fat saturation. With time, muscle atrophy and fatty infiltration occurs (▶ Fig. 2.115). With chronic atrophy, abnormal enhancement is not seen.

Lymphoma can be unilateral or bilateral in the neck, typically involving nodal chains. Enlarged nodes are usually nonnecrotic. In Hodgkin lymphoma, extranodal involvement is rare. In non-Hodgkin lymphoma, nonnodal disease can occur in the palatine, lingual, and pharyngeal (adenoids) tonsils. MRI and CT cannot differentiate Hodgkin from non-Hodgkin lymphoma. Diffuse nodal involvement with bilateral grossly enlarged, homogeneous, nonenhancing (by CT), well delineated lymph nodes within the neck is suggestive of chronic lymphocytic leukemia (▶ Fig. 2.116), although other lymphomas and leukemias may have this appearance.

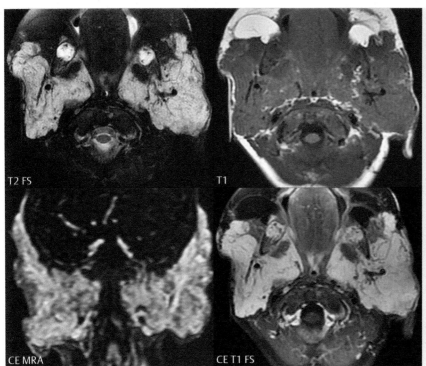

Fig. 2.111 Bilateral infantile hemangioma, parotid space. Axial MR images reveal relatively homogeneous, bilateral masses in the parotid space with uniform, prominent enhancement, in this 5-month-old girl. Of note, the lesions are hyperintense on the T2-weighted scan. Most infantile hemangiomas are solitary, but on occasion (20%) can be multifocal, as in this patient. The coronal contrast-enhanced MRA exam depicts the proliferative endothelial nature of this benign tumor, reflected by intense early enhancement.

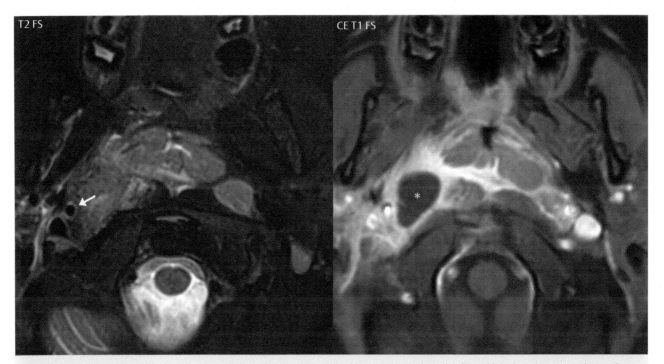

Fig. 2.112 Retropharyngeal abscess, MR. On the T2-weighted scan in this pediatric patient, enlarged, inflamed lymph nodes appear distinct from muscle, with intermediate to high signal intensity. Enhancement around the internal carotid artery—seen as a flow void (*white arrow*)—is noted but the caliber of the vessel is not reduced. Compromise and mild shift to the left of the nasopharynx are also present. This abscess demonstrates a very characteristic appearance for a soft tissue infection, with a nonenhancing, central necrotic region (*asterisk*), a suppurative lateral retropharyngeal space lymph node, surrounded by extensive enhancing inflamed/infected tissue.

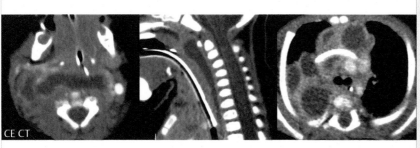

Fig. 2.113 Retropharyngeal abscess, CT. On an axial enhanced CT image, fluid with a faint rim of abnormal enhancement distends the retropharyngeal space and flattens the prevertebral muscles. The sagittal midline reformatted scan reveals that this prevertebral fluid collection extends inferiorly to the mediastinum. An axial CT image at the level of the carina depicts the mediastinal involvement, together with multiple pleural-based empyemas. This 2-month-old infant presented with staphylococcus aureus septicemia.

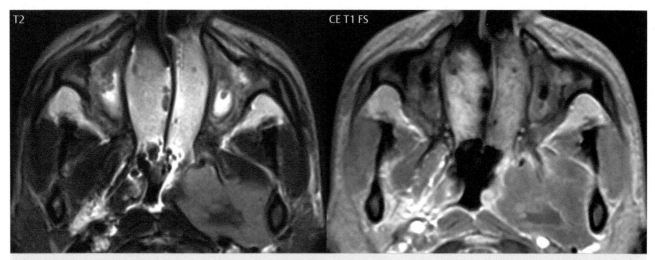

Fig. 2.114 Burkitt lymphoma. There is an enhancing mass lesion, in this 18-year-old patient, with its epicenter in the left parapharyngeal space. There is extension to the masticator space. The mass causes posterior displacement of the internal carotid artery. Centrally, there is a lack of enhancement, consistent with necrosis.

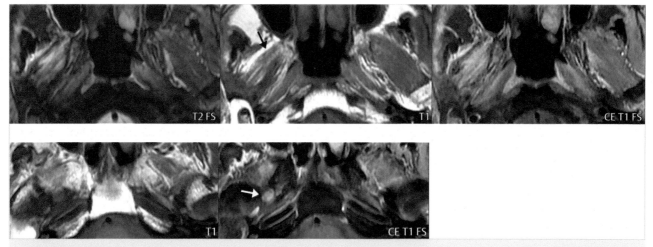

Fig. 2.115 Denervation atrophy. There is mild hyperintensity of the right lateral pterygoid muscle on the T2-weighted scan (neurogenic edema), with mild fatty atrophy demonstrated on the T1-weighted scan (*black arrow*), and mild enhancement postcontrast, with both edema and enhancement typical in the acute and subacute phases (**part 1**). The cause for denervation is evident on a more caudal section (**part 2**), with enhancing perineural tumor (*white arrow*), involving the mandibular division of the trigeminal nerve, seen within the foramen ovale.

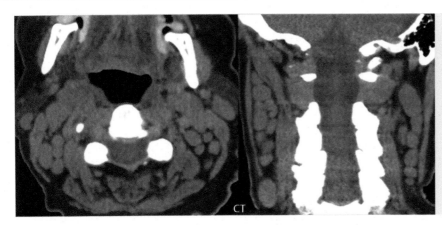

Fig. 2.116 Chronic lymphocytic leukemia. There are grossly enlarged lymph nodes bilaterally throughout the neck, at essentially all levels. This appearance is nonspecific, with differential diagnosis including the viral lymphadenitises and the lymphoproliferative disorders (specifically lymphoma and leukemia).

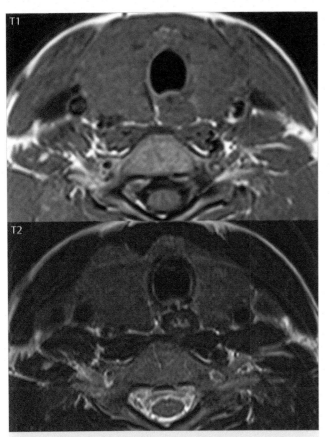

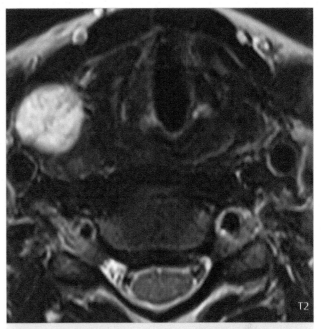

Fig. 2.118 Thyroid adenoma. A large, well-defined, hyperintense thyroid nodule is noted on the right, on a T2-weighted axial image. In the thyroid, however, these characteristics are unfortunately not specific for a benign lesion. For example, papillary carcinoma, the most common thyroid cancer, can present either as a benign appearing nodule or as a mass with irregular margins.

Fig. 2.117 Multinodular goiter. There is diffuse enlargement of the thyroid gland, seen on axial scans, with a mildly heterogeneous, nodular appearance.

MR and CT are rarely used as a primary imaging modality for evaluation of the thyroid gland. However, the thyroid is often incidentally included within the anatomic region covered on all neck examinations. Benign disease involving the thyroid gland is common, including multinodular goiter (▶ Fig. 2.117) and benign adenomas (▶ Fig. 2.118). In regard to a goiter, size and extent should be described, together with any tracheal deviation or compression. Multinodular goiters are characterized by nodularity, focal calcifications, cysts, and scarring. Ultrasound and nuclear medicine remain the primary imaging modalities for the evaluation of thyroid disease, with fine-needle aspiration used to evaluate palpable nodules and specifically to exclude malignancy. Nodule size does not correlate with malignancy. Papillary and follicular thyroid carcinomas are the most common malignant thyroid neoplasms, and have a favorable prognosis. A further, more in depth description of thyroid disease and neoplasms is beyond the scope of this book.

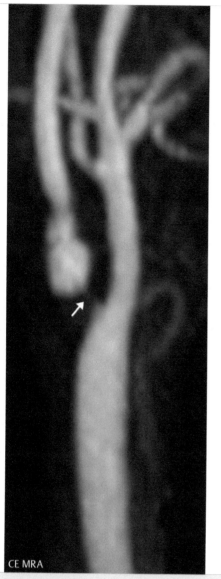

Fig. 2.119 Atherosclerotic disease of the internal carotid artery (ICA), CE-MRA. There is a string sign (*arrow*) at the origin of the right internal carotid artery, indicating greater than 95% stenosis. There is also irregularity noted involving the proximal 1.5 cm of the ICA, consistent with additional atherosclerotic disease.

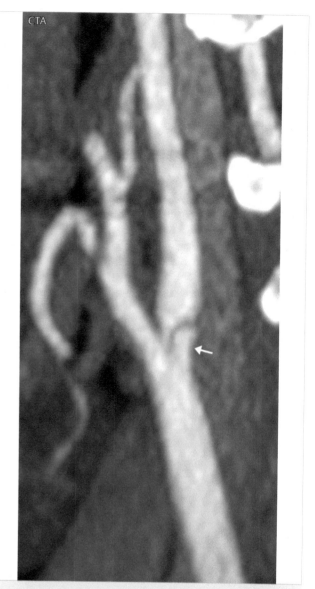

Fig. 2.120 Ulcerated plaque, internal carotid artery origin, CTA. There is a large ulcerated plaque (*arrow*) involving the proximal right internal carotid artery at the bifurcation, resulting in a 90% or greater stenosis.

2.14.5 Vascular Lesions

CT angiography (CTA) and contrast-enhanced MR angiography (CE-MRA) are commonly used today for evaluation of the carotid and vertebral arteries. The most frequent indication is atherosclerotic disease, with evaluation, in particular, focused on the carotid bifurcation. Critical to this assessment is evaluation of stenosis involving either the distal common carotid artery or the proximal internal carotid artery (▶ Fig. 2.119). Stenosis of the latter is reported, preferably using cross-sectional area measurements, relative to (percentage wise) a more distal normal section of the internal carotid artery.

Ulcerated plaques are well-visualized by either modality, and are important to recognize, as such, and included in the report (▶ Fig. 2.120 and ▶ Fig. 2.121). CE-MRA is typically performed with a field of view that extends from the aortic arch to the

skull base, providing a broad assessment of atherosclerotic disease, with close inspection of all the major arteries visualized important, due to the generalized nature of atherosclerotic disease (▶ Fig. 2.122). Time resolved CE-MRA enables assessment of the vascularity of mass lesions and provides information regarding arterial and venous flow. The latter is important for evaluation of vascular malformations and other vascular lesions such as subclavian steal syndrome.

Dissection of the internal carotid artery can be spontaneous, posttraumatic, or due to an underlying predisposing arteriopathy. CTA and CE-MRA both well depict the luminal narrowing, together with (if present) focal aneurysmal dilatation (▶ Fig. 2.123). The latter occurs in 30%, typically immediately prior to the internal carotid artery entering the carotid canal at the skull base. The dissection itself can extend for a variable length, usually originating a few cm distal to the carotid bulb. The intramural hematoma itself is well delineated on

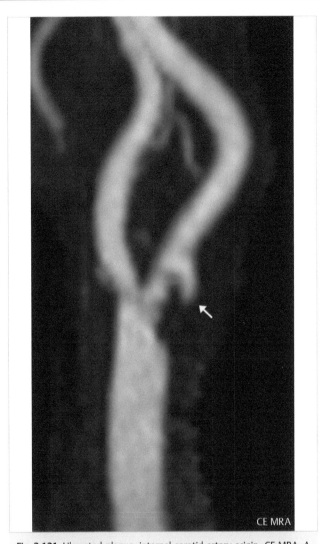

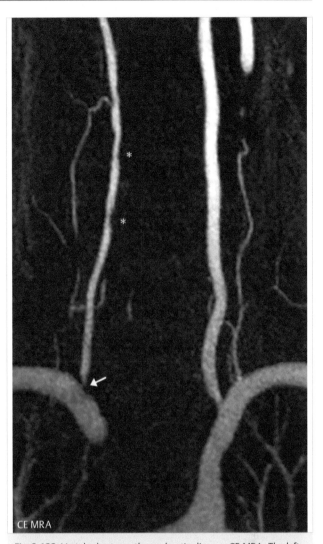

Fig. 2.121 Ulcerated plaque, internal carotid artery origin, CE-MRA. A prominent ulcerated plaque (*arrow*) is present involving the proximal right internal carotid artery, 1 cm distal to the bifurcation. There is approximately 50% stenosis of the proximal right ICA, with additional mild atherosclerotic irregularity.

Fig. 2.122 Vertebral artery atherosclerotic disease, CE-MRA. The left vertebral artery is noted to be dominant, in this thick section coronal MIP image. There is a severe stenosis at the origin of the right vertebral artery (*arrow*). There is also luminal irregularity (*asterisk*) seen at multiple levels involving the right vertebral artery, consistent with additional atherosclerotic disease. There is mild atherosclerotic narrowing present at the origin of the left vertebral artery.

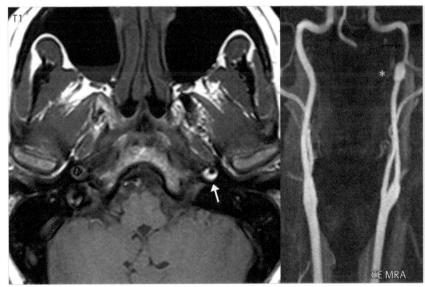

Fig. 2.123 Internal carotid artery dissection. A crescent of abnormal high signal intensity (*white arrow*), partially encasing the internal carotid artery, is noted, at the skull base, on a precontrast T1-weighted scan, consistent with a mural (methemoglobin) hematoma. The ICA lumen is reduced in caliber, which is also evident (*black arrow*) on the 3D contrast-enhanced MRA exam. Just proximal to this short segment of luminal stenosis is a pseudoaneurysm (*asterisk*).

precontrast axial T1-weighted MR scans with fat saturation, on which the methemoglobin in the hematoma will be seen as a hyperintense crescent adjacent to the residual patent lumen. The treatment of dissection involving the internal carotid artery is medical, specifically anticoagulation.

Venous thrombosis, in particular that of the internal jugular vein, has many etiologies, including drug abuse, central venous catheterization, compression by benign or malignant disease, hypercoagulable states, and infection. The thrombosed vein is typically enlarged in the acute and subacute time frame, with peripheral enhancement of the vessel wall and surrounding inflammation. Collateral venous channels may develop with chronic thrombosis, with the (occluded) internal jugular vein itself small.

3 Spine

3.1 Normal Anatomy, Imaging Technique, and Common Variants

3.1.1 Anatomy of the Normal Spine

There are seven cervical vertebral bodies and eight cervical nerves. C1 is the atlas, a bony ring. C2 is the axis, with the dens extending superiorly. From C3 to C7 there is a gradual increase in size of the vertebral bodies. The uncinate processes are bilateral superior projections from the C3 to the C7 vertebral bodies that indent the disk and vertebral body above (posterolaterally), forming the uncovertebral joints. Laterally, the transverse foramen lies within the transverse process, and contains the vertebral artery. There is a normal slight increase in spinal cord size extending from C4 to C6. The neural foramina course anterolaterally at a 45-degree angle with a slight inferior course. These thus lie oblique to the standard sagittal and axial imaging planes. In the cervical region, the epidural venous plexus is prominent, with sparse epidural fat, the opposite to some extent of that in the lumbar spine. In regard to dermatomes, the hand is innervated by C6 (the thumb), C7 (the middle finger), and C8 (the little finger). Within any specific neural foramen, the nerve within the foramen is that corresponding numerically to the level below—for example, the C5 nerve lies within the foramen at C4–5.

There are 12 thoracic vertebral bodies. The ribs articulate with the vertebrae both at the disk level and at the transverse process (although for the latter only at T1-T10). The exit foramina for the basivertebral veins (part of the internal vertebral venous plexus) lie posteriorly within the mid-vertebral body, with the channel within the vertebral body itself often visualized as a Y in the axial plane (in both the thoracic and lumbar regions). In the thoracic region, epidural fat is often prominent posterior to the thecal sac and dura. Transitional type vertebrae are not uncommon at the thoracolumbar junction.

In the lumbosacral spine, there are five lumbar segments (vertebral bodies), five (fused) sacral segments, and four coccygeal bones (the coccyx). At all levels in the spine, the intervertebral disks are composed of a central gelatinous core (the nucleus pulposus, high signal-intensity [SI] on T2-weighted scans) with surrounding dense fibrous tissue (the annulus fibrosus, with low SI on T1- and T2-weighted scans). Because of the increased size of the intervertebral disks in the lumbar region, differentiation of the hydrated nucleus from the annulus fibrosus is easily recognized in normal disks. The bony parts of the lumbar vertebrae include the pedicles, transverse processes, articular pillars (pars interarticularis, superior and inferior articular facets), laminae, spinous processes, and vertebral body. The facet joints are diarthrodial synovial-lined and richly innervated.

On axial imaging the superior articular facet forms a "cap" anterolaterally with the inferior articular facet posteromedial connecting to the lamina. The ligamenta flava (bilateral paired ligaments, which connect the lamina of adjacent vertebrae, and are present from C2 to S1) extend from the anterior aspect of the upper lamina to the posterior aspect of the lower lamina. The epidural venous plexus is less prominent than in the cervical spine. In regard to dermatomes, the foot is innervated by L4 (medial big toe), L5 (midfoot), and S1 (little toe). Within any specific neural foramen (for both the thoracic and lumbar spine), the nerve within the foramen is that corresponding numerically to the level above—for example, the L4 nerve lies within the foramen at L4–5. Transitional vertebrae at the lumbosacral junction are quite common, with an incidence near 10%.

A single anterior spinal artery and two paired posterior spinal arteries supply the spinal cord. These vessels are fed by anterior and posterior radiculomedullary arteries. The major anterior radiculomedullary artery in the thoracic and lumbar region is the artery of Adamkiewicz, which usually arises between T9 and L1. There are typically no substantial anterior radiculomedullary feeders inferior to the artery of Adamkiewicz.

In the sagittal plane, the conus is commonly described in textbooks and in the anatomy literature to be located at L1–2. This statement is somewhat misleading. Looking specifically at the location of the tip of the conus, from published studies, this ranges in normal individuals from 10% occurring at the upper third of L1 to 10% occurring at the upper third of L2, with the maximum percentage (25%) occurring at the lower third of L1. A common clinical statement from magnetic resonance (MR) is that the conus in normal patients should lie at the T12-L1 level, with this statement referring to the conus itself and not specifically the tip. The posterior longitudinal ligament (which extends from the body of the axis to the sacrum) lies posterior to the vertebral bodies and anterior to the thecal sac, being in the lumbar region about 1 mm thick (anteroposterior [AP]) and 5 mm wide (left to right). The facet joints of the upper lumbar spine are oriented predominantly in the sagittal plane, while those of the lower lumbar spine are oriented more in the coronal plane.

On off-midline sagittal images, the dorsal root ganglion (and ventral root) is seen to lie in the superior portion of the neural foramen. In the lumbar region in particular, the sagittal plane is important for evaluation of foraminal narrowing, equal or greater in value than the axial plane. In regard to the neural foramen, the margins are composed of the disk and vertebral body anteriorly, the pedicles superiorly and inferiorly, and the facet joints posteriorly. In the axial plane, the bony canal and the thecal sac are well visualized, with the vertebral body anteriorly, pedicles laterally, and lamina posteriorly.

3.1.2 Imaging Technique

Because of its complexity, a description of the normal appearance of the spine on MR, specifically looking at the different sequences and parameter weighting, is important. T1-weighted images depict fat (and specifically the vertebral body marrow) as high SI, the spinal cord and intervertebral disks as intermediate SI (on very high quality images, gray and white matter within the cord can be distinguished on the basis of SI, on both T1- and T2-weighted scans), and cerebrospinal fluid (CSF) as low SI. Normally hydrated (nondegenerated) disks will appear slightly hypointense to the vertebral marrow. The normal ligamentum flavum is well seen, with intermediate SI. On thin section axial imaging, particularly in the lumbar spine, positioning of the slice relative to the vertebral body, endplate, and disk can be differentiated on the basis of signal intensity, which changes from slightly high signal intensity (the fatty marrow of the vertebral body), to low (the endplate), to intermediate (the intervertebral disk). These structures can also be differentiated in a similar fashion on axial T2-weighted scans. Sagittal T1-weighted images (obtained without any obliquity) depict the neural foramina poorly due to their oblique orientation (except in the lower lumbar spine). T1-weighted scans typically can be acquired in a short scan time (2 to 4 minutes), with high signal-to-noise ratio (SNR) and high spatial resolution. Their general utility is for detection of structural abnormalities, marrow infiltration, degenerative disease, and abnormal contrast enhancement (following administration of a gadolinium chelate).

On T2-weighted images (specifically as typically acquired today, with fast spin echo technique), CSF and hydrated disks will have high SI, spinal cord intermediate SI, muscle low SI, and fat (including specifically that within the vertebral body marrow) intermediate to high SI. In the sagittal plane in adults, a central band of low SI is seen in normal disks, best visualized in the lumbar region due to the size of the disks. This structure, the "intranuclear cleft," is due to fibrous transformation and is observed in all normal disks in patients over the age of 30. Lack of visualization of the intranuclear cleft should be considered abnormal, with such absence common in early degenerative disk disease. For improved visualization of soft tissue and marrow abnormalities on the basis of T2 changes, fat saturation should be employed in combination with T2-weighted fast spin echo imaging. The thecal sac is well assessed on T2-weighted images, with this scan technique also important for detection of spinal cord abnormalities (edema, gliosis, demyelination, and neoplasia).

Low flip angle gradient echo imaging is commonly employed in the cervical spine for axial T2-weighted imaging. On these scans, CSF and the intervertebral disks have high SI, the cord intermediate SI, and the marrow usually low SI (due to magnetic susceptibility effects, unless the scan is acquired with three-dimensional [3D] technique and a very short echo time [TE]). Good gray-white matter differentiation is seen within the cord. The utility of these scans is for detection of degenerative changes (disk herniation, canal compromise, foraminal stenosis) and evaluation of intrinsic cord abnormalities (multiple sclerosis [MS], tumors, edema, and hemorrhage). There may be a slight exaggeration of canal and foraminal stenosis due to magnetic susceptibility effects, in particular if the TE is substantially greater than 10 msec. This technique is (as with all gradient echo techniques) sensitive to, and commonly markedly degraded by, the presence of metal.

On MR there is a complex temporal evolution of vertebral body and disk appearance, in the infant, which is beyond the scope of this textbook. In the time frame from young adulthood to advanced age, the appearance of vertebral body marrow on MR is determined by the combination of red and yellow marrow, the former hematologically active marrow with lower T1

signal intensity when compared to yellow (fatty) marrow. With normal aging, there is a conversion from red to yellow marrow, which is reflected by higher signal intensity on T1-weighted scans of the vertebral marrow. With increasing age, both diffuse and focal replacement of red by yellow marrow occurs. Focal fat, as the latter is termed, is easily seen (due to its high signal intensity), and commonly encountered, on T1-weighted scans. Focal fat is seen more often in the elderly, and is identified as such by its isointensity to fat on all MR pulse sequences.

Attention should be paid to a few additional specifics in regard to MR acquisition technique, in order to obtain high-quality images. For both sagittal and axial acquisitions, if the phase encoding gradient is in the AP dimension, placement of a coronal saturation pulse (presaturation slab) is necessary to eliminate motion artifacts that might otherwise substantially degrade the image. In the cervical spine this includes motion of the mouth and swallowing. In the thoracic spine, cardiac motion can otherwise be a substantial problem. And in the lumbar spine motion artifacts originate from the aorta, vena cava, internal organs, and anterior abdominal fat (with respiration). For spine imaging the maximum slice thickness that should be acquired in any plane and any portion of the spine is 3 mm (▶ Fig. 3.1). On fast spin echo T2-weighted scans, signal loss within the thecal sac is common due to CSF pulsation, with this problem being most prominent in the cervical region (on axial images) and to a lesser extent in the thoracic region (on both axial and sagittal images). Axial images for optimal clinical interpretation should be angled parallel to the disk space, with state-of-the-art MR systems offering accurate and automatic vertebral body numbering as well as angling of axial images parallel to the disk space in both the AP and right to left dimensions. Image normalization is advocated in the lumbar spine in particular for routine use on axial images. Because of the use in MR of surface coils for spine imaging, structures located superficially, and thus close to the coil, will have artifactual high SI. When the window and center are chosen for display of the spinal canal, the posterior soft tissue structures are often obscured, being depicted with very high signal intensity due to their proximity to the surface coil. Image normalization is a post-processing feature that takes into account the sensitivity of the coil and enables the visualization of structures both close and distant relative to the receiver coil, providing more homogeneous signal intensity across the field of view. It is important also to realize that today receiver coil coverage is integrated and continuous, allowing imaging of the spine in its entirety without gaps or image registration problems. Signal intensity drop off at the edge of the field of view, in the craniocaudal dimension, should not occur, and is indicative of an operator error. Thus, anatomic regions that were difficult to image in the past due to technical issues, including specifically the cervicothoracic and the thoracolumbar junctions, are well visualized on modern scanners (▶ Fig. 3.2).

Following intravenous contrast enhancement, normal enhancing structures include, in particular, the venous plexus. The external vertebral plexus is a network of veins along the anterior vertebral body, laminae, and spinous, transverse, and articular processes. The internal vertebral plexus is a network of veins in the epidural space (the "epidural venous plexus"), both anteriorly and posteriorly. The basivertebral veins, seen on sagittal

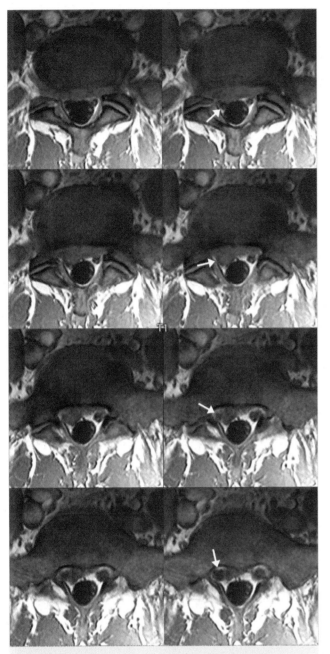

Fig. 3.1 Right paracentral disk herniation at L5–S1, evaluated on high-resolution thin section imaging at 3 T. One problem in MR regarding the evaluation of disk herniations is the large thickness of the slice relative to the disk and relevant portion of the affected nerves. Illustrated are contiguous high in-plane spatial resolution 2-mm thick axial images. Here, the right S1 nerve root (*arrows*) can be followed on each section, initially exiting from the thecal sac, subsequently being compressed and displaced (both posteriorly and laterally) to varying degrees by the adjacent disk herniation, and subsequently recovering its normal shape just prior to its exit in the neural foramen.

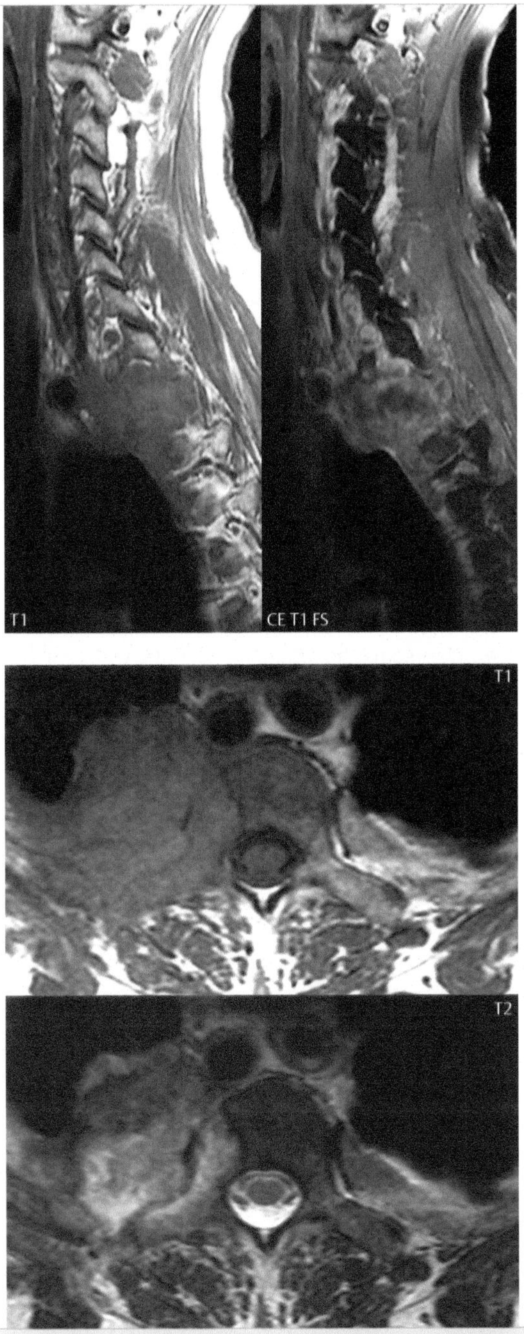

Fig. 3.2 Pancoast (superior sulcus) tumor. An apical soft tissue lung mass is noted, seen both in the sagittal (**part 1**) and axial (**part 2**) planes, with extensive involvement of the chest wall, ribs, and adjacent spine (specifically the facets, transverse process, pedicle, and lateral vertebral body). There is no spinal canal compromise. The lesion demonstrates inhomogeneous contrast enhancement, with the suggestion of a central necrotic (nonenhancing) component. An apical lung mass with adjacent bone involvement should be considered to be bronchogenic carcinoma unless otherwise proven.

imaging centrally within the vertebral body, drain posteriorly into the anterior internal vertebral plexus. The anterior plexus is larger, with longitudinal veins on each side of posterior longitudinal ligament, which taper at the disk space level. Displacement and engorgement often accompany a disk herniation. These venous structures all drain via intervertebral veins that accompany spinal nerves within the neural foramina. An additional normal enhancing structure is the dorsal root ganglion.

The most common indication for administration of intravenous contrast in spine MR imaging is in the postoperative back (predominantly the lumbar spine) for the differentiation of scar from disk. On scans obtained within 20 minutes following contrast injection, scar enhances whereas recurrent or residual disk material does not. There will be prominent enhancement of the normal epidural venous plexus, which also improves depiction of the neural foramina and abnormal soft tissue therein. Contrast enhancement is also used routinely for evaluation of intradural, and soft tissue extradural, neoplastic disease. For extradural neoplasia, acquisition of post-contrast scans using fat saturation markedly improves recognition of abnormal contrast enhancement. Contrast enhancement is not normally administered when the clinical question is that of vertebral metastatic disease. This pathology is well-delineated in most cases without intravenous contrast administration. In certain instances, contrast administration can improve the depiction of vertebral metastatic disease. However, when used for this indication, scans must be performed with fat saturation. Otherwise the low signal intensity of a metastatic lesion (on a T1-weighted scan) may enhance to near isointensity with the adjacent high signal intensity of fatty marrow, reducing conspicuity. Contrast enhancement is also routinely used for other disease processes that involve the spinal cord, in particular ischemia and demyelination. Infection, whether intradural or extradural, is an additional major indication for contrast administration on MR.

Imaging of the spine in CT is typically performed without intravenous contrast administration. Depending on clinical symptoms and indications, intrathecal contrast administration may be performed prior to CT for improved depiction of the thecal sac, cord and nerve roots therein, and nerve root sleeves.

It should be kept in mind that spine imaging by both CT and MR is acquired in non-load bearing and on occasion may not reflect the positioning and pathology that would be present if the patient were imaged in an erect position. Flexion and extension views, which are extensively used in plain radiography, could be obtained with both computed tomography (CT) and MR but only in a limited fashion, and are not part of routine clinical practice.

It is also important to be familiar with the following terminology in spine imaging, which applies to lesion localization. An extradural (epidural) mass is one that is located outside the dura, and thus can cause, when of sufficient size, compression of the thecal sac. An intradural-extramedullary mass is one located within the thecal sac, but external to the cord. Such a lesion produces a filling defect in the CSF, outlined by a sharp meniscus above and below, with the ipsilateral subarachnoid space enlarged up to the level of the mass and the spinal cord deviated away from the mass. An intramedullary mass is one that involves (arises within) the spinal cord, and produces smooth cord enlargement with gradual effacement of the subarachnoid space. A block, which is an old term originating from myelography, is a level at which the subarachnoid space is obliterated. Depending on the location of the lesion causing the block, the thecal sac may be displaced (if extradural), and there can be cord compression (if the compression occurs at the level of, or above, the conus).

3.1.3 Common Normal Variants and Incidental Findings

Transitional vertebrae are a common anomaly at the lumbosacral junction, occurring in 5 to 10% of patients. There can be lumbarization of S1, or sacralization of L5 (▶ Fig. 3.3). Key identifying features include a disk at L5–S1 that is small (the L5–S1 disk should be the largest of the lumbar disks), and the absence of a normal sacral curvature in the sagittal plane. Also helpful is the position of the conus. With modern MR scanners, a relatively high-resolution sagittal scout can be obtained of the entire spine, allowing a count from the dens (C2), which is readily recognizable, and providing the most reliable count of the vertebrae. On CT, articulation or fusion of an enlarged transverse process of the lowest lumbar segment to the sacrum can be seen (unilaterally or bilaterally). There will be decreased mobility at the affected level, with increased mobility and stress at the interspace immediately above. A not uncommon appearance on MR of the lumbar spine, well seen in the sagittal plane, is an apparent normal L5–S1 with degenerative findings at L4–5. This likely reflects, in some patients, the lack of normal mobility at L5–S1, and thus in a sense a transitional vertebra. In the literature, a transitional lumbosacral spine is reported as a known cause of back pain.

In a more broad sense, transitional vertebrae or variants therein can also be seen in the cervical and thoracic spine. Although much less common than variants at the lumbosacral

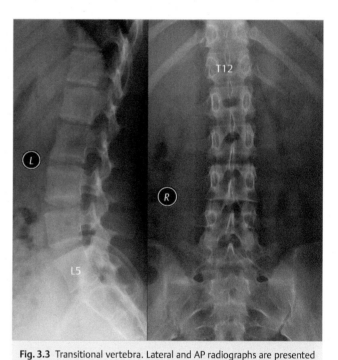

Fig. 3.3 Transitional vertebra. Lateral and AP radiographs are presented in a patient with a sacralized L5. The count was established on the basis of the chest X-ray. There were 12 rib-bearing vertebral bodies, with the left rib at T12 small, and the right rib vestigial (and poorly visualized on the AP view). Nonsegmentation of L5 and the sacrum bilaterally is well seen on the AP radiograph. The lateral radiograph demonstrates the L5–S1 disk space to be small, and absence of the normal sacral curvature. Both findings can be key to recognition on MR of a transitional vertebra at the lumbosacral junction.

junction, variants involving the dens and the thoracolumbar junction are well known. In a very small number of patients, a fusion anomaly of C2 and C3 can be seen, with its most apparent feature been the unusually long craniocaudal dimension of the dens. With regard to the thoracolumbar junction, the presence of either 11 or 13 thoracic vertebral bodies, as opposed to the normal 12, is known. Vestigial ribs at L1 are a common incidental finding on CT.

A single level, congenital, cervical vertebral nonsegmentation can also be considered in a sense a normal variant (▶ Fig. 3.4). Although a nonsegmentation will predispose the patient to accentuated degenerative disease at the levels above and below (due to slightly greater than usual motion at those levels), by itself the entity is asymptomatic and an observed variant in patients imaged by MR and CT for other reasons. On MR a small vestigial disk is commonly visualized. The shape of the nonsegmentation is distinct, as seen in the sagittal plane, with the two vertebrae not appearing as a rectangle, but rather with a smooth inward curvature toward the fusion level (seen with a narrow "waist" in the AP dimension). By shape, this entity can easily be distinguished from a postsurgical fusion, in which both vertebrae retain their normal rectangular shape.

Craniovertebral junction anomalies include failure of segmentation between the skull base and C1, also referred to as atlantooccipital assimilation (or occipitalization of the atlas), which can be partial or complete (with assimilation of the lateral masses of C1 and the adjacent occipital condyles). Another

distinct entity, a midline posterior cleft in the bony arch of the atlas, is quite common, in autopsy series seen in 4% (▶ Fig. 3.5). An anterior arch cleft is much less common (▶ Fig. 3.6), and is typically seen in association with a cleft posteriorly (split atlas).

An os odontoideum is a well-corticated ovoid ossicle, located superior to a hypoplastic odontoid. Its etiology is controversial, and has been ascribed to both congenital and acquired causes. Current thinking is that an os odontoideum results from an undiagnosed fracture through the C2-odontoid growth plate before the age of 5 or 6. A common secondary finding is a hypertrophic appearance of the anterior arch of C1, as seen in the mid-sagittal plane, appearing rounded as opposed to the typical crescent shape (▶ Fig. 3.7) Differentiation from an acute high type II odontoid fracture is important, which can be made on MR on the basis of the absence of associated soft tissue edema and on CT by the absence of a well-defined fracture line (extending through the cortex) and the absence of a hypertrophic anterior C1 arch.

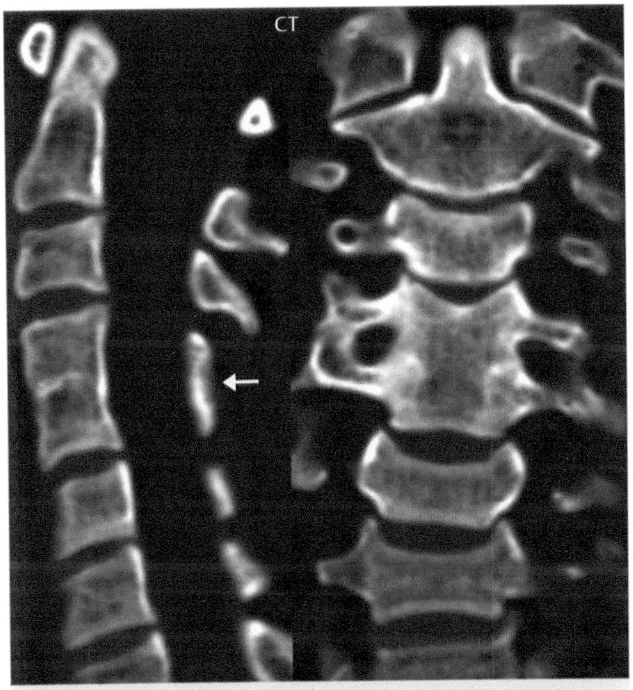

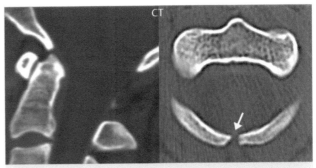

Fig. 3.5 Posterior fusion defect of C1. There is incomplete ossification of the arch of C1 posteriorly along the midline (*arrow*), seen on sagittal and axial CT. The margins of the defect are well corticated. This common congenital variant should not be mistaken for a fracture.

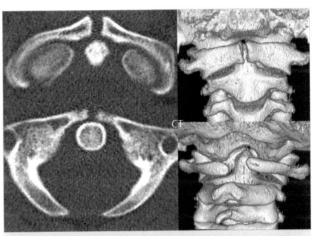

Fig. 3.6 Anterior and posterior fusion defects of C1. Note the well corticated margins and absence of a discrete fracture line. Such fusion defects are congenital in nature, and are primarily incidental findings. Incomplete posterior fusion can be seen in normal children up to the age of 10, with bony fusion typically occurring by age 5. Clefts of the anterior arch are much rarer than those of the posterior arch, occurring in 0.1% of the population.

Fig. 3.4 Congenital cervical vertebral body nonsegmentation (single level). Well seen on sagittal and coronal CT is nonsegmentation of C4–5. Note in this instance that there is nonsegmentation both anteriorly (vertebral body) and posteriorly (*arrow*, spinous process). The vertebral body segment is slightly narrowed in the AP dimension at the level of nonsegmentation, a characteristic finding. On CT there is little evidence of a residual disk space, which is typically more evident on MR.

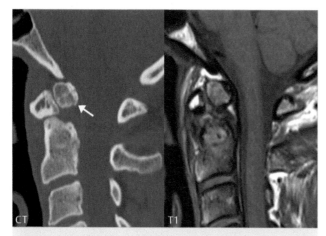

Fig. 3.7 Os odontoideum. This anatomic variant is illustrated on both sagittal CT and MR images. The well-corticated os (*arrow*) lies above a hypoplastic odontoid process. Note the corticated margins on CT, the lack of edema on MR, and the hypertrophic anterior arch of C1, all characteristic for this variant, and distinguishing it from an acute type II odontoid fracture.

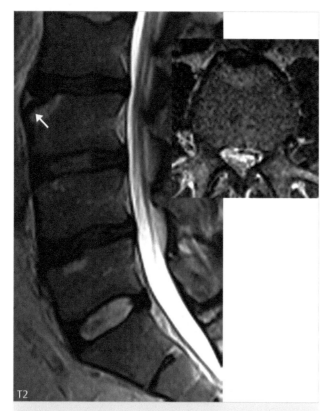

Fig. 3.8 Congenital lumbar spinal stenosis. Despite evidence of mild degenerative changes, including disk dehydration and loss of disk space height, there is no compromise of the canal due to disk disease. The spinal canal is, nevertheless, small in AP dimension. Congenitally shortened pedicles—the etiology of this finding—are evident in the axial image. For the clinician recognition of this entity is important, as a congenitally narrowed canal will amplify the severity of any degenerative findings or trauma. Note the incidental limbus vertebra (*arrow*), involving L3 anteriorly and superiorly.

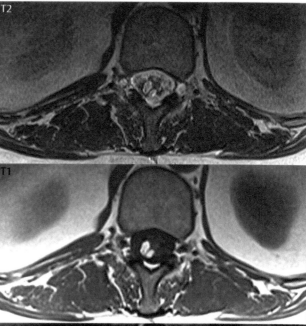
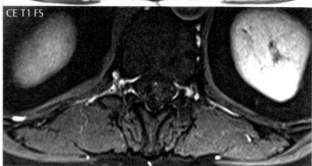

Fig. 3.9 Lipoma, incidental, of the conus. A small mass adjacent to the conus is seen, isointense to fat on both T2- and T1-weighted scans. Its identity as a lipoma is confirmed on the post-contrast image with fat saturation, both due to the suppression of signal intensity from the lesion itself and the lack of abnormal contrast enhancement. Small lipomas intimately associated with the conus medullaris are seen on occasion, and need not be symptomatic.

A limbus vertebra is a small, triangular corticated bone fragment, corresponding to the anterosuperior (most common) or anteroinferior corner of a vertebral body, caused by herniation of nucleus pulposus beneath the apophysis. The most common location is midlumbar, with no treatment indicated (▶ Fig. 3.8).

The filum terminale extends from the tip of the conus to the end of the thecal sac, where it inserts on the first coccygeal segment. A diameter < 2 mm is normal, and the average filum measures about 1 mm in thickness. It is easily seen on high-resolution axial MR images. In < 5% of patients, a small amount of fat can be seen blending in with and extending along the filum terminale, without focal enlargement. This entity, a fatty filum terminale, is well seen on MR on T1-weighted scans, and is a normal variant. On occasion, a small focal collection of fat, incidental to any clinical symptomatology, can be observed adjacent to the conus (▶ Fig. 3.9).

Lumbosacral nerve root anomalies are seen in 1 to 3% of the population. The most common anomaly involves the roots of L5 and S1 unilaterally, with two roots arising from a single

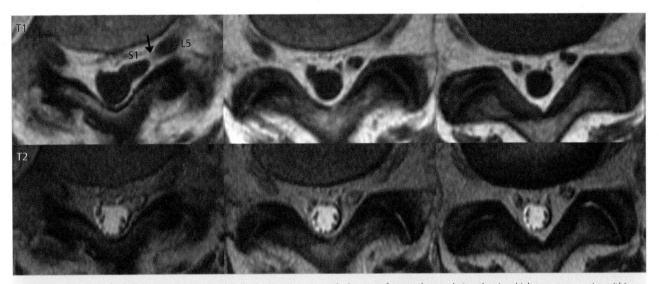

Fig. 3.10 Conjoined nerve root. This common entity has many variants, with the most frequently seen being that in which two nerves arise within a single root sleeve, which subsequently divides, with the respective nerves then exiting separately in the appropriate foramina. Illustrated is a conjoined L5–S1 nerve root sleeve on the left. The sections chosen show the two nerves (L5 and S1, labeled) on the left just after separation (*arrow*), on the slice just caudal to this (middle column), and then on a final more caudal axial slice (right column) where relative symmetry of right and left has been reestablished.

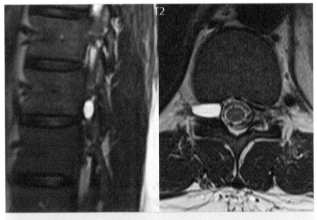

Fig. 3.11 Type II spinal meningeal cyst (Tarlov perineural cyst, thoracic). Small cysts such as that illustrated are commonly noted on cervical and thoracic MR exams, as seen on the right at a lower thoracic level, and are incidental findings.

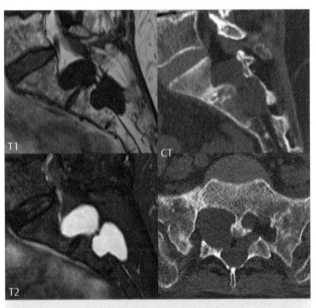

Fig. 3.12 Type II spinal meningeal cysts (Tarlov perineural cysts). Tarlov cysts are the most frequently encountered spinal meningeal cysts in clinical practice. Such lesions typically involve the sacral nerve roots, and demonstrate CSF SI on all pulse sequences. In the example presented, Tarlov cysts involve the S2 and S3 nerve root sleeves on the right. Foraminal enlargement and posterior scalloping of the vertebral bodies are common.

(conjoined) root sleeve, but then exiting separately in the appropriate foramina (▶ Fig. 3.10). This entity is asymptomatic, but noteworthy for two reasons. On MR, when a disk herniation is identified at the level of a conjoined nerve root, description of this is important for operative planning. Alternatively, on CT due to poor soft tissue contrast, a conjoined nerve root can be mistaken for a herniated disk, if the film reader is not familiar with this normal variant.

3.1.4 Incidental Cystic Lesions

The Nabors classification differentiates three types of spinal meningeal cysts. Types I and II are both extradural, with type I not containing and type II containing nerve roots. Type I includes IA, extradural arachnoid cysts, and IB, sacral meningoceles. Type II includes the commonly visualized Tarlov cysts, so

prevalent in the sacrum, and the common very small foraminal cysts seen incidentally in the cervical and thoracic spine on MR (▶ Fig. 3.11). Tarlov cysts are frequently large, multiple, and bilateral. When large, there will be scalloping of the surrounding bone (▶ Fig. 3.12).

Type III spinal meningeal cysts are intradural-extramedullary in location (and include arachnoid cysts, which can present with cord compression) (▶ Fig. 3.13), and are most often seen in

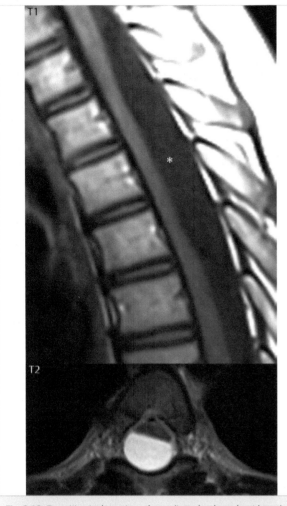

Fig. 3.13 Type III spinal meningeal cyst (intradural arachnoid cyst). These cysts (*asterisk*) are most commonly thoracic in location and dorsal to the cord, as illustrated. They can cause substantial displacement of, and mass effect upon, the cord. In this instance the cord is displaced anteriorly, and markedly compressed/flattened (with the latter well seen on the axial scan). The thin wall of the cyst, as in this instance, is usually not visualized on MR.

the thoracic spine dorsal to the cord. Spinal meningeal cysts (other than type IA) communicate with the subarachnoid space and contain CSF, and on MR will thus demonstrate CSF signal intensity on all pulse sequences. Clinically, spinal meningeal cysts, with the exception of type III, are usually asymptomatic.

Lateral meningoceles are included in the discussion of incidental lesions, since most are asymptomatic. Eighty five percent are seen in neurofibromatosis. With a lateral meningocele, there is protrusion laterally of the dura and arachnoid through an enlarged neural foramen, with scalloping of the pedicles, lamina, and dorsal surface of the vertebral body (▶ Fig. 3.14). The lesions are usually solitary. A lateral meningocele will have CSF signal intensity on all MR pulse sequences.

3.2 Congenital Disease

3.2.1 Congenital Spinal Stenosis

No measurements are absolute; however, AP dimensions of the spinal canal less than 10 mm in the cervical region (▶ Fig. 3.15) and 12 mm in the lumbar region (see ▶ Fig. 3.8) are considered to be stenotic. To some extent canal dimensions are more critical in the cervical spine, due to the presence of the cord, and in this region AP diameters of 10 to 13 mm are considered to represent relative spinal stenosis. It should be noted that the normal dimensions of the cervical spinal canal vary according to anatomic level, sex, age, and height. One easily recognized imaging finding in congenital spinal stenosis of the lumbar region is tapering of the canal dimension from the upper to the lower lumbar levels, with this region normally equal in size or greater in dimensions when compared to the thoracic spine. Patients with congenital cervical spinal stenosis are predisposed to traumatic spinal cord injury. Clinical presentation with congenital cervical spinal stenosis is typically due to myelopathic symptoms. However, radicular symptoms may be present, in either cervical or lumbar congenital stenosis, due to nerve root impingement with narrowing of the lateral recesses or neural foramina. A major element of congenital spinal stenosis is short pedicles. Achondroplasia is well known for symptomatic lumbar stenosis, with the entire spine stenotic in some

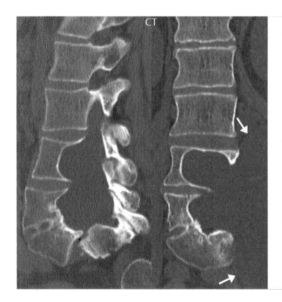

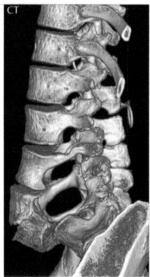

Fig. 3.14 Lateral meningoceles, neurofibromatosis type 1, CT. Sagittal and coronal reformatted CT scans **(part 1)** depict prominent scalloping of the L4 and L5 vertebral bodies, which can be identified as chronic in nature due to the thin sclerotic bony margin. The density therein was fluid (CSF) by attenuation measurement. In this patient, the meningoceles extended far beyond the spine into the adjacent soft tissues, with only the medial margin (*white arrows*) of their soft tissue extent identified on this cropped image. Volume rendering of the CT dataset **(part 2)** demonstrates both the vertebral body scalloping as well as thinning and deformity of the pedicles.

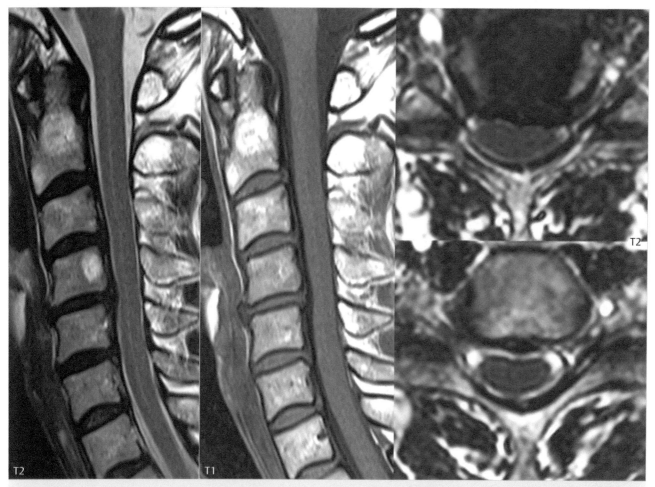

Fig. 3.15 Congenital cervical spinal stenosis. Sagittal images identify a reduced AP dimension to the cervical spine, with little CSF either anterior or posterior to the cord. Axial images are presented at the C4–5 and mid C5 levels. At C4–5 a broad-based disk osteophyte complex leads to moderate spinal canal stenosis with moderate cord flattening, which otherwise in a patient with a normal diameter canal would have had little impact. Note also that even at the mid C5 level there is markedly reduced CSF anterior and posterior to the cord, on axial imaging, with mild to moderate cord flattening.

patients. Down syndrome is known for congenital stenosis of both the cervical and lumbar spine.

3.2.2 Scoliosis

Scoliosis is simply lateral curvature of the spine. Ninety percent of cases are idiopathic with no underlying cause. The typical idiopathic scoliosis is an S-shape curve, with the thoracic curvature convex to the right. The remaining 10% are congenital (▶ Fig. 3.16), neuromuscular, and posttraumatic in etiology. In congenital scoliosis, vertebral anomalies can be seen (e.g., a hemivertebra) (▶ Fig. 3.17) and in other instances the scoliosis is associated with a congenital abnormality such as diastematomyelia or a Chiari I malformation (with hydromyelia). Neuromuscular causes include cerebral palsy, with an incidence as high as 50% in patients with severe disability as assessed by the gross motor function classification system. Posttraumatic etiologies include prior fracture, chronic osteomyelitis, prior surgery, and radiation therapy. Plain films are utilized for quantitation of the curvature and monitoring for possible progression. MR is the imaging modality of choice for evaluation of atypical or progressive scoliosis, specifically to exclude an underlying abnormality, with coronal imaging important (in addition to the more routinely acquired sagittal and axial scans).

3.2.3 Tethered Cord

This congenital anomaly is defined by a low position of the conus, with the conus being tethered (held in that position) due to an additional abnormality. Causes include a tight (often slightly thickened) filum terminale, lipomyelomeningocele (and variants thereof), diastematomyelia, and retethering following meningomyelocele repair (▶ Fig. 3.18). The clinical presentation is typically that of a young child with progressive neurologic dysfunction, specifically gait disturbance, motor and sensory loss in the lower extremities, and bladder dysfunction (all presumably due to cord traction and ischemia). In a tight filum terminale there will be an identifiable conus. The most common appearance of a tethered cord, however, is that of the cord extending without change in caliber to the lumbosacral region, tethering posteriorly with an associated lipoma and dysraphic posterior spinal elements. There may be associated hydromyelia. Treatment is surgical with release

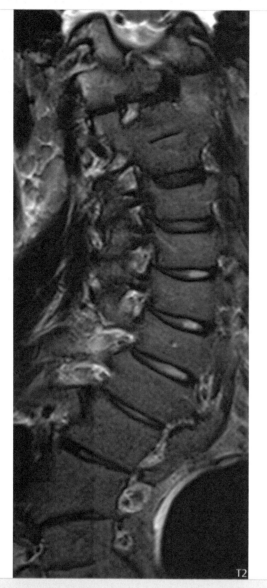

Fig. 3.16 Congenital scoliosis. Two curves are present, the first convex to the left in the cervical spine, and the second convex to the right in the thoracic spine. However, this is different from the more common idiopathic S-shaped scoliotic curvature, which is thoracolumbar in location, with the thoracic component convex to the right. There are nonsegmentation anomalies involving the skull base and upper cervical spine, together with an anomalous upper thoracic vertebral body (representing nonsegmentation of a normal vertebra and a hemivertebra) at the apex of the lower curvature.

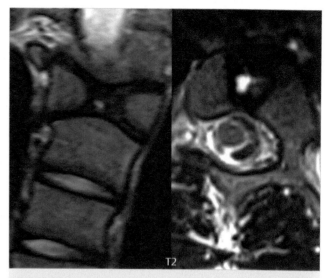

Fig. 3.17 Butterfly vertebral body. Coronal and axial images well depict a not uncommon vertebral body anomaly, a "butterfly" vertebral body. In this entity, there is failure of fusion of the two halves of the vertebral body due to persistent notochordal tissue centrally.

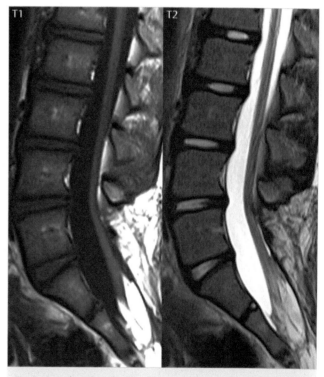

Fig. 3.18 Tethered cord with a lipoma (retethering). This 12-year-old child had surgery at 2 years of age, with release of a tethered spinal cord and excision of a lipomeningocele. On the current exam, there is retethering, with the cord taunt and extending to a residual lipoma in the low sacral region. There is evidence of bony spinal dysraphism posteriorly.

of the tether, for prevention of symptom progression. Following release, the level of the conus/distal cord typically will not change.

3.2.4 Syringohydromyelia

Hydromyelia is strictly defined as dilatation of the central canal of the spinal cord, lined by ependyma. Syringomyelia is defined strictly as the presence of a fluid-filled cavity within the spinal cord, lined by gliotic parenchyma, specifically not representing dilatation of the central canal. Unfortunately, these terms are commonly confused, and used interchangeably, by physicians. Thus the term syringohydromyelia has emerged, being less specific and including both hydromyelia and syringomyelia. Syringobulbia refers to the extension of a fluid collection into the brainstem, often accompanied by cranial nerve findings

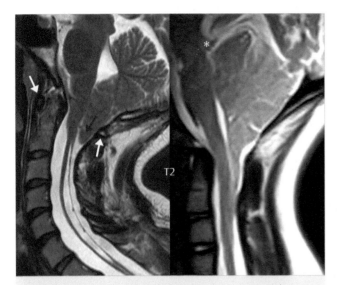

Fig. 3.19 Chiari I and II. Although sharing a common name, these two entities are distinct. A Chiari I is defined by herniation (*small black arrow*) of the wedge-shaped cerebellar tonsils >5 mm below the foramen magnum (first patient, left image). Note in this instance the tonsils extend well below the level of C1 (*white arrows*). In symptomatic Chiari I patients there may be accompanying dilatation of the central spinal canal (hydromyelia), also present in this patient. A Chiari II is however a hindbrain dysgenesis, with many distinctive features involving the brain (second patient, right image). Note the fused, beaked (*asterisk*) tectum (colliculi), the slitlike fourth ventricle, the foreshortening of the pons in the AP dimension, and the low tentorial insertion. The tonsillar herniation is more peglike than wedged, often extending a much greater distance than seen with a Chiari I malformation.

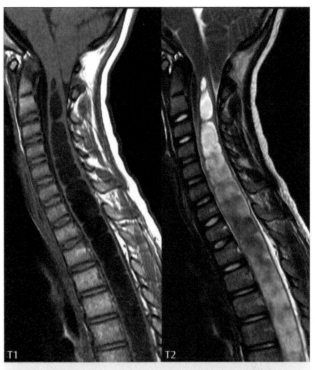

Fig. 3.20 Chiari I with extensive, marked hydromyelia. Wedge-shaped cerebellar tonsils are noted extending well below the C1 level. There is little if any CSF surrounding the brainstem at the level of the foramen magnum. There is marked dilatation of the central canal of the spinal cord, with a characteristic haustral-like appearance and the cord substance itself compressed peripherally. Complete evaluation of the cord from the foramen magnum to the conus is important in such cases, to establish the caudal extent of the central canal dilation, which may extend to the conus.

(due to compression). These entities are all difficult to visualize on CT. MR well depicts the cord and any pathology therein, and specifically abnormal fluid collections. The sagittal plane is commonly used to define the extent of syringohydromyelia, with the axial plane providing localization relative to the cross-section of the cord. Axial images also better identify very small cavities, and can determine with greater certainty the true extension of hydromyelia (with minimal dilatation of the central canal difficult to assess on sagittal images due to partial volume effects). Neoplastic disease and trauma are common etiologies for syringomyelia, whereas the Chiari I and II malformations account for the majority of cases of hydromyelia (▶ Fig. 3.19 and ▶ Fig. 3.20).

Intravenous contrast administration is strongly recommended in patients with syringomyelia, improving the sensitivity for detection of neoplastic disease. In the patient population at large, hydromyelia is much more commonly encountered, congenital in etiology, than syringomyelia due to either neoplasia or trauma. Both syringomyelia and hydromyelia can be treated by direct shunting of the cavity, amongst other options. An enlarging syrinx in a posttraumatic patient, for example following cervical cord injury, can cause neurologic deterioration unless so treated. With MR imaging at 3 T now commonly available clinically, the normal central canal of the spinal cord is routinely visualized on high-resolution images, with the canal slightly smaller or larger (specifically with a range of normal diameters) depending on the individual (▶ Fig. 3.21).

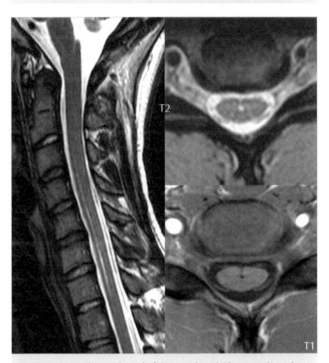

Fig. 3.21 Normal central canal of the spinal cord. The central canal can be visualized on high-resolution MR images in some individuals, as seen on sagittal and axial images, appearing slightly prominent size wise but within the spectrum of normal.

3.2.5 Meningomyeloceles and Lipomyelomeningoceles

In a meningomyelocele and a meningocele, there is incomplete closure of the posterior bony elements, with the contents of the spinal canal extending through the defect (open spinal dysraphism) (▶ Fig. 3.22). A meningocele, by definition, contains only dura and arachnoid, with neurologic deficits uncommon. A meningomyelocele, by definition, contains neural tissue within the expanded posterior subarachnoid space, with cord tethering. Imaging studies are rarely acquired at presentation in the newborn, with the exposed neural placode readily evident (in a meningomyelocele) and surgery typically performed within 48 hours (▶ Fig. 3.23). MR and CT are often obtained many years following surgery, and demonstrate a wide dysraphic defect with an accompanying CSF-filled sac covered by skin. Retethering is a common long-term complication. It is important to note that Chiari II malformations are virtually always associated with a meningomyelocele (▶ Fig. 3.24).

Lipomyelomeningoceles (and lipomyeloceles) differ from the two entities just described by the presence of a lipoma attached to the dorsal surface of the cord termination and intact skin overlying the defect (closed spinal dysraphism) (▶ Fig. 3.25). The lipoma extends through the dysraphic spinal canal merging with and becoming indistinguishable from, subcutaneous fat. The distal cord is tethered by the lipoma. When a mass is present posteriorly, it presents clinically under the age of 6 months (▶ Fig. 3.26). If the mass is subtle, presentation may not be until 5 to 10 years of age when neurologic or urologic deficits are noticed. Occasionally this entity goes undetected until adulthood, since the lesion is skin-covered.

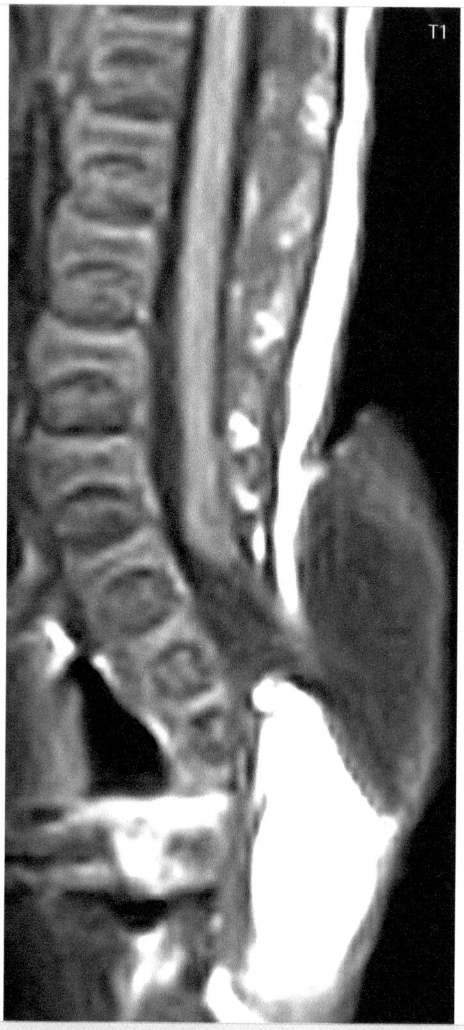

3.2.6 Diastematomyelia

In diastematomyelia the spinal cord is split into two hemicords, each invested by pia and each with a central canal, and dorsal

Fig. 3.22 Tethered cord with a meningomyelocele. In distinction to spina bifida, a meningomyelocele consists of not only a posterior arch defect but also herniation of the meninges and neural structures through this defect. Here, the midline sagittal image reveals a CSF-filled sac posteriorly in the lower lumbar region communicating with the normal thecal sac. The spinal cord extends to at least the level of the lumbosacral junction and dysraphic posterior osseous elements are present from L4 to S1. Abundant fatty tissue inferior to the defect is also seen, with high SI. Note the hypointensity of the vertebral bodies relative to the intervertebral disks, characteristic for an infant.

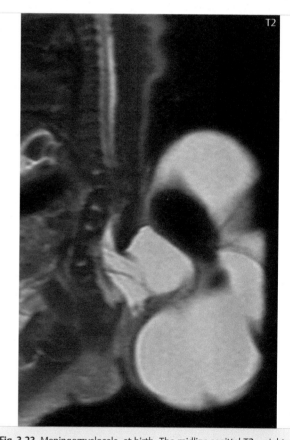

Fig. 3.23 Meningomyelocele, at birth. The midline sagittal T2-weighted image from the MR exam of this newborn, on the first day of life, is presented. A large spinal defect is noted posteriorly in the low lumbar region, with a CSF-filled sac protruding dorsally. It is very rare to ever see such a case on MR, given that surgery (repair with closure) is performed almost immediately. By definition, this defect lacks a skin covering, with neural tissue (and specifically the CSF sac) exposed to air.

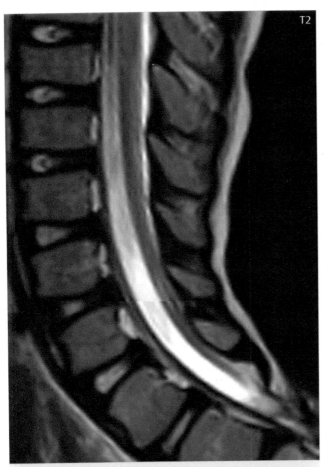

Fig. 3.24 Tethered cord in a patient with a Chiari II malformation. The typical tethered cord patient presents with neurologic dysfunction early in life, with many cases repaired at birth. Retethering may occur, as illustrated. The cord gradually tapers until reaching the end of the thecal sac, with no distinct conus—a typical appearance for either simple tethering or retethering. Nearly all Chiari II patients present at birth with a meningomyelocele, as was the case with this child.

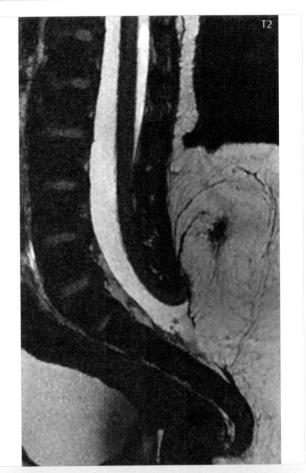

Fig. 3.25 Lipomyelocele. A single sagittal midline T2-weighted image demonstrates the cord extending to and tethered in the sacral region, without a change in caliber. There is an extensive posterior bony sacral defect, through which the cord continued terminating in a neural placode (visualized on adjacent off midline images, not presented) within the large dorsal lipoma.

and ventral horns. The two hemicords may lie within the same dural sac, or in separate sacs. A fibrous band or osteocartilaginous spur is often present at the most caudal aspect of the split (▶ Fig. 3.27). Most cases are lower thoracic or lumbar in location. Vertebral segmentation anomalies are common, and the presence of multiple nonsegmented vertebrae in the thoracic region is a clue to the possible presence of diastematomyelia. Clinical presentation is often nonspecific. There may be signs related to cord tethering, and cutaneous stigmata may be present along the back. As with all congenital anomalies involving neural structures, MR is the modality of choice, with imaging in all three orthogonal planes mandated.

3.2.7 Caudal Regression

In caudal regression (sacral agenesis), there is absence of sacrococcygeal vertebrae, which in more severe cases extends to include a portion of the lumbar spine. The agenesis is limited to

the sacrum in about half of cases. As might be expected, associated anomalies of the gastrointestinal and genitourinary systems are common, in particular anal atresia. Clinical findings range from mild deformities of the feet or distal muscle weakness to lower extremity paralysis, depending on the extent of vertebral involvement. Associated cord tethering is common. MR well depicts the level of regression together with the vertebral anomalies. In about half of patients (and specifically in patients without tethering) there is a characteristic, hatchetlike appearance (blunting, with the terminus slightly shorter along its ventral aspect) to the cord termination (▶ Fig. 3.28). In this instance the cord terminus is usually above L1.

3.2.8 Anterior Sacral Meningocele

An anterior sacral meningocele is a protrusion of the dura and leptomeninges, of varying size, anteriorly through a defect in the sacrum. The neck of the lesion is typically narrow. On sagittal CT or MR (or lateral plain film), the residual sacrum will be

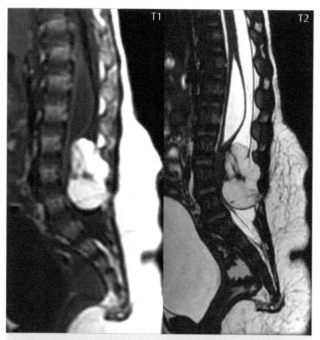

Fig. 3.26 Tethered cord with a lipoma. The spinal cord (visualized on sagittal images) extends at least to the L4–5 level, where it is tethered posteriorly to a large intraspinal lipoma. There is a prominent hydromyelic cavity in the terminal section of the cord, just proximal to the lipoma. Note that this is a closed (occult) spinal anomaly.
For the clinician, the prominent superficial fatty tissue in the lower lumbar region dorsally should raise the question of an underlying abnormality.

scalloped anteriorly and beneath the defect (in a semicircular manner), leading to the appearance of a scimitar or sickle (▶ Fig. 3.29). On MR, the contents will be isointense with CSF on all pulse sequences. It is important to delineate on imaging whether nerve roots traverse the sacral defect to lie within the meningeal sac, which negates simple ligation of the neck of the meningocele.

3.2.9 Dorsal Dermal Sinus

A dorsal dermal sinus is a midline epithelial-lined tract that extends from the skin inward to a variable distance. The tract extends to the spinal canal in about half of cases (a dorsal dermal sinus may terminate in soft tissue, at the dura, or within the thecal sac) (▶ Fig. 3.30). Most are either lumbosacral (the largest percentage) or occipital in location. A dimple or small ostium may be seen on the skin, frequently associated with a hairy nevus, hyperpigmented patch, or capillary angioma. Symptoms occur due to infection or neural compression, the latter with an associated dermoid or epidermoid cyst (about half of cases have a dermoid or epidermoid cyst at the tract termination). Cord tethering is common in lumbosacral lesions. When infected, intravenous contrast enhancement on MR is recommended, and improves delineation of the sinus tract and visualization of associated inflammation.

3.2.10 Intraspinal Enteric Cyst (Neurenteric Cyst)

Most patients present as adolescents or young adults with pain, and, on imaging, marked compression of the cord. The cyst itself can have variable contents, and thus a spectrum of signal intensity on MR (including that of CSF). The cyst is usually single, smooth, unilocular, intradural-extramedullary in location, and ventral or ventrolateral to the cord, occurring either in the cervical or thoracic region. There are associated vertebral anomalies in about half of patients (▶ Fig. 3.31). The bony spinal canal may be focally expanded (due to local pressure effects). There will be no abnormal contrast enhancement, differentiating this lesion from neoplasia. An important additional differential diagnostic consideration is that of an arachnoid cyst (type III spinal meningeal cyst), which will have CSF signal intensity on all pulse sequences and is not associated with vertebral anomalies.

3.2.11 Spinal Cord Herniation

Idiopathic spinal cord herniation is a rare, known entity in the thoracic spine, and a cause of thoracic myelopathy. On sagittal MR scans there will be an abrupt ventral deviation of the cord, due to prolapse through an anterior or lateral dural tear (▶ Fig. 3.32). An important diagnosis to exclude in this instance is a type III spinal meningeal arachnoid cyst, with both *CT* myelography and MR CSF flow studies permitting differentiation. Although of unknown etiology, a congenital origin has been postulated.

3.2.12 Dermoid and Epidermoid Cysts

These are not true neoplasms, and can be congenital (e.g., associated with a dorsal dermal sinus) or acquired (after surgery, lumbar puncture, or trauma) in origin. These cystic lesions are lined by squamous epithelium, with the presence of hair and skin elements (dermal appendages) defining a dermoid (as opposed to an epidermoid). Cyst rupture can occur, and can be asymptomatic or cause chemical meningitis. They are most commonly intradural-extramedullary, or intramedullary in location. Most spinal dermoid and epidermoid cysts arise in the lumbosacral region (▶ Fig. 3.34). They are typically well-circumscribed round lesions.

On both CT and MR, the fat component of a dermoid can be readily recognized, although the proportion of fat varies markedly. Unless infected, these lesions do not enhance on MR (other than subtle enhancement of the capsule). On CT and MR, epidermoid cysts (which do not contain fat) have an appearance similar to CSF (and thus an arachnoid cyst), with diffusion-weighted imaging (DWI) (an epidermoid has marked hyperintensity on DWI) critical for differential diagnosis, and often for detection as well. An epidermoid cyst can also be differentiated from CSF on FLAIR, although the difference in signal intensity can be subtle (and, FLAIR scans are typically utilized only in the

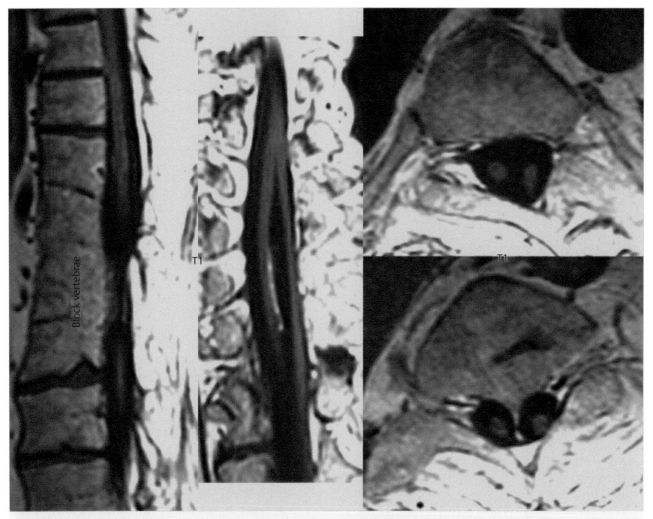

Fig. 3.27 Diastematomyelia. Sagittal, coronal, and axial MR images depict multiple nonsegmented midthoracic vertebral bodies, two hemicords, and on the final axial image a bony spur separating the two cords. Vertebral segmentation anomalies are common with diastematomyelia, in particular block vertebrae, and thus the presence of the latter finding (on plain film or CT) should raise the question of diastematomyelia.

brain). In large dermoid and epidermoid cysts, there may be remodeling of the bony spinal canal.

3.2.13 Neurofibromatosis

Spine manifestations in neurofibromatosis type 1 include posterior scalloping of the vertebral bodies (▶ Fig. 3.33), lateral meningoceles, and neurofibromas of exiting nerve roots (with enlargement therein of the neural foramina) (▶ Fig. 3.35). Multiple cutaneous neurofibromas are the hallmark of this disease. Plexiform neurofibromas of the paraspinal and sacral regions are also common. Neurofibromatosis type 1 occurs in about 1 in 3,000 births. On MR, neurofibromas characteristically are markedly hyperintense on T2-weighted scans. As with other neural origin tumors, enhancement is also seen following gadolinium chelate injection (▶ Fig. 3.36).

The incidence of neurofibromatosis type 2 (NF2) is approximately 5% that of type 1. Bilateral vestibular schwannomas are pathognomonic for this disease. Tumors involving the spine, and specifically intradural lesions, are very common in NF2. Extramedullary lesions include schwannomas and meningiomas, with neurofibromas less common. Intramedullary lesions include astrocytomas and ependymomas, although these are less common (in comparison with extramedullary lesions) (▶ Fig. 3.37).

3.2.14 Klippel-Feil

Today Klippel-Feil is broadly defined to include any patient with failure of segmentation of two or more cervical vertebrae (most commonly C2–3 or C5–6) (▶ Fig. 3.38). Most patients do not exhibit the classic clinical triad of short neck, low posterior hairline, and limited neck motion. Commonly associated anomalies include deafness, congenital heart disease, Sprengel deformity (elevation and rotation of the scapula), and urologic abnormalities. Nonsegmentation at one or two cervical levels is

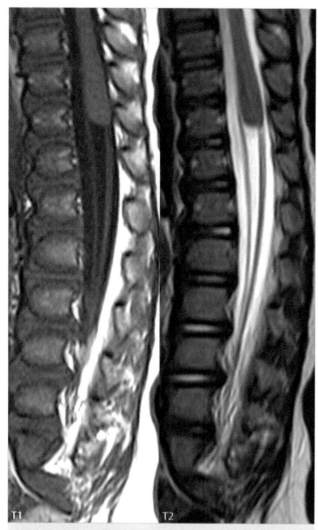

Fig. 3.28 Caudal regression (sacral agenesis). The conus medullaris of this 7-month-old infant is wedge- or hatchet-shaped and terminates at T11. There is hypoplasia of the S1 and S2 vertebral bodies, with no evidence of the more caudal portions of the sacrum or coccyx.

most common (▶ Fig. 3.39), and there may be associated occipitoatlantal nonsegmentation. Less common are patients with extensive cervical and thoracic nonsegmentation anomalies (▶ Fig. 3.40). Patients are often asymptomatic. There can be cord and nerve root compression. Patients with more extensive abnormalities are predisposed to spinal cord injury following minor trauma. Diastematomyelia is present in a small percentage of patients with Klippel-Feil.

3.2.15 Achondroplasia

Achondroplasia, an autosomal dominant disorder, is the most common cause of dwarfism. In the lumbar spine, the interpedicular distance characteristically decreases from L1 to L5 and the pedicles will be short, leading to spinal stenosis. In the cervical spine there can be generalized spinal canal stenosis, with stenosis at the foramen magnum also known to be associated (potentially resulting in cervicomedullary compression).

3.3 Trauma

In regard to the mechanisms of spine injury, and in particular referencing the cervical spine, flexion injuries lead to anteriorly wedged vertebral body fractures (▶ Fig. 3.41). In a severe flexion injury there can be disruption of the posterior longitudinal ligament and the interspinous ligaments (▶ Fig. 3.42), facet distraction, and anteroposterior subluxation (posterior ligament complex disruption). In the most severe cases, bilateral facet dislocation can occur. Extension injuries lead to posterior element fractures, and in a severe extension injury there can be disruption of the anterior longitudinal ligament and subluxation. In axial load injuries (e.g., from diving into shallow water), vertebral body compression (burst) fractures and lateral element fractures occur (▶ Fig. 3.43).

In high velocity auto accident injuries, axial load injury may result in compression of multiple contiguous vertebral bodies, in particular involving the thoracic spine (▶ Fig. 3.44). Rotational injuries rarely occur in isolation, rather typically with flexion, and result in lateral mass fractures and unilateral facet subluxations or dislocations.

Fractures can be classified as stable or unstable on the basis of the three-column concept. The anterior column is defined as the anterior two-thirds of the vertebral body, the middle column the posterior one-third, and the posterior column extending from the posterior vertebral body margin to the tip of the spinous process. Injury of two of the three columns, or the middle column, is considered an unstable fracture. CT with multiplanar reformatted images is critical for the evaluation of osseous injury (including the assessment of bony canal compromise and the presence of bone fragments therein), with MR extremely valuable for evaluation of the spinal cord and injuries involving, or in which the important element is, soft tissue (e.g., an epidural hematoma, or acute disk herniation). Acquisition of T2-weighted scans with fat suppression (or alternatively the use of STIR) is important for the demonstration of marrow edema (and improved detection, as compared to CT, of vertebral body microfractures) and soft tissue injury (e.g., involving the paraspinal musculature). Although marrow edema is commonly seen on MR in acute fractures, it is not always present. In the cervical spine on CT, review of high-resolution reformatted sagittal and coronal images is mandatory, in addition to thin section (source) axial images.

3.3.1 Cervical Spine Trauma

Specific osseous injuries in the cervical spine are subsequently discussed. Atlantooccipital dislocation (dissociation) occurs due to disruption of the ligaments between the occiput and C1. Increased distance is seen on coronal and sagittal reformatted CT images between the occipital condyles and the lateral masses of C1. MR visualizes both this finding and edema in the region of the disrupted stabilizing ligaments, reflecting the ligamentous injury itself. Atlantooccipital dislocation is often fatal.

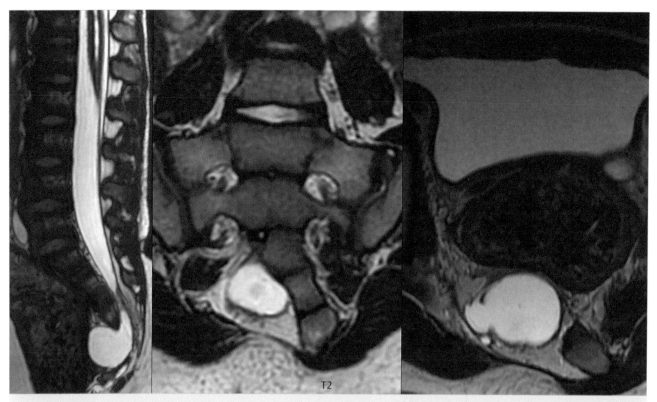

Fig. 3.29 Anterior sacral meningocele. Sagittal, coronal, and axial T2-weighted scans demonstrate a small presacral CSF collection contiguous with the thecal sac. There is also mild hydromyelia involving the distal cord, seen on the sagittal image. Characteristic accompanying findings include hypoplasia of the sacrum and, in the coronal plane, a curved "scimitar" shape to the sacrum. The Currarino syndrome (triad), present in this patient, consists of an anorectal malformation (typically with constipation), bony sacral defect, and presacral mass (anterior meningocele or benign teratoma). Note the dilated stool-filled rectum, reflecting the third part of the triad in this patient.

A Jefferson fracture is a burst fracture involving both the anterior and posterior arches of C1 (the atlas) (▶ Fig. 3.45). Unless the transverse atlantal ligament is disrupted, the patient is usually neurologically intact. Odontoid fractures occur with both flexion and extension injuries, and are primarily transverse in orientation (and thus can be difficult to detect on axial images). They are classified according to the location of the fracture line. Type I involve the upper portion of the odontoid (▶ Fig. 3.46), type II involve the junction of the odontoid and the body of C2 (these are the most common, and have the highest rate of nonunion, ▶ Fig. 3.47), and type III extend into the body of C2 (▶ Fig. 3.48).

A Hangman fracture is a bilateral fracture of the C2 ring, which has many variants (▶ Fig. 3.49). The pedicles and even the vertebral body may be involved. Extension of the fracture into the transverse foramen, as with all such fractures, raises the question of damage to the vertebral artery. The C2 vertebral body will be displaced anteriorly relative to C3—sometimes this is minimal—(but with the laminae still aligned) on the lateral plain film, and on sagittal CT or MR. As opposed to other fractures of the cervical spine that often compromise the spinal canal, these fractures often widen the canal and neurologic symptoms may be absent or minimal (autodecompression). A Clay-shoveler fracture is an avulsion fracture of a spinous process, involving a lower cervical or upper thoracic vertebra, classically C6 or C7 (▶ Fig. 3.50).

A teardrop fracture occurs due to flexion in combination with axial compression, resulting in a fracture involving the anteroinferior aspect of a cervical vertebral body (▶ Fig. 3.51). Bilateral facet fractures or dislocation occur due to flexion. A unilateral facet fracture involves both flexion and rotation. Vertebral body compression fractures can occur due to flexion (▶ Fig. 3.52). Hyperflexion typically involves injury to the posterior musculature and posterior ligamentous complex (detected in part on MR due to the accompanying edema), together with facet fracture/subluxation/dislocation (▶ Fig. 3.53 and ▶ Fig. 3.54). If the injury to the posterior paraspinal musculature is unilateral, the injury involved flexion with rotation.

3.3.2 Burst Fracture

A burst fracture occurs secondary to axial loading, with vertical compression. Typically a single vertebral body is involved, with radial displacement of fragments. Burst fractures are most common in the lower thoracic and lumbar regions. Neurologic deficits result due to retropulsion of bone fragments into the spinal canal (▶ Fig. 3.55). CT is the study of choice for initial evaluation, with MR providing potentially important supplemental information regarding the cord (and specifically damage therein, including edema and hemorrhage) and ligamentous injury (see ▶ Fig. 3.43).

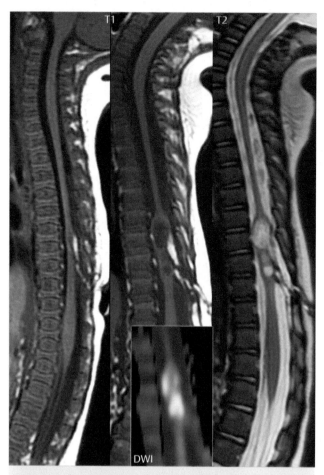

Fig. 3.30 Dorsal dermal sinus. Sagittal midline images are presented in this infant, the first being at 2 months of age (left most image). Additional images (T1- and T2-weighted, and DWI - insert) are provided from a second exam at 9 months of age. On the initial exam a sinus tract is noted extending from the skin, posteriorly, to the thoracic cord. There is a small associated intradural lipoma. On the follow-up exam, the sinus tract is again noted, but now well seen is an intramedullary lesion, with low and high SI respectively on T1- and T2-weighted images, and restricted diffusion (high SI on DWI). This abnormality corresponds to a growing epidermoid (with an epidermoid or dermoid found, in association, in 50% of dermal sinus cases), which was resected a few weeks following the second exam.

3.3.3 Flexion Injury

Flexion injuries of the spine, other than those involving the cervical spine, occur most commonly from T12 to L2. The injury is termed a Chance fracture, and consists of an anterior vertebral body compression fracture in combination with an injury involving the posterior elements (with a spectrum from ligamentous disruption to transverse fracture). There will be anterior wedging of the involved vertebral body. In the past this occurred due to the use of seat belts (prior to the introduction of shoulder belts), due to passenger restraint with sudden forward flexion in a head on collision. This injury is also seen in unrestrained occupants in a major motor vehicle accident.

3.3.4 Benign Osteoporotic Fractures

Osteoporotic compression fractures occur in the elderly, and are more common in postmenopausal women, due to bony insufficiency (▶ Fig. 3.56 and ▶ Fig. 3.57). Although loss of height of a vertebral body is well identified on CT, discrete fractures (through cortical bone) are often not visualized, making CT poor for differentiation of acute from chronic changes (▶ Fig. 3.58). MR readily identifies both the loss of height and edema therein, in acute benign vertebral body compression fractures. STIR is the favored imaging technique, with images acquired in the sagittal plane, for the detection of edema in an acute benign compression fracture (▶ Fig. 3.59).

The edema is also well seen on T1-weighted and fat suppressed T2-weighted scans, but is more striking on STIR images, likely due to the combined T1- and T2-weighting of this sequence, with edema producing an increase in signal intensity by the change in both T1 and T2. The edema within the vertebral body also demonstrates abnormal contrast enhancement on scans acquired with fat suppression (▶ Fig. 3.60).

In an acute vertebral body compression fracture, the entire vertebral body may be involved, or simply a portion of the body immediately adjacent to, and parallel with, the intervertebral disk (e.g., involvement of the upper or lower one-third of a body). Surprisingly, in cases that involve the entirety of the vertebral body, identification of a discrete fracture line on MR (as a low signal intensity irregular line extending through the vertebral body) can be made on occasion, improving further diagnostic confidence.

Sacral insufficiency fractures can occur unilaterally or bilaterally, with marrow edema seen in the sacral alae. Although fracture lines and sclerosis may be seen on CT, MR is the imaging modality of choice for diagnosis, with substantially improved detection. A moderate in size, patchy area of edema will be visualized, and is typically well seen on T1-weighted, T2-weighted (with fat saturation) and STIR images (▶ Fig. 3.61).

Contrast enhancement will be present in the area of edema, and well seen on images acquired with fat saturation. Usually no other findings are present, and specifically there will not be an associated mass lesion. In an elderly woman with pain (often with a history of minor trauma), specific attention should be paid to the sacrum, which may be only in part visualized on sagittal and axial images that are otherwise obtained for disk disease. Coronal imaging is recommended specifically through the sacrum. The differential diagnosis for a sacral insufficiency fracture is a metastasis to the sacrum, with clinical presentation and imaging appearance (specific portion of the sacrum involved, and the lack of an associated mass) providing differentiation. Although restricted diffusion strongly favors a malignant lesion, it should not be considered definitive in the differentiation of a malignant from a benign (compression) fracture, whether of a vertebral body or the sacrum.

Chronic compression fractures on MR will demonstrate loss of height with normal hematopoietic marrow or replacement with fatty marrow (▶ Fig. 3.62). Vertebroplasty which involves the injection of bone cement percutaneously via either one or both pedicles, and which is used in many centers for treatment of the severe pain associated with acute vertebral collapse, produces an irregular area of low signal intensity within the vertebral body on all MR pulse sequences (▶ Fig. 3.63). Resolution of

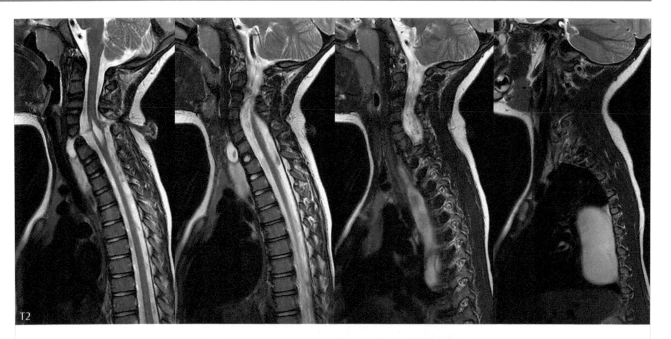

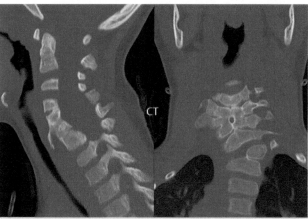

Fig. 3.31 Neurenteric cyst On sagittal T2-weighted images (**part 1**), a large cystic lesion is noted anterior to the spine, extending from the midcervical region to the mediastinum. Continuity of the lesion is demonstrated with the spinal canal, together with extension to involve the cord itself (with a small intramedullary component). On sagittal reformatted CT (**part 2**), the bony spinal canal is seen to be focally enlarged, with nonsegmentation of the C5–C7 vertebral bodies. The coronal reformatted CT demonstrates a midline circular vertebral defect, the persistent canal of Kovalevsky.

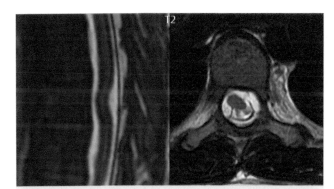

Fig. 3.32 Idiopathic spinal cord herniation. The sagittal T2-weighted scan demonstrates focal anterior displacement (kinking) of the cord in the midthoracic region. On the axial scan, the cord is noted to have prolapsed through an anterolateral dural defect. The patient presented with spastic monoparesis of the right leg. Findings were confirmed at surgery, with reduction of the herniation.

the edema is slow, in an acute benign compression fracture, with months transpiring before the signal intensity within the vertebral body returns to normal.

3.3.5 Spinal Cord Injury

MR is employed in acute trauma to screen for and assess spinal cord injury. The exam should include both T1- and T2-weighted scans (including T2* gradient echo imaging), in part due to the importance of detection of hemorrhage within the cord. Methemoglobin is easily detected on T1-weighted scans, with deoxyhemoglobin well visualized on T2-weighted scans, in particular T2*-weighted scans. Evaluation for the presence of edema on T2-weighted scans, and its extent within the cord, is an additional important aspect, with this adequately assessed on fast spin echo scans (▶ Fig. 3.64), but with higher sensitivity using fast STIR. Substantial hemorrhage within the cord carries a poor prognosis, with little neurologic recovery likely (▶ Fig. 3.65).

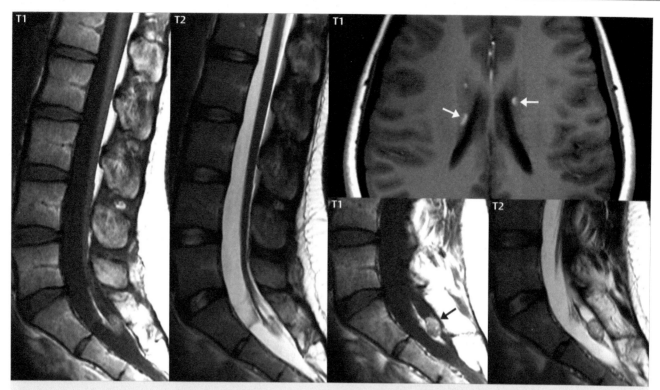

Fig. 3.33 Dermoid cyst. The cord is tethered in the sacral region, with a gradual reduction in diameter and no distinct conus. A small soft tissue mass (*black arrow*) is noted in the sacral portion of the thecal sac, of intermediate signal intensity with interspersed fat (high signal intensity on the T1-weighted scan). This dermoid has ruptured, with typical small fat globules (*white arrows*) identified in the ventricular system on the axial T1-weighted scan of the brain.

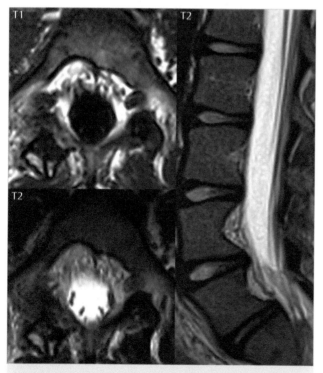

Fig. 3.34 Vertebral body scalloping, neurofibromatosis type 1, MR. There is posterior scalloping of L4, and to a lesser degree L5 (without any associated mass), seen on axial and sagittal images. Spine manifestations of NF1 include scoliosis, bony dysplasia, dural ectasia (with vertebral scalloping), and lateral meningoceles.

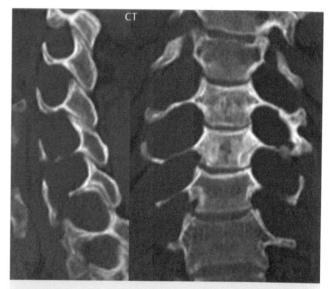

Fig. 3.35 Neurofibromatosis type 1, CT. Sagittal and coronal reformatted CT sections demonstrate the neural foramina of the cervical spine to be diffusely enlarged, due to the presence of plexiform neurofibromas.

Edema, unaccompanied by hemorrhage, carries an excellent prognosis, with substantial neurologic recovery, often complete. Cord compression in acute injury leads to myelomalacia, which early on may simply manifest as edema. Cystic necrosis subsequently develops, commonly within central gray matter due to

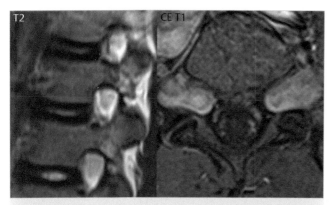

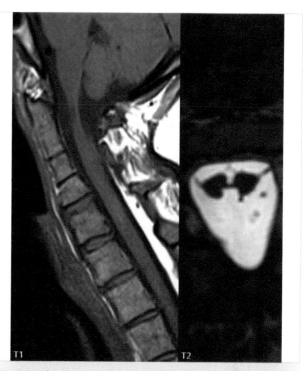

Fig. 3.36 Neurofibromatosis type 1, MR. There is diffuse enlargement of lumbar nerve roots within the neural foramina (which are also slightly enlarged), consistent with a diagnosis of NF1. The lesions are hyperintense on the T2-weighted scan, and demonstrate moderate contrast enhancement. This adolescent male patient has extensive plexiform neurofibromas, meeting the clinical criteria for diagnosis on this basis together with the presence of multiple café-au-lait spots.

Fig. 3.38 Klippel-Feil. On the sagittal MR image, the C2–C4 vertebral bodies are hypoplastic and nonsegmented, with absence of normal intervening disk spaces. Diastematomyelia is identified on the axial scan at C1–2, with the two hemicords tethered by a fibrous band and enveloped in a single arachnoid-dural sheath.

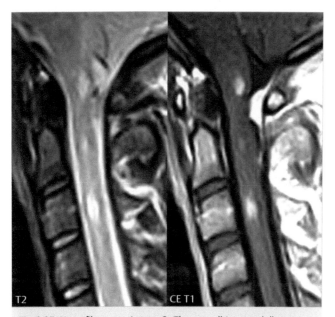

Fig. 3.37 Neurofibromatosis type 2. Three small intramedullary lesions, with high signal intensity on the T2-weighted scan and abnormal enhancement post-contrast, are noted within the cervical cord, consistent with either small astrocytomas or ependymomas, both which occur in NF2. Note also the small enhancing meningioma, with a broad dural base adjacent to the posterior arch of C1.

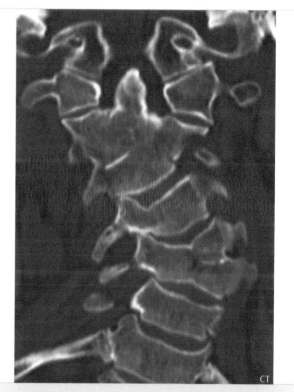

Fig. 3.39 Klippel-Feil. Nonsegmentation is noted at two levels on a coronal reformatted CT image. Hemivertebra are present in both instances, at C2–3 and C5–6, together with prominent scoliosis of the cervical spine.

its greater metabolic needs. In a chronic cord injury, there may be syringomyelia (a result of necrosis within the cord) or simply cord atrophy.

Traumatic disk herniations are most common in the cervical spine, and less common in the thoracic and lumbar regions (▶ Fig. 3.66). In the cervical spine, these may occur following relatively minor trauma; however, the incidence increases with severity of trauma. Cervical disk herniations are most common with hyperextension injury (e.g., whiplash), with the C5–6 level most often involved. Posterolateral disk herniations are

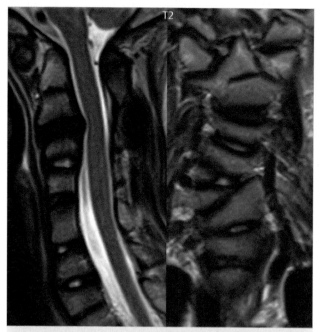

Fig. 3.40 Multiple cervical vertebral anomalies (Klippel-Feil). Seen on sagittal and coronal MR these include hemivertebrae (C5, C6), nonsegmentation of the posterior elements (C1–2), and a wedge-shaped vertebral body (C7). A large osteophyte at C2–3 reflects accentuated movement at this level, with mobility of the cervical spine otherwise evidently restricted.

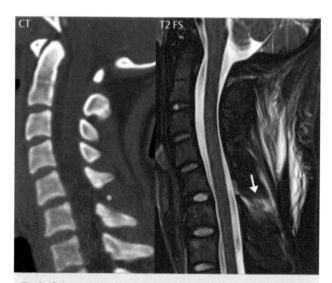

Fig. 3.42 Interspinous ligament injury. On CT, this injury is visualized only indirectly by widening of the interspinous distance (*asterisk*). On MR, edema within the ligament can be directly visualized (*arrow*), with the extensive posterior paraspinous edema/hemorrhage an additional indication of the severity of the injury in this patient.

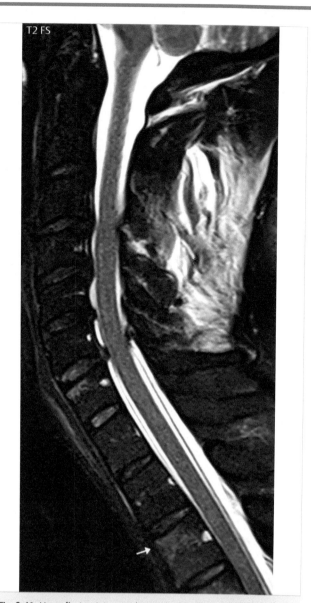

Fig. 3.41 Hyperflexion injury with vertebral body fractures and posterior soft tissue injury. There is extensive abnormal high signal intensity in the posterior paraspinous musculature/ligamentous complex (*asterisk*), consistent with a more severe flexion injury. There is minimal loss of height (and anterior wedging) of the C7 vertebral body with abnormal high signal intensity in the superior portion, consistent with an acute compression deformity. A similar injury involves the superior portion of T3 (*arrow*). Beginning at the C6–C7 level and extending caudally, there is a large posterior extradural fluid collection. This had the signal intensity characteristics of CSF on all pulse sequences, and was felt to represent an extradural CSF collection due to a dural tear.

3.3.6 Epidural Hemorrhage

Most spinal epidural hemorrhages are either "spontaneous" (with no known cause) (▶ Fig. 3.67) or posttraumatic, the latter occurring principally in conjunction with spinal fractures (▶ Fig. 3.68 and ▶ Fig. 3.69). Other etiologies are much less common, but do include coagulopathies. The signal intensity of such a hemorrhage will depend on its temporal stage, and the severity of neurologic symptoms upon the location and degree

prevalent, with symptoms including immediate neck and arm pain. In patients with cervical fractures, a disk herniation is most common immediately below the fracture. Acute epidural hematomas are the other main cause, in the setting of trauma, of soft tissue cord compression.

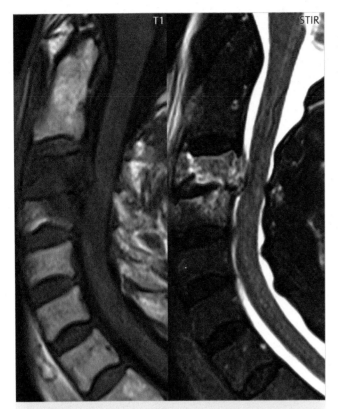

Fig. 3.43 Traumatic C3 burst fracture. An axial load injury has resulted in a burst fracture of C3, with mild loss of height and edema seen throughout the vertebral body. A vertically oriented, fracture plane is seen on the sagittal T2-weighted image extending through the C3 vertebral body. Retropulsion of the posterior portion of the C3 vertebral body into the spinal canal results in mild spinal canal compromise with mild cord flattening. There is no evidence of cord edema in this region. Edema in the posterosuperior portion of the C4 vertebral body is consistent with an additional acute fracture. Prevertebral soft tissue edema (only partially depicted) extended from the skull base to the C4 level.

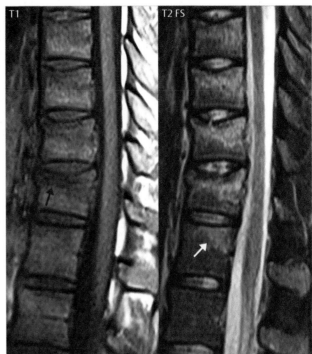

Fig. 3.44 Compression fractures, acute (traumatic), thoracic spine (MR). Edema within the superior half of every visualized thoracic vertebral body is consistent with microfractures, with the clinical history being that of a motor vehicle accident with an axial load injury. Note that the edema is better demonstrated on the T2-weighted image with fat saturation (as abnormal high signal intensity), for example within T12 (*white arrow*) *than* on the T1-weighted spin echo scan (with low signal intensity). This difference is accentuated due to the age of the patient, 17 years old, with a predominance of hematopoietic marrow. There is mild loss of vertebral body height at T11 with a suggestion of a discrete fracture line (*black arrow*) and minimal retropulsion. There is no significant spinal canal compromise at any level. There is minimal loss of vertebral body height involving the superior portion of the T8 and T10 vertebral bodies.

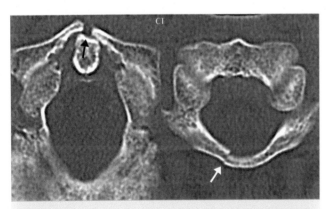

Fig. 3.45 C1 fracture. Because C1 is a ring, when fractured there will typically be at least two fracture lines (as in this instance, with fractures of both the anterior [*black arrow*] and posterior [*white arrow*] arches). The Jefferson fracture, of which this is an example, is a burst fracture due to axial loading.

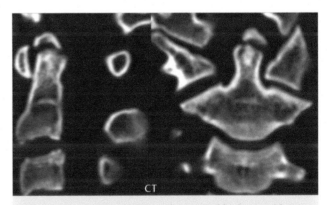

Fig. 3.46 Type I odontoid fracture. There is a mildly distracted fracture involving the tip of the odontoid, seen on sagittal and coronal reformatted images. A type I fracture involves only the superior portion of the dens, as distinguished from a type II fracture that involves the base of the dens. In this patient, there is likely an additional atlantoaxial dissociation injury, with increased distance between the articular facets of C1 and C2 on the right.

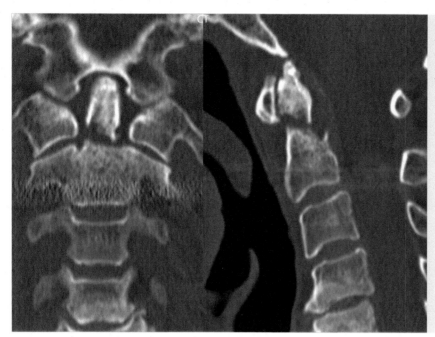

Fig. 3.47 Chronic type II odontoid (dens) fracture. Coronal and sagittal reformatted images of the upper cervical spine are presented. There is non-union (pseudoarthrosis) of this chronic fracture.

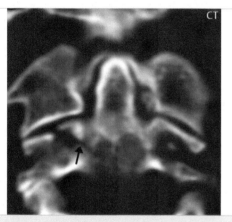

Fig. 3.48 Type III odontoid fracture. In type III, the fracture extends into the body of C2 (*black arrow*), as illustrated on a coronal reformatted image.

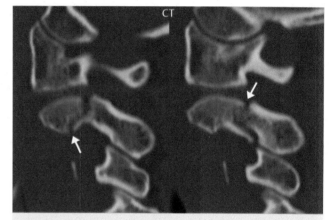

Fig. 3.49 Traumatic spondylolisthesis of C2 (hangman fracture). Sagittal images reveal coronally oriented fractures (*arrows*) bilaterally of the pars interarticularis of the axis (C2). In this instance there is little displacement or angulation.

of spinal cord compression. The clinical presentation is often emergent, with spinal cord compression and (in the absence of prompt treatment) permanent neurologic impairment. Symptoms often include focal pain, motor and sensory loss, and bowel and bladder dysfunction. Most epidural hematomas extend over several vertebral segments. Treatment in cases with neurologic compromise is by prompt surgical evacuation. MR is the imaging modality of choice, due to its excellent depiction of soft tissue, specifically of the spinal cord, adjacent soft tissues, and the hematoma itself.

Symptomatic postoperative epidural hematomas are very infrequent (occurring in less than 0.2% of surgical patients) and, as with all spinal epidural hemorrhages, are likely due to disruption of the rich venous plexus within the epidural space. Clinical presentation can be within the first 24 hours following surgery or with a several day delay. In young children with high-speed (motor vehicle) craniocervical junction injuries, retroclival epidural hematomas can occur, the majority with

accompanying tectorial membrane injury. Overt disruption of the tectorial membrane (which is simply a superior extension of the posterior longitudinal ligament), or stretching and detachment can be seen.

3.3.7 Brachial Plexus Injury

The brachial plexus is formed from the anterior nerve roots (ventral rami) of C5–C8 and T1, and innervates the arm and hand. In adults, most brachial plexus injuries are due to high velocity trauma. Symptoms range from pain to paralysis. Avulsion injuries occur (in preganglionic plexus injuries), with or without pseudomeningoceles (▶ Fig. 3.70).

Clinically patients may present with a "dead arm" and imaging is performed to assess whether there is complete nerve root avulsion from the cord (not surgically amenable to repair) or damage is within the more distal plexus, in which case

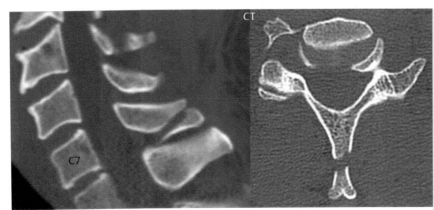

Fig. 3.50 Clay-shoveler fracture. Sagittal and axial CT images **(part 1)** depict a slightly displaced acute fracture of the C7 spinous process. Note the very sharp discontinuity of cortical bone, best seen on the axial section, defining this fracture as acute. On sagittal MR **(part 2),** the fracture of the spinous process can be identified (*white arrow*), but is more difficult to detect than on CT. Note the relative absence of edema within the bone adjacent to the fracture line, a common but nonintuitive finding in acute trauma. What CT does not depict however is the extensive nature and severity of the injury, reflected by the diffuse edema in the posterior paraspinal tissues (*asterisk*) and the prevertebral edema/fluid (*black arrow*).

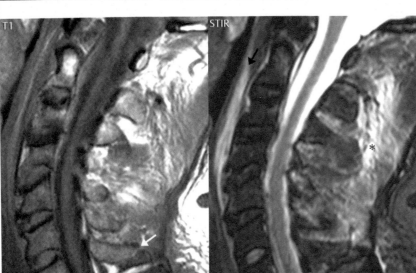

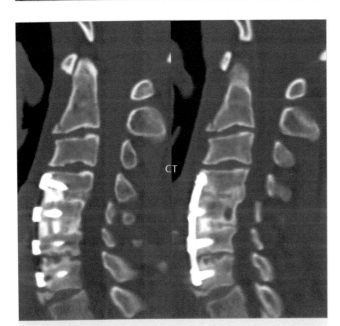

Fig. 3.51 Hyperflexion teardrop fracture. Teardrop fractures of both C2 and C7 are seen on sagittal reformatted images, with displacement of the fracture fragments from the anteroinferior corner of the respective vertebral bodies. There has been a prior anterior plate and screw fusion of C4–C7.

re-anastomosis may be possible. On MR imaging, increased signal intensity on T2-weighted fat suppressed images (an early sign of denervation) and contrast enhancement of the affected paraspinal muscles (denervation injury) are considered the most reliable indirect diagnostic signs. Postganglionic injuries include stretch injuries and avulsion injuries, the latter with nerve disruption. Stretch injuries are more common, and are visualized in the acute setting with thickening of the nerves and hyperintensity on T2-weighted scans (▶ Fig. 3.71). Fibrosis is seen in the chronic phase. Completed avulsion results in an appearance of discontinuity and distal nerve retraction. For a complete discussion of brachial plexus pathology, the reader is referred to the musculoskeletal literature. It should, however, be noted in imaging of the brachial plexus for pain that, due to the incidence of apical lung carcinoma and the proximity to the brachial plexus, the lung apices must be included in one's search pattern (see ▶ Fig. 3.2).

3.4 Degenerative Disease

3.4.1 Degenerative Spinal Stenosis

Degenerative spinal stenosis can be central, subarticular (lateral recess) in location (the space between the posterior margin of

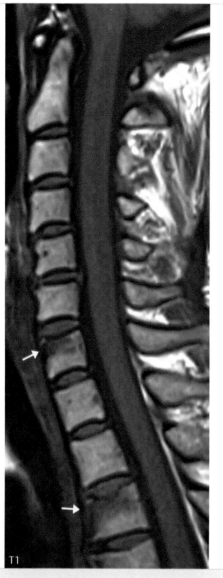

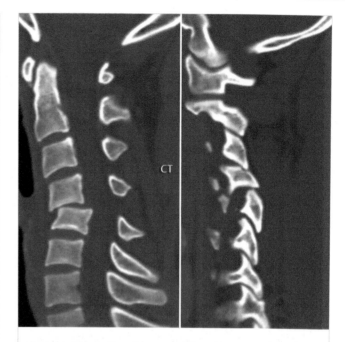

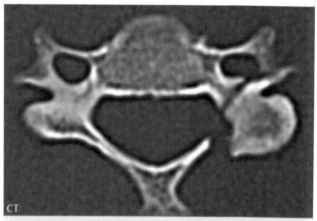

Fig. 3.52 Compression fractures, acute, cervical spine. In trauma, a vertebral body may wedge anteriorly due to flexion. Or, with excess axial load, a compression (burst) fracture may result—this being the most common traumatic injury in the thoracic spine. The latter may manifest as a loss of vertebral body height, as seen in the T3 vertebral body (*lower white arrow*). However, body height may be maintained, rendering visualization impossible on plain film or CT With MR these microfractures are easily identified due to marrow edema, in this instance with low signal intensity (*upper arrow*) on the T1-weighted scan within C7.

Fig. 3.53 Severe hyperflexion injury, CT. Midline and right lateral sagittal reformatted CT images are presented **(part 1)**, along with a single axial image at the C4 level **(part 2)**. There is a fracture involving the left C4 lamina extending into the articular pillar and transverse foramen. The C4–C5 facet on the right is perched. Splaying of the C4–C5 spinous processes, consistent with interspinous ligament injury and instability, is also noted. Together these result in 4 mm of anterolisthesis of C4 on C5 with a mild acute kyphotic angulation at this level. This anterolisthesis and a broad-based disk bulge at the C4–5 level (not well seen on the images presented) result in mild AP dimension spinal canal narrowing at this level. Given the extent of injury, likely the entire posterior ligamentous complex is disrupted at C4–5.

vertebral body and the anterior margin of superior facet, bounded by the thecal sac medially and the pedicle laterally), or foraminal. Degenerative disease anteriorly (a disk bulge with or without accompanying osteophyte), posteriorly due to ligamentum flavum buckling or thickening, and posterolaterally due to facet joint hypertrophy can all contribute to spinal canal stenosis. In the lumbar spine, it is very common to have all three elements contributing (▶ Fig. 3.72).

The ligamenta flava are paired, thick ligaments (predominantly composed of elastic fibers) that connect the lamina of adjacent vertebral bodies. They extend from the anteroinferior aspect of the superior lamina to the posterosuperior aspect of the inferior lamina. The ligamenta flava increase in thickness normally from the cervical to the lumbar regions. They are situated posterolaterally in the canal, and anterolaterally are contiguous with the capsule of the facet joint. In degenerative disease, the ligamentum flavum becomes visibly thickened, and thus may cause narrowing of either the lateral recess or spinal canal. In regard to facet joint hypertrophy, hypertrophy of the superior articular facet is a primary cause of lateral recess stenosis, and resulting nerve compression. Epidural lipomatosis is simply excessive fat deposition in the epidural space. It is seen in chronic steroid use and in morbid obesity, and is usually thoracic and lumbar in distribution. It is reported that patients can become symptomatic, due to compression of the thecal sac.

The neural foramen is bounded by the pedicles superiorly and inferiorly, the vertebral body and disk anteriorly, and the facets posteriorly. Nerve roots exit from the thecal sac, pass

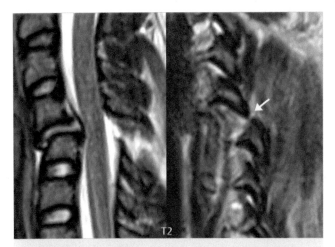

Fig. 3.54 Severe hyperflexion injury, MR. On the midline sagittal MR image, there is a traumatic anterolisthesis of C4 on C5, with an acute disk herniation, leading to mild canal narrowing and cord compression. There is splaying of the C4–5 spinous processes, and edema between, consistent with disruption of the interspinous ligament. On the off-midline image, a perched facet is also noted (*arrow*), implying at least an additional tear of the interfacetal ligaments.

through the lateral recess, and enter the neural foramen. Degenerative disease of the disk, endplates, and facets can all contribute to neural foraminal narrowing (▸ Fig. 3.73).

Imaging of the neural foramina, specifically for evaluation of narrowing, is best performed in the sagittal plane, but more specifically in the true cross-section to the foramen. In the lumbar spine, direct sagittal imaging approximates this plane. However, in the cervical spine, acquisition (or reconstruction) of planes that are oblique in two dimensions are necessary. This is required due to the course of the neural foramina in the cervical spine, which is both anterolateral and superoinferior. Neural foraminal narrowing in the lumbar spine, as viewed on the basis of sagittal MR, is specifically assessed by evaluation in both the craniocaudal and AP directions for perineural fat obliteration, and (for the most severe disease) by direct nerve root compression or morphologic change. Evaluation of foraminal stenosis should thus include a description of the specific fat planes that are obliterated, together with any changes in morphology of the nerve itself (due to compression). Although degenerative neural foraminal narrowing is commonly seen in patient exams, the correlation between clinical symptomatology and MR imaging appearance is generally poor.

3.4.2 Disk, Endplate, Foraminal, and Spinal Canal Disease

Cervical Spine

The cervical spine is most mobile at C4–5, 5–6, and 6–7, with most disk herniations occurring at these levels. The age of presentation is commonly the third to fourth decades. MR is the

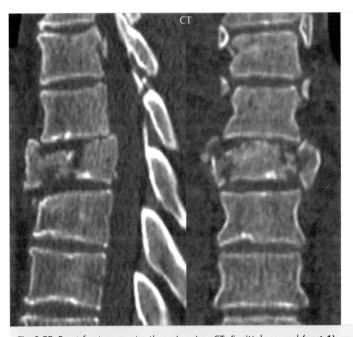

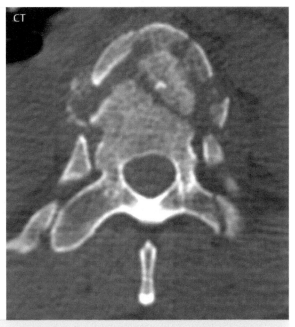

Fig. 3.55 Burst fracture, acute, thoracic spine, CT. Sagittal, coronal (**part 1**), and axial (**part 2**) reformatted CT images are presented of the midthoracic spine, in the acute time frame following trauma. There is moderate loss of height of T7, with mild anterior wedging. Portions of the vertebral body are displaced (on the sagittal image) both anteriorly and posteriorly, and (on the coronal image) both to the left and right. Note the centrifugally located vertebral body fragments, best appreciated on the axial image.

examination of choice. Thin section axial gradient echo T2-weighted scans are critical for diagnosis, supplemented by sagittal imaging. A very thin rim of low signal intensity can often be visualized on axial T2-weighted scans along the posterior aspect of the disk (in both normal patients and in the presence of a herniation), corresponding to the dura, volume averaged together with the posterior longitudinal ligament. Thin section post-contrast axial T1-weighted scans are usually not acquired in patients with radiculopathy; however, these do substantially improve visualization of foraminal disk herniations due to

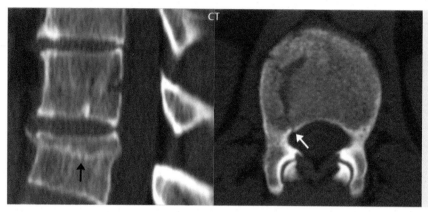

Fig. 3.56 Compression fracture, acute, L1 (CT). On the sagittal reformatted image, a mild anterior wedge compression deformity is noted, with an acute fracture suggested only indirectly (in this plane) by the sclerotic line (*black arrow*). This corresponds to compressed trabecular bone. CT is excellent for demonstration of acute fracture lines, in particular where they intersect cortical bone (*small white arrow*, axial plane), but insensitive to marrow edema and microfractures, which are well depicted by MR.

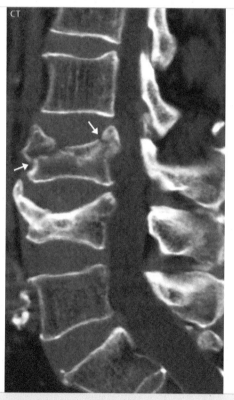

Fig. 3.57 Compression fracture, acute and chronic, lumbar spine (CT). There is generalized osteopenia. There is an acute compression fracture of L3 with discrete fracture lines identified (*arrows*). There is approximately 50% loss of vertebral body height. There is moderate retropulsion of the posterior superior portion of the L3 vertebral body into the spinal canal. This leads to approximately one-third to one-half loss of bony central spinal canal dimensions in the AP direction. However, the level of canal compromise should be well below the termination of the conus, which could not be determined on this CT. Also demonstrated is a chronic anterior wedge compression deformity of L4, with the time frame of this deformity established by its presence on a prior exam. There is mild retropulsion of the superior posterior portion of this vertebral body into the spinal canal.

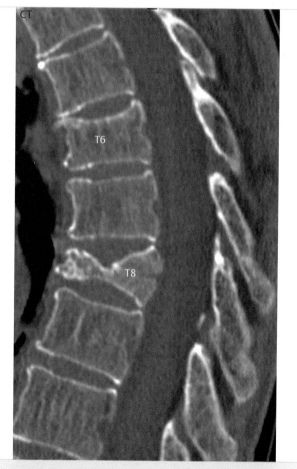

Fig. 3.58 Compression fractures, osteoporotic (CT). There is mild loss of vertebral body height involving T6, with a prominent wedge compression deformity of T8. The accentuated vertical trabeculae and the demineralization of the spine reflect generalized osteoporosis. Note the accentuated kyphotic deformity of the thoracic spine. However, without demonstration of a discrete fracture line, neither compression deformity can be classified in regard to time frame.

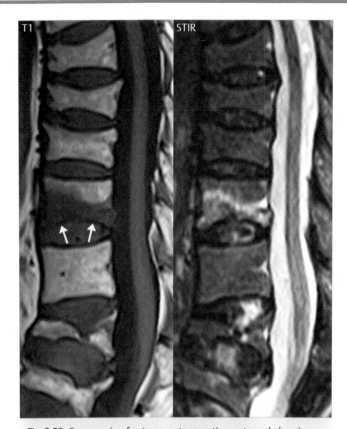

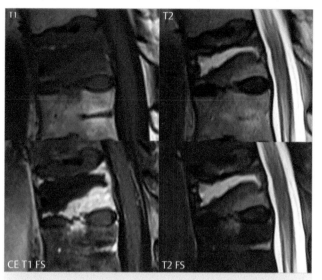

Fig. 3.59 Compression fractures, osteoporotic, acute and chronic (MR). There are compression deformities of T7–T10, T12, and L1. With the exception of T10, there is uniform high signal intensity (SI) fatty marrow within these vertebral bodies seen on the T1-weighted scan, with no edema (which would be seen as abnormal high SI) noted on STIR. These compression deformities are thus chronic. However, the inferior half of T10 demonstrates abnormal low SI on T1 (*small white arrows*) and corresponding high SI on STIR, consistent with edema and an acute compression fracture. The scan is typical of an osteoporotic elderly woman, with compression fractures at multiple levels.

Fig. 3.60 Compression fracture, osteoporotic, acute, the use of fat saturation and contrast enhancement. STIR and pre-contrast T1-weighted scans are most commonly used to detect marrow edema, with STIR being especially sensitive. Vertebral edema, as well as focal marrow replacement, is however not well demonstrated on T2-weighted fast spin echo (FSE) scans. This is due to both entities being high signal intensity (SI), and thus difficult to differentiate from normal high SI fatty marrow. With the application of fat saturation, T2-weighted FSE scans become sensitive to marrow edema, and provide higher in plane resolution and less sensitivity to motion artifacts as compared to STIR. Despite this improvement, STIR may still better demonstrate marrow edema, and is favored by many radiologists. Illustrated is an acute compression fracture of T12, with a large fluid collection (hemorrhage) therein, an uncommon finding but one occasionally seen with acute compression fractures. The marrow edema within T12 is well seen due to its low SI on the T1-weighted image, yet is isointense to normal marrow on the T2-weighted image. On the T2-weighted scan with fat saturation the edema is also easily recognized, due to the abnormal high signal intensity as compared to normal marrow. Note also that marrow edema enhances strikingly post-contrast, and is well identified on the post-contrast T1-weighted scan with fat saturation.

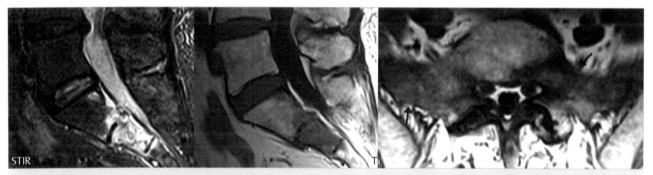

Fig. 3.61 Sacral insufficiency fracture. These fractures also occur in osteoporotic patients, typically with mild trauma. The fracture can be unilateral or bilateral, with marrow edema seen as low signal intensity on T1-weighted images and high signal intensity on STIR. In this instance the fracture is well seen on sagittal midline images, which is not always the case. A classic imaging presentation is edema bilaterally within the sacral alae, although often asymmetric, as seen on the axial T1-weighted scan (bilaterally, with low SI, *arrows*) at the S1 level. Dedicated imaging of the sacrum provides improved visualization, as opposed to the typical scan protocol as presented for lumbar imaging.

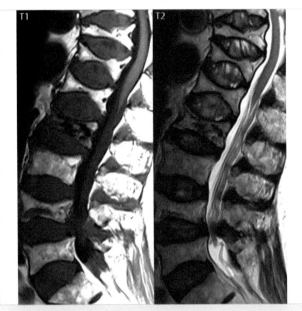

Fig. 3.62 Multiple compression fractures, chronic, lower thoracic and lumbar spine (MR). This 83-year-old woman has severe degenerative spine disease and has presented clinically on many occasions with intractable back pain. Chronic compression fractures are noted from T11–L5, with sparing in part of L3 and with varying loss of height of the remaining vertebral bodies. Note the very high SI marrow on the T1-weighted scan, reflecting fatty marrow. Evidence of prior vertebroplasty is noted at L2 and L4, with visualization of low SI bone cement on both pulse sequences, although more readily evident at this slice position within L2.

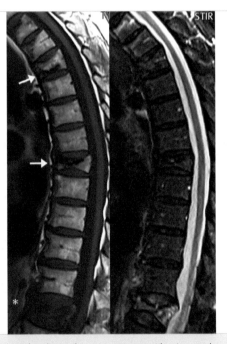

Fig. 3.63 Vertebroplasty. Changes consistent with prior vertebroplasty (*arrows*) are identified within T4 and T8. Bone cement, due to the lack of mobile protons, appears very low signal intensity (*black*) on all pulse sequences. Note that there is no edema demonstrated within either treated vertebral body, which is best confirmed by the lack of abnormal high SI on STIR. However, an acute compression fracture with edema is present at L1 (*asterisk*), with abnormal low SI marrow on T1 and high SI on STIR.

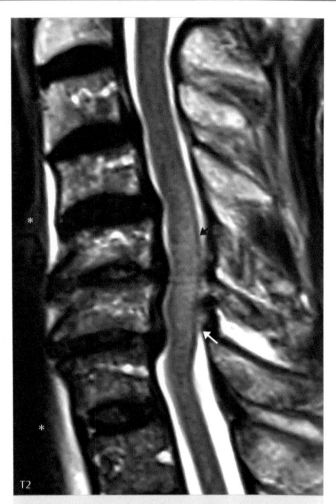

Fig. 3.64 Cord contusion, cervical spine. Extensive degenerative changes, and specifically narrowing of the spinal canal on that basis, can predispose a patient to cervical cord injury. This elderly patient presented with a traumatic cord injury, and on MR demonstrated extensive cord edema (*arrow*) in the mid- to lower cervical region, where the canal dimensions had been previously compromised by multilevel disk osteophyte complexes. The cord is also minimally expanded in this region. Note the presence of pre-vertebral fluid/hemorrhage (*asterisk*), confirming that substantial trauma occurred.

enhancement of the epidural venous plexus. In the cervical spine, the normal epidural venous plexus is prominent, and can be dilated adjacent to a disk herniation. Foraminal disk herniations in particular can be difficult to visualize, due to the relative isointensity of the disk to epidural venous plexus on axial gradient echo T2-weighted scans.

Symptoms from an acute cervical disk herniation can be radicular, due to a posterolateral or foraminal location (▶ Fig. 3.74), or myelopathic, with large central herniations. On high-resolution thin section axial gradient echo T2-weighted scans, the dorsal and ventral nerve roots, as they exit from the cervical cord, can be identified. Paired denticulate ligaments can also be commonly identified, interposed between the nerve roots. These consist of triangular ligament extensions with a broad base along the lateral margin of the cord and their apex attaching laterally to the dura.

As previously discussed, but worth repeating, there are seven cervical vertebrae and eight cervical nerves, C1–C8. The cervical nerves exit through the foramina above the corresponding numbered vertebrae, with C8 exiting in the foramen below the C7 vertebra. Thus, a posterolateral or foraminal disk herniation at C6–7 will cause compression of the C7 cervical nerve. Knowledge of the cervical dermatomes is important for correlation of

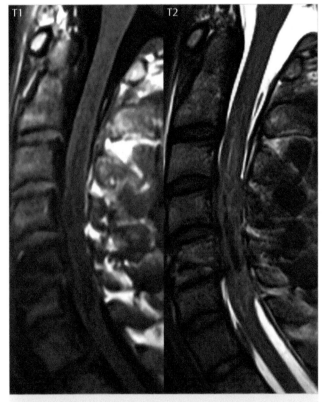

Fig. 3.65 Severe cord trauma, cervical spine. This young man became quadriplegic following a motor vehicle collision in which he was an unrestrained back seat passenger. There is cord swelling and abnormal cord signal consistent with edema spanning the levels of C2–C7. The subarachnoid space is effaced from C2–C6. Hypointense signal within the cord at the C4 and C5 levels on the T2-weighted scan is consistent with acute spinal cord hemorrhage. Patients with cord hemorrhage in acute injury typically do not improve clinically from that of their initial presentation. Fractures of the C5 and C6 vertebral bodies are identified, due to abnormal signal and loss of height, and were better characterized by CT (not shown).

clinical symptoms with anatomic findings, with pain diagrams distributed commonly to patients prior to the exam in many clinics. These are also very helpful in the thoracic and lumbar spine. The anatomic distribution of C6, C7, and C8 is easy to remember, with the C7 distribution including the middle finger, C6 including the thumb, and C8 including the fourth and fifth fingers.

An acute cervical disk herniation will be visualized as an anterior (or anterolateral or foraminal) epidural soft tissue mass (▶ Fig. 3.75). Close inspection of the cervical foramina is mandated, since a disk herniation in this position (▶ Fig. 3.76) is often much less evident than those that are central or paracentral in location. The abnormal soft tissue will be contiguous with the disk space, with the only exception being that of a free disk fragment. It should be noted, however, that the majority of free disk fragments will lie immediately adjacent to, and be inseparable from, the native disk. Disk herniations have signal intensity similar to, on both T1- and T2-weighted scans, the native disk. The focal nature of a disk herniation is used to differentiate this process from a disk bulge, with the latter often defined as a process involving 180 degrees or more of the disk circumference. In older patients, and those also involved long term in activities associated with marked motion of the cervical spine, asymptomatic chronic disk herniations are commonly observed (▶ Fig. 3.77).

Although often difficult in an individual patient to differentiate from an acute disk herniation, the presence of associated bony spurs extending from the vertebral body endplates can be used to identify a chronic disk herniation (▶ Fig. 3.78). These bony spurs occur due to bone remodeling, with elevation of the periosteum by a disk herniation and subsequent bone deposition. Myelopathic symptoms are more common with chronic disk herniations, with radicular symptoms common in acute disk herniations (▶ Fig. 3.79).

Hypertrophic endplate spurs, also referred to as diskosteophyte complexes, are commonly seen on both MR and CT, and are typically asymptomatic. Given how frequent these are—most older patients have at least mild multilevel disease—it is not surprising that these do not correlate well with symptoms. Disk-osteophyte complexes are felt to be the end result of a disk bulge, which is defined as circumferential expansion of the disk, specifically greater than 180 degrees (and not focal, as with a chronic disk herniation). In many instances the chronic nature of this process can be identified on MR, due to the presence of

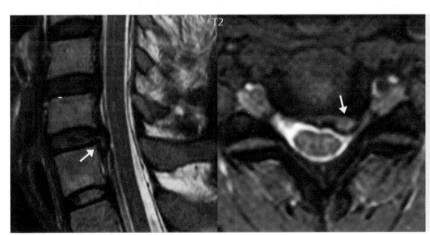

Fig. 3.66 Traumatic disk herniation, cervical spine. A posttraumatic disk herniation is noted (*arrows*) at a lower cervical level, paracentral and foraminal in position, with slight inferior migration relative to the disk space level seen best on the sagittal scan. There is mild deformity of the adjacent anterolateral cord seen on the axial scan.

associated broad based osteophytes (which manifest low signal intensity on all MR sequences) (▶ Fig. 3.80).

These osteophytes are well identified on CT, albeit the associated disk bulge is often poorly visualized. One special area of note in the cervical spine involves the uncovertebral joints. These small synovial lined joints (also known as the joints of Luschka) lie between the uncinated processes of the lower cervical vertebrae posteriorly and laterally, and allow for flexion and extension, while limiting lateral flexion. Uncovertebral joints are present from C3 to C7, with encroachment upon the foramina anteriorly due to degenerative involvement occurring from C2–3 to C6–7. Hypertrophy of the uncovertebral joint is not uncommon in older patients, often asymmetric when comparing side to side and, together with facet osteoarthritis (posteriorly), causes foraminal narrowing in the AP dimension

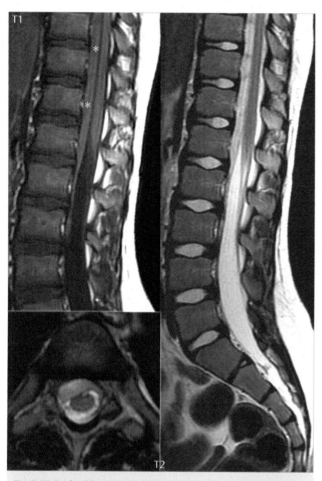

Fig. 3.67 Epidural hematoma, thoracolumbar spine. Sagittal images reveal a fluid collection (*asterisk*) anterior to the cord, causing posterior displacement and mild compression therein, which extends caudally to the L1–2 level. Superiorly, this extended to the C2–3 level (images not shown). The hematoma is nearly isointense with CSF on the T2-weighted scan, but well seen on the T1-weighted scan due to its intermediate signal intensity. The gradual tapering of the fluid collection in the lumbar region defines the fluid as extradural in location. On the axial T2-weighted scan at the level of the conus, there is a sufficient difference in signal intensity between the epidural hematoma and more posterior CSF to allow good delineation. There is only mild compression/deformity of the cord at this level. This epidural hematoma was spontaneous, with an acute clinical presentation and no known etiology.

(▶ Fig. 3.81). Disk space narrowing is an additional cause of foraminal narrowing, decreasing the height of the neural foramen, with the end result of all these factors being nerve root compression.

Degenerative foraminal narrowing is common in older patients. The bony encroachment of the foramina is well visualized on CT, with sagittal reformatted images important in this regard. On CT it is readily evident that the osteophyte commonly extends into the mid-portion of the foramen, dividing the foramen into an upper and lower portion. Keeping this in mind, it is not surprising that, on thin section axial MR images, depiction of the foramen can be limited and misleading. With a large osteophyte lying in the mid-portion of the foramen, unless axial imaging is performed with very thin sections, partial volume imaging will lead to poor visualization of the encroachment. In the cervical spine, the standard MR sequences used for evaluation of the neural foramina include thin section T2*-weighted gradient echo imaging in the axial plane (▶ Fig. 3.82) and fast spin echo T1- and T2-weighted imaging in the sagittal plane. Due to the anterolateral, and slight inferior, course of the neural foramina, oblique sagittal images are, however, best for visualization of the foramina on MR, and should be routinely acquired.

Ossification of the posterior longitudinal ligament is an uncommon cause of acquired cervical spinal stenosis. There is an increased incidence in Asian patients, in particular Japanese. Other, more common etiologies of cervical spinal stenosis include ligamentous infolding and facet joint hypertrophy. As with all cases of spinal stenosis, patients are at greater risk for traumatic spinal cord injury. The posterior longitudinal ligament is prominent, with low signal intensity on both T1- and T2-weighted scans (▶ Fig. 3.83), and in some instances with intermediate signal intensity centrally within focally prominent areas of ligamentous infolding. Involvement is multilevel and can be continuous or segmental. Spinal cord compression is seen with more prominent disease involvement.

Degenerative (acquired) spinal stenosis, previously discussed in general terms, is caused by advanced degenerative disk

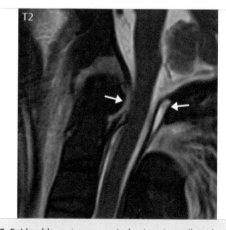

Fig. 3.68 Epidural hematoma, cervical spine. A small epidural hematoma (*arrows*) is seen both anterior and posterior to the cord, at the level of the foramen magnum, on a midline sagittal image. There is mild posterior displacement of the cord, which is compressed anteriorly. Note also the extensive abnormal prevertebral soft tissue, representing a combination of hemorrhage and edema.

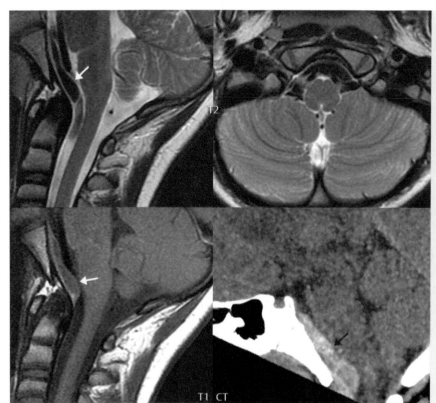

Fig. 3.69 Retroclival epidural hematoma, tectorial membrane injury. A moderate in size epidural hematoma is seen just posterior to the clivus, with low signal intensity on T2- and intermediate signal intensity on T1-weighted images, consistent with deoxyhemoglobin (*white arrows*). CSF flow voids make recognition more difficult on the axial T2-weighted image. The epidural hemorrhage is also well visualized on sagittal reformatted CT, with high density (*black arrow*). No overt tear of the tectorial membrane is seen. This injury occurs in the pediatric population, with high speed motor vehicle accidents the most common cause. In this instance, CT and MR are relatively equivalent for diagnosis of the epidural hematoma, with MR superior for detection of accompanying tectorial membrane injury.

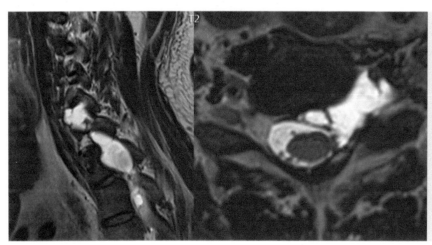

Fig. 3.70 Brachial plexus injury, chronic. Sagittal and axial T2-weighted scans demonstrate focal abnormal high signal intensity within the neural foramina on the left at two levels, consistent with CSF. Pseudomeningoceles occur as a result of trauma due to a tear in the meningeal sheath surrounding the nerves, with resultant CSF extravasation. In this instance there has been bone remodeling (with enlargement of the fluid spaces) due to the long-standing nature, with the injury having occurred at birth in this 49-year-old patient.

disease, with the latter process also referred to by the term spondylosis (▶ Fig. 3.84). Contributing factors include decreased disk height with thickening and buckling of the intraspinal ligaments, prominence of the posterior longitudinal ligament and ligamentum flavum, disk bulges, herniations, and osteophytic spurs (anterior to the thecal sac), and hypertrophy of the facet joints (posterior to the thecal sac). Symptom onset is skewed toward the older population, and to some degree thus differentiated from acute disk herniations. Symptoms are myelopathic and include progressive/intermittent numbness, weakness of the upper extremities, pain, abnormal reflexes, muscle wasting (involving the interosseous muscles of the hand), and staggering gait. Although commonly not quantified, defined measurements are established for spinal stenosis, with evaluation best on axial images. Normal is defined as >13 mm, borderline being 10 to 13 mm (these patients may experience symptoms), and <10 mm diagnostic of cervical spinal canal stenosis. The most commonly affected levels are C4–5, 5–6, and 6–7, with multilevel involvement common. In mild spinal canal stenosis the ventral subarachnoid space will be effaced. With more severe disease there will be cord flattening. In advanced disease, myelomalacia, specifically edema, gliosis, and cystic changes can be present.

Thoracic Spine

Disk herniations in the thoracic region are less common, as compared to their counterparts in the cervical and lumbar regions. Clinically, radicular symptoms with a dermatomal distribution may be seen (▶ Fig. 3.85). From published literature

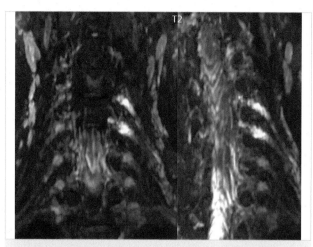

Fig. 3.71 Traumatic brachial plexus injury. This 17-year-old male adolescent presents 5 months following shoulder trauma, with mild dysfunction. A stretch injury is identified on the left, involving the proximal C5 and C6 anterior rami of the brachial plexus, with prominence (thickening) and high signal intensity on T2-weighted images due to fluid and edema. Thick section MIP images are presented, in both the coronal and sagittal oblique planes.

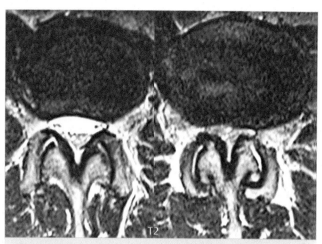

Fig. 3.72 Degenerative spinal stenosis, lumbar spine. At L2–3, the first axial level illustrated, there is mild facet osteoarthritis without significant spinal canal stenosis. At L3–4, the second axial level illustrated, there is moderate to severe spinal canal stenosis due to a combination of moderate bilateral facet osteoarthritis, ligamentum flavum buckling/infolding, and a mild disk osteophyte complex. In regard to the latter, note the much larger diameter of the L3–4 disk as compared to L2–3.

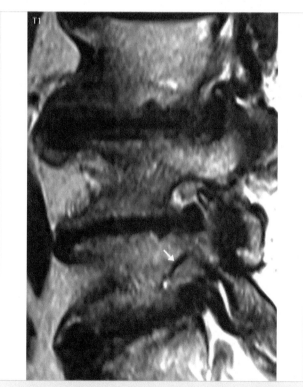

Fig. 3.73 Degenerative neural foraminal narrowing, lumbar spine. On sagittal imaging at L5–S1, a disk osteophyte complex extends posteriorly and obliterates the inferior portion of the neural foramen, resulting in compression of the L5 nerve (*arrow*). Note the lack of normal fat (circumferential to the nerve), which is obliterated in both the anteroposterior or superoinferior dimensions. At L4–5, one level above, a similar process is seen, but less severe with only mild compromise of the neural foramen, with fat preserved both anteriorly and inferiorly to the nerve.

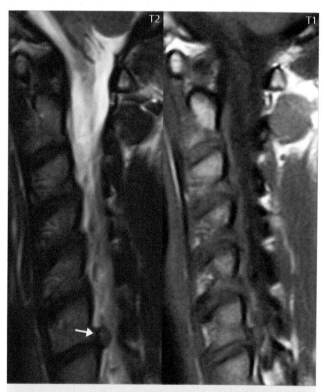

Fig. 3.74 Foraminal disk herniation, cervical spine (sagittal plane). Close inspection of sagittal images can substantially improve detection of foraminal herniations, which may otherwise go unrecognized. A C6–7 disk extrusion, foraminal in location, is easily identified in this patient both on T2- (*arrow*) and T1-weighted off-midline sagittal images. Oblique foraminal views offer a further improvement in depiction and detection of cervical foraminal disease, although unfortunately not performed by most sites.

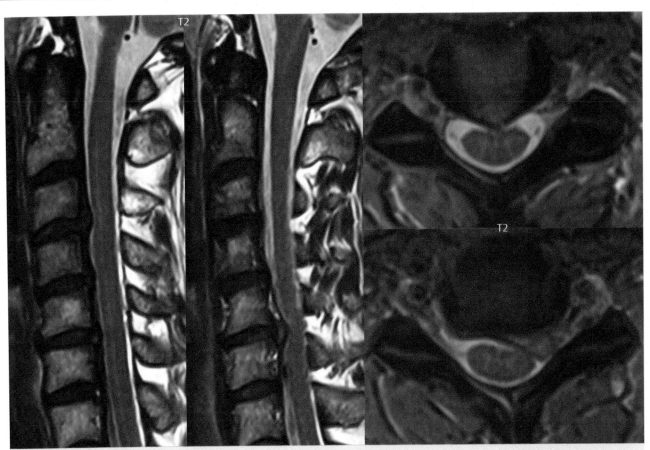

Fig. 3.75 Central and paracentral disk herniations, cervical spine. Sagittal and axial images reveal presumed acute (recent) disk herniations at C3–4 and C5–6. Note the relative absence of associated osteophytes on the sagittal images. The herniation at C3–4 is central in location, that at C5–6 paracentral with some extension into the foramen on the left. Both disk herniations are likely extrusions on the basis of the sagittal images.

series, symptomatic thoracic disk herniations are most commonly present in the lower thoracic spine, from T9–10 to T11–12. Acute cord compression with myelopathy is rare.

The imaging evaluation of thoracic disk herniations is the province of MR. Diagnosis requires thin sections with high image quality, and specifically implementation of strategies to minimize motion artifacts due to the heart, respiration, and CSF pulsation (▶ Fig. 3.86). With excellent image quality, sensitivity is high even to very small disk herniations. In the past, specific level localization on MR was difficult; however, today, high-quality sagittal scout images of the cervicothoracic region can be acquired, with these mandatory for correct level identification (see ▶ Fig. 3.85).

There is a high incidence of chronic asymptomatic small thoracic disk herniations on routine MR imaging (▶ Fig. 3.87). Deformity of the cord contour is also common, often in the absence of any clinical symptoms and occurring even with very small herniations. In this regard it should be kept in mind that the MR evaluation is performed in only one position (supine), and is not physiologic, with disk herniations when the patient is upright, and particularly in flexion, likely causing impact upon nerves and the cord not seen by MR.

Lumbar Spine

Tears of the annulus fibrosus are of three types. Concentric tears (type I) are parallel to the curvature of the outer margin of the disk. Radial tears (type II) involve all layers of the annulus from the nucleus to the surface. Transverse tears (type III) cross Sharpey fibers, which lie at the periphery of the annulus adjacent to the vertebral endplate. There is a tendency to interpret any focus of abnormal high signal intensity within the annulus as a tear. In the absence of definitive studies, this likely is overcalling annular tears. From clinical experience, all three types of tears are seen on MR imaging, although a tear that is easily identifiable as a distinct type is less common. Enhancement of annular tears is noted following intravenous contrast administration, due to enhancement of granulation tissue that forms as part of the normal reparative process. Larger concentric tears are well seen on thin section axial images, both due to T2 hyperintensity (▶ Fig. 3.88) and abnormal enhancement.

A disk bulge is broad based and circumferential, and thus differentiated from a disk herniation which is defined as a focal lesion. Often the definition used to differentiate the two entities is that the extent of a disk bulge (circumference wise) is greater than 180 degrees. A disk bulge will extend beyond the margin of the adjacent vertebral endplates. These findings occur early in disk degeneration, due to laxity within the annulus fibrosus. A disk bulge can narrow the spinal canal and the inferior part of the neural foramen. In chronic disease, the bulge is often accompanied by an osteophyte along its margins, thus the term "disk osteophyte complex."

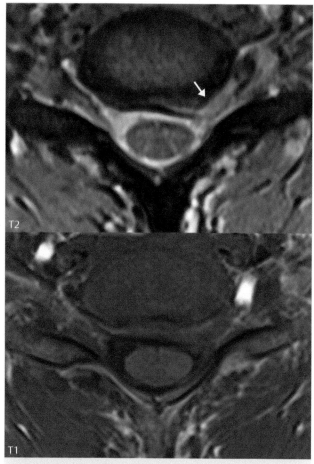

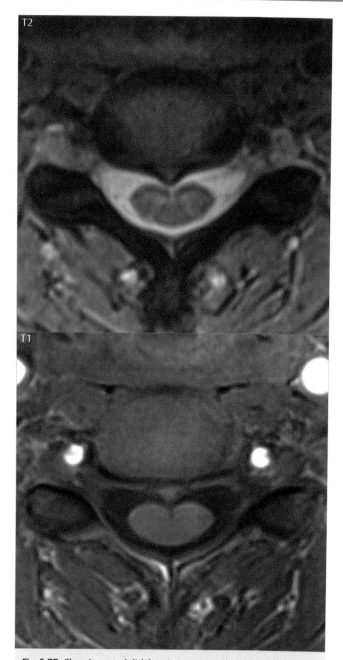

Fig. 3.76 Foraminal disk herniation, cervical spine (axial plane). Foraminal disk herniations in the cervical spine may be difficult to detect, due to isointensity with the venous plexus within the neural foramen on gradient echo T2-weighted scans. Careful image inspection, including all sequences and planes, is mandatory, together with a high sensitivity to abnormal soft tissue (disk material) within the foramen. In this instance, the disk herniation with high signal intensity (*arrow*) on the gradient echo T2-weighted scan and intermediate signal intensity on the corresponding T1-weighted scan is relatively well visualized. Although seldom used in this application, post-contrast scans allow exquisite visualization of cervical foraminal disk herniations, which appear as nonenhancing soft tissue easily differentiated from the intense enhancement of the abundant venous plexus.

Fig. 3.77 Chronic central disk herniation, cervical spine. Asymptomatic small and large chronic cervical disk herniations are a common finding on screening MR examinations. Illustrated is one such small central disk herniation. Without inspection of axial images above and below, or the sagittal images for accompanying osteophytes, it is not possible to confirm such a herniation as either acute or chronic. There is mild associated cord flattening. Note that the central "H" of gray matter is well identified with higher signal intensity than more peripheral white matter on this axial gradient echo T2-weighted scan obtained at 3 T.

A disk protrusion is herniation of the nucleus pulposus through a (small) tear in the annulus, contained by the outer fibers of the annulus. It is easily differentiated from a bulge on axial imaging, with focal extension of disk material visualized beyond the margin of the vertebral endplates. A disk protrusion will be largest at its base, the major differentiating point from a disk extrusion (which is narrower at the base than the dome).

A disk extrusion is herniation of the nucleus pulposus through a ruptured annulus. Extruded material remains in contiguity with the parent disk. With an extrusion, the largest diameter of the herniation will be distant from the native disk, with the neck (the area immediately contiguous to the native disk) smaller in diameter (see ▶ Fig. 3.88). Even without surgery, granulation tissue forms surrounding such a disk herniation, with a thin line of enhancement seen depicting this tissue

on post-contrast scans. In time, with conservative therapy only, there can be a substantial reduction in size of the disk herniation, and in many cases complete resorption (▶ Fig. 3.89).

The term disk herniation is used to encompass both disk protrusion and extrusion. Ninety percent of lumbar disk herniations occur at L4–5 or L5–S1 (▶ Fig. 3.90), with the majority of the remainder at L3–4. Disk herniations are further defined

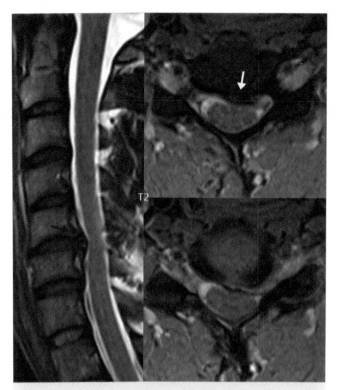

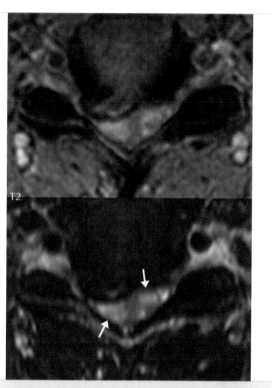

Fig. 3.78 Disk herniation, chronic, cervical spine. The presence of an osteophyte just superior or inferior to a disk herniation, often visualized best on sagittal images, implies that the herniation is chronic. On the axial gradient echo T2-weighted scan, at C5–6, a left paracentral and foraminal herniation is visualized with high signal intensity disk material surrounded by a thin low signal intensity rim. This herniation is bordered superiorly by a prominent osteophyte (*small black arrow*), visualized both on the sagittal FSE T2-weighted scan and—as low signal intensity (*white arrow*)—on the axial gradient echo T2-weighted scan, covering the high signal intensity disk material immediately below.

Fig. 3.79 Chronic cervical disk herniation with cord compression and signal abnormality. The chronic herniation seen on FSE (upper) and gradient recalled echo (GRE) (lower) T2-weighted images severely narrows the neural foramen on the right. There is moderate narrowing of the foramen on the left, degenerative in nature and unrelated to the disk herniation. The cord is deformed (compressed), with focal abnormal high signal intensity (*small white arrows*) consistent with gliosis seen on both scans.

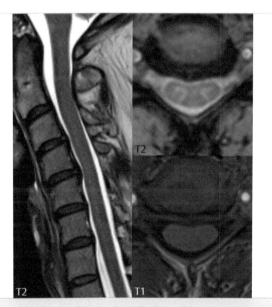

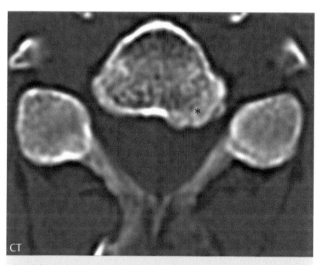

Fig. 3.81 Uncovertebral hypertrophy. Degeneration of the uncovertebral joint is common, leading to a broad osteophyte (*asterisk*) in a characteristic position, as illustrated on axial CT. This process can lead both to foraminal narrowing and mild effacement of the thecal sac, the latter in a paracentral location.

Fig. 3.80 Mild cervical degenerative findings. There is reversal of the normal cervical lordosis. Minimal disk osteophyte complexes are noted at C4–5, C5–6, and C6–7. There is mild to moderate flattening of the cord (versus its normal elliptical appearance in cross-section), at the C4–5 level, a finding well seen on axial images.

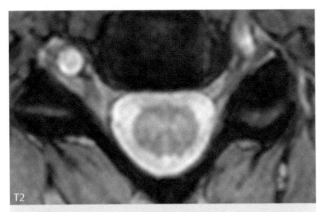

Fig. 3.82 Degenerative neural foraminal narrowing, cervical spine. On this gradient echo axial T2-weighted scan, the right neural foramen is widely patent, with moderate neural foraminal narrowing on the left. Mild facet osteoarthritis and disk degenerative disease (an osteophyte) contribute in this instance to the foraminal narrowing.

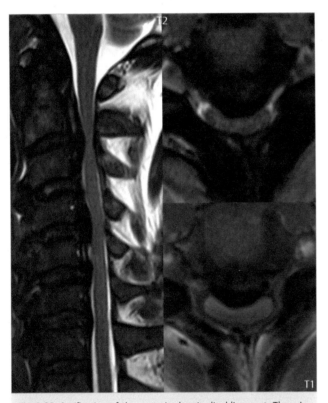

Fig. 3.83 Ossification of the posterior longitudinal ligament. There is multilevel effacement of the thecal sac, with cord compression, most prominent at C2–3 and C4–5. Axial imaging well depicts the densely ossified posterior longitudinal ligament (with low signal intensity on both T2- and T1-weighted scans), which at the level illustrated (C2–3) produces marked cord deformity and moderate to severe central spinal canal stenosis.

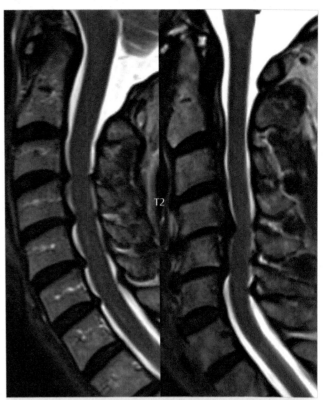

Fig. 3.84 Moderate to severe cervical spondylosis. Osteophyte distribution within the cervical spine directly varies with spinal axis mobility. The more mobile lower cervical spine is affected initially with superior spread as disease worsens. Exams from two patients are illustrated, with the first demonstrating moderately advanced degenerative disease with disk osteophyte complexes at the C3–C7 levels. The osteophytes in this instance result in mild central spinal canal stenosis—note the lack of CSF surrounding the cord at the involved levels. In the second patient, there is severe central spinal canal stenosis at C4–5. An osteophyte compresses the thecal sac, obliterating the CSF space both anterior and posterior to the cord, and markedly flattens the cord. Additional common degenerative findings, present in this patient, include disk space height loss at the C4–5 and C5–6 levels and a slight anterolisthesis of C2 on C3.

by their location: central, paracentral, subarticular (lateral recess), foraminal, and extraforaminal (far lateral). A small central protrusion may cause no symptoms, with the exiting nerve roots unaffected. A paracentral protrusion or extrusion causes symptoms due to compression of the exiting nerve root, for example S1 with an L5–S1 disk herniation (▶ Fig. 3.91).

Foraminal disk herniations commonly compress the root above, numerically in the lumbar spine, for example L5 with an L5–S1 disk herniation. Extraforaminal (far lateral) disk herniations may or may not impinge upon the spinal nerves. A lateral osteophyte is commonly mistaken for an extraforaminal disk herniation, and should always be kept in mind. Central and paracentral disk herniations are most common, with a foraminal herniation slightly less common, and lateral herniations the least common of all. Findings involving the nerves themselves include posterior displacement (whether within the thecal sac itself, or subsequent to the exit of the nerve), compression, nerve root swelling (edema; which can be seen by either size of the nerve or slight high signal intensity on a T2-weighted scan), and abnormal contrast enhancement. Intravenous contrast is not commonly administered for evaluation of disk herniations preoperatively, and thus experience is limited. However, with a disk herniation acutely compressing upon a nerve, enhancement of a relatively long segment of the nerve within the thecal sac is not uncommon. This enhancement may persist, with the long-term temporal appearance not well studied. The presence of enhancement does, regardless, provide supporting evidence for the clinical significance of a compressive lesion.

The term free disk fragment is used interchangeably with sequestered disk. A free disk fragment is defined as herniated disk material that is separate from the parent disk. Migration of

disk material can occur either superiorly or inferiorly relative to the level of the parent disk (▶ Fig. 3.92), or into the neural foramen. A distinctive finding on MR is that a free disk fragment will have slight hyperintensity on T2-weighted scans when

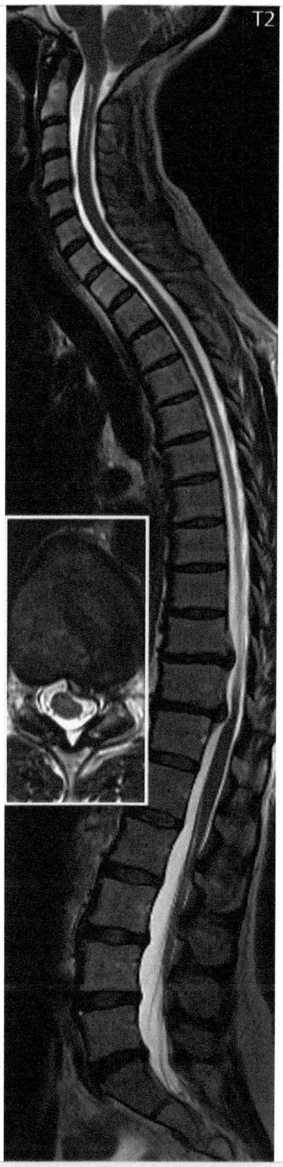

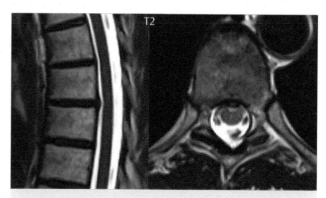

Fig. 3.86 Small central thoracic disk herniation, pitfalls of imaging technique. A small central disk herniation is seen in the midthoracic spine on thin section (3-mm) sagittal and axial T2-weighted FSE images, a standard imaging approach at both 1.5 T and 3 T. Such findings are commonly incidental, representing chronic small disk herniations without any clinical correlate, although in any one case it cannot be determined whether the lesion is acute or chronic. However, detection by the radiologist demands close attention to and inspection of the images, given that the lesion is small and that CSF pulsation artifact leads to an inhomogeneous appearance to adjacent CSF (CSF "flow voids"), in particular on axial scans.

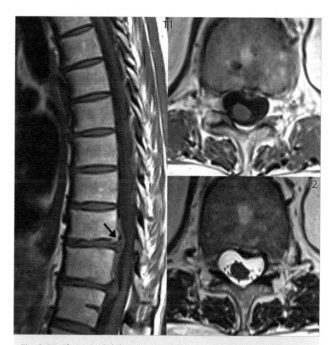

Fig. 3.87 Thoracic disk herniation, chronic. A sagittal T1-weighted image of the thoracic spine, along with axial T1-and T2-weighted images at T10–11 are illustrated. Note the small osteophyte (*arrow*) superior to the herniation at T10–11, favoring that the disk herniation is chronic. This small chronic left paracentral herniation also causes mild deformity of the adjacent cord, seen on the axial images. Attention to imaging technique is particularly critical in the thoracic spine, in order to achieve high quality, artifact free, images.

Fig. 3.85 Thoracic disk herniation, definitive vertebral body count, and level localization. Modern MR scanners can provide rapidly a sagittal scout of the entire spine, as illustrated. High-resolution images can also be fused from the cervical, thoracic, and lumbar regions, a process known as image composing. This has the advantage of definitive identification of vertebral body count. In the example shown, disk herniations are seen at T10–11 and T11–12, with a high-resolution axial image of the left paracentral disk herniation at T11–12 also presented. Note the mild deformity/flattening of the adjacent cord. Prior to the availability of these techniques, definitive vertebral body identification was often not possible on MR in the thoracic spine, due to the absence of a true count from C1, and in the lumbar spine due to the relatively high incidence of transitional vertebrae (and difficulty thus in defining the L5–S1 level).

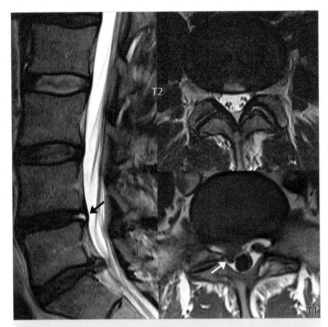

Fig. 3.88 Right paracentral L5–S1 disk extrusion. There is partial disk desiccation at L3–4, which demonstrates lower signal intensity on the sagittal T2-weighted scan than the disk above and a less well-defined intranuclear cleft. There is both disk desiccation and mild loss of disk space height at L4–5 and L5–S1. An annular tear (*small black arrow*), with high signal intensity on T2-weighted scans in both the sagittal and axial planes, is noted at L4–5. At L5–S1, seen in both planes, a disk extrusion (defined by the broadest diameter of the herniation being distant from the otherwise normal disk margin) compresses and posteriorly displaces the right S1 nerve root *(white arrow)*.

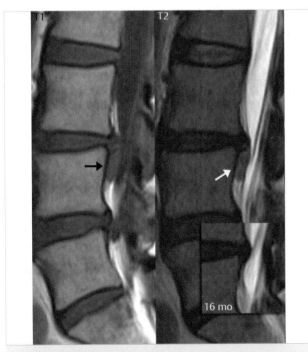

Fig. 3.89 Resorption of a disk herniation with conservative therapy. An inferiorly migrated disk herniation is identified at L3–4 (*black arrow*). This likely represents a sequestered disk due to the slight high signal intensity on the T2-weighted scan (*white arrow*). On the follow-up scan, obtained 16 months later, there is a return to near normal appearance, with little residual disk herniation identified.

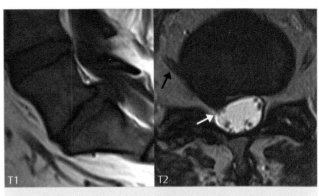

Fig. 3.90 Mild compression of the thecal sac and the adjacent nerve therein by a paracentral disk herniation, lumbar spine. In this patient, the thecal sac extends more caudally than usual. On the axial image, a right paracentral disk herniation at L5–S1 displaces posteriorly the right S1 *nerve* (*white arrow*) within the thecal sac. Dorsal and ventral nerve roots can be identified for both S1 and S2 bilaterally, within the thecal sac, and L5 (*black arrow*) is identified already having exited the neural foramen.

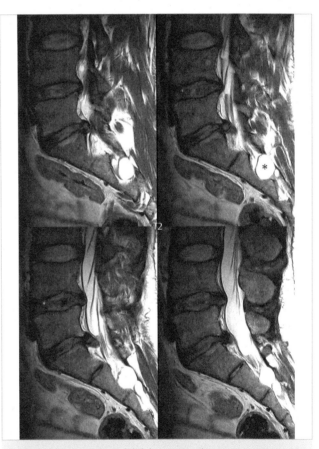

Fig. 3.91 L5–S1 paracentral disk herniation, thin section imaging. T2-weighted sagittal images (four contiguous sections) at 3 T are illustrated, with voxel dimension of $0.6 \times 0.5 \times 2.4$ mm^3. The SNR at 3 T makes possible high in-plane resolution, thin-section imaging, with improved depiction of disk herniations (which are generally small in size, compared to the slice thickness employed in MR), together with their relationship to adjacent nerves. For example, the disk herniation (*white arrow*) is adjacent to, but does not substantially displace (in this view), the S1 nerve, seen just posteriorly (on the third image). Incidentally noted are several type II spinal meningeal cysts (Tarlov cysts, *asterisk*) involving sacral nerve roots.

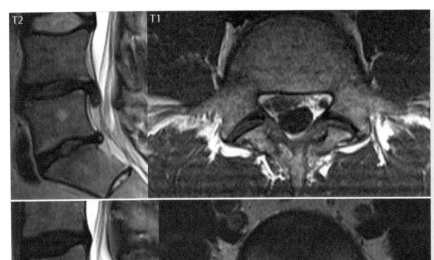

Fig. 3.92 Disk extrusion with inferior migration, lumbar spine. In the first patient (upper set of images), a disk extrusion is noted at L4–5 on the sagittal image, with inferior migration. The axial scan localizes the herniation to a right paracentral location, with the L5 nerve on the right difficult to identify, due to displacement laterally by disk material, which obliterates the normal epidural fat planes. In the second patient (lower set of images), a disk extrusion with inferior migration is identified at L5–S1, with slight hyperintensity to the native disk on the sagittal T2-weighted scan, suggestive of a disk fragment (sequestered disk). On the axial scan this disk herniation is noted to be both central and right paracentral in location, compressing the right S1 nerve as it exits the thecal sac.

compared with the native disk. Granulation tissue surrounding the fragment will demonstrate enhancement post-contrast (▶ Fig. 3.93). It should be noted that a fragment will typically lie immediately contiguous to the parent disk (or the nonsequestered portion of the disk herniation), and is almost never seen to be physically separate. Thus, when there is extensive migration of disk material, the possibility of a free fragment is likely, and should be suggested.

Degenerative changes of the intervertebral disk and adjacent endplates can occur at any level in the spine, but they are most often encountered in the lumbar spine (on MR) with the discussion focusing therein. The earliest visualized degenerative change in a disk is the loss of a distinct intranuclear cleft as seen on sagittal T2-weighted scans. Subsequent changes include loss of hydration (decreased signal intensity on T2-weighted scans, a sensitive indicator of early disk degenerative disease) and loss of disk height. With the exception of trauma, disk herniation in the absence of degenerative changes is very unusual. A vacuum intervertebral disk is a degenerated disk that contains gas within clefts of the annulus fibrosus and nucleus pulposus. These are more common in the lumbar spine and in elderly patients. Vacuum disks are visualized on CT as very low-density (gas) collections within the disk. On MR, corresponding linear areas of low signal intensity (signal void) on T1- and T2-weighted scans are seen.

A synovial cyst is a small, round or ovoid, fluid-containing lesion associated with (and immediately adjacent to) a degenerated facet joint, most often seen in the lumbar region. When located medially, these can cause radicular pain by compression of a nerve root (thus mimicking a disk herniation clinically), and commonly cause some compression of the thecal sac (▶ Fig. 3.94). Recognition of the relationship to the facet joint is

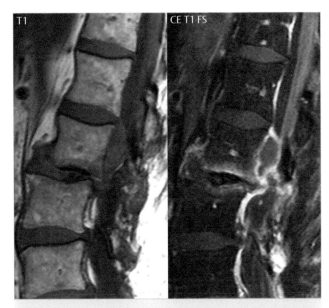

Fig. 3.93 Large sequestered (free) disk fragment. In this postoperative case, disk material has migrated from the parent disk (L2–3) superiorly to lie posterior to the L2 vertebral body. There is compression of the thecal sac, with peripheral enhancement of this sequestered disk delineating surrounding granulation tissue. There is a mild retrolisthesis of L2 on L3, with the prior bilateral laminectomy at both L3 and L4 not well visualized on the images presented.

important for diagnosis. On MR, the appearance is variable due to the specific fluid content. Enhancement of the cyst capsule is characteristic. On CT, synovial cysts can appear hypo- to hyperdense, and may be calcified.

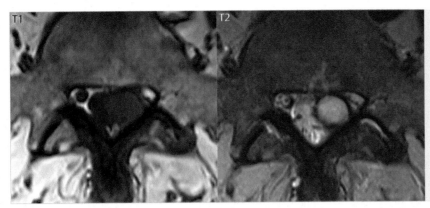

Fig. 3.94 Synovial cyst. On axial images, a large cystic lesion is seen medial to the left facet joint at L5–S1, compressing both the adjacent thecal sac as well as the left S1 nerve root in the lateral recess.

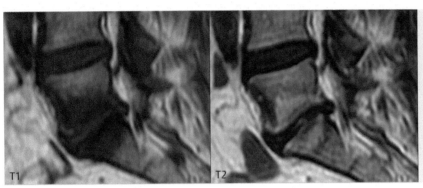

Fig. 3.95 Endplate degenerative changes, type 1. On sagittal images, there is low signal intensity involving the vertebral endplates adjacent to the L5–S1 disk space on the T1-weighted scan, with corresponding high signal intensity on the T2-weighted scan. These findings are consistent with edema, as seen in type 1 endplate degenerative disease. Note the accompanying loss of disk space height, also degenerative in nature.

Endplate Degenerative Changes

Endplate degenerative changes are common, and occur immediately adjacent to the disk space. These may involve only a segment of the endplate, or its entirety. At degenerative levels there is typically involvement of both the endplate above and below, although mild changes on one side only can be seen. Type 1, 2, and 3 endplate degenerative changes were described in the late 1980s by Michael Modic, one of the early pioneers in spine MR, and so are often referred to as Modic type changes. The discussion that follows is specifically tailored to the evaluation of the spine on T2-weighted scans with fat saturation.

Otherwise, type 1 and 2 endplate changes may be difficult to visualize on T2-weighted scans, and do not show the findings subsequently described. Decreased signal intensity on T1- and increased on T2-weighted scans characterize type 1, which represent edematous changes (▶ Fig. 3.95). Type 1 endplate changes enhance postcontrast. Two important entities should be considered in differential diagnosis. Metastatic disease has a similar signal intensity appearance (low on T1-, and high on T2-weighted scans), but is typically a more focal lesion, with isolated involvement of the endplate uncommon (and the disease characterized by the multiplicity of lesions). There is also some resemblance on imaging between type 1 endplate degenerative disease and disk space infection with accompanying osteomyelitis. Both entities exhibit edema within the endplate. However, in infection, the involvement of the adjacent vertebral body strictly parallels the disk, the demarcation between the disk and vertebral body is often lost, fluid pockets (pus) should be present within the disk, and a paraspinous mass will also be present.

Increased signal intensity on T1- and signal intensity paralleling fat on T2-weighted scans characterize type 2 endplate changes, which correspond to fatty infiltration (▶ Fig. 3.96). Type 2 endplate changes are much more common than type 1. A mixed pattern, with both type 1 and 2 changes in the same endplate is common. Type 3 corresponds to bony sclerosis, which is much less common than the other two endplate changes and has low signal intensity on both T1- and T2-weighted scans. Vertebral endplate signal intensity changes are a common finding in patients with low back pain; however, the correlation between clinical symptoms and imaging findings is poor.

Schmorl Node

A Schmorl node is a prolapse of the nucleus pulposus through the vertebral body endplate into the medullary space of the body (due to axial loading). In a sense, it represents herniation of disk material in the craniocaudal dimension, through the vertebral endplate, as opposed to that more traditionally considered posteriorly, involving the annulus fibrosus. Schmorl nodes are typically asymptomatic. On CT, they are depicted with a sclerotic rim, contiguous with the endplate. The signal intensity of the central portion of the lesion is somewhat variable on MR, although always with lower signal intensity on T1-weighted images relative to nearby normal fatty marrow. The sclerotic rim is typically well identified on MR, as a thin irregular low signal intensity line (on all pulse sequences) (▶ Fig. 3.97). Contrast enhancement along the periphery is typical, likely due to the presence of granulation tissue. An essential feature is the location immediately adjacent to the disk space. Surrounding focal endplate changes (edema) are common.

Scheuermann Disease

In Scheuermann disease there is an accentuated thoracic kyphosis, with multiple (three or more contiguous levels) mildly wedged thoracic vertebrae (▶ Fig. 3.98). These findings are accompanied by endplate irregularity, multiple Schmorl nodes, and disk space narrowing, with the latter greatest anteriorly. Disk desiccation will be present on MR. Multiple disk herniations may also be noted. This entity is felt to be due to chronic repetitive trauma in skeletally immature individuals.

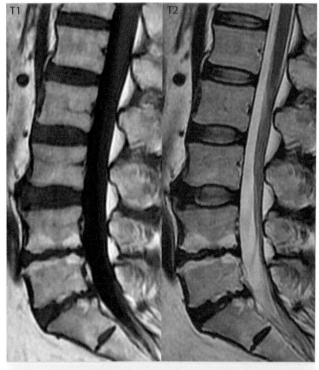

Fig. 3.96 Endplate degenerative changes, type 2. Sagittal T1- and T2-weighted images reveal abnormal high signal intensity, reflecting fatty replacement, within the vertebral endplates adjacent to the L4–5 disk, consistent with type 2 endplate degenerative disease. Note the additional degenerative changes at this level including loss of disk space height and endplate irregularity.

3.4.3 Abnormalities of Vertebral Alignment

Spondylolisthesis (Anterolisthesis)

Spondylolisthesis is the forward slippage of one vertebral body relative to the adjacent more inferior (distal) body (▶ Fig. 3.99). It is very easy to evaluate vertebral alignment on sagittal reformatted CT or sagittal MR images, and this is an important part of every diagnostic read. The common causes of spondylolisthesis include degenerative disease (specifically involving the facet joints), spondylolysis, and surgery or trauma. Attention should be paid to evaluation of the neural foramina on off midline sagittal images, with the anterior slippage narrowing the neural foramen (causing a more horizontal orientation) and potentially causing nerve root impingement. Narrowing of the spinal canal is also seen with degenerative spondylolisthesis, although usually not severe unless the slippage is great. Anterolistheses are routinely graded in regard to the degree of subluxation, with grade 1 being up to one-fourth of the vertebral body, grade 2 between one-fourth and one-half, grade 3 between one-half and three-fourths, and grade 4 (which is rare) greater than three-fourths (▶ Fig. 3.100). Not surprisingly, most anteriolithesesare grade 1.

Spondylolysis

Spondylolysis is defined as interruption of the bony pars interarticularis, with controversy over the years in terms of the etiology of this lesion (congenital vs. traumatic). On the basis of our experience, spondylolysis is the result of trauma. Most cases are chronic, and observed in adults. On rare occasion, acute lesions are noted in the adolescent population, typically an athletic injury. In this instance the imaging appearance is quite different, with the fracture line often indistinct, and on MR edema seen in the pars on both sides of the fracture line. Although reported to be either unilateral or bilateral, spondylolysis is most common to be bilateral (in its chronic presentation), and to involve the lower lumbar spine. Bilateral involvement allows motion of the posterior elements relative to the adjacent vertebrae, specifically the superior and inferior facets at the involved level move independently. The superior facet remains attached to the vertebral body, and the inferior facet moves with the more inferior level. The interruption of the bony pars is best seen on sagittal reformatted CT (▶ Fig. 3.101).

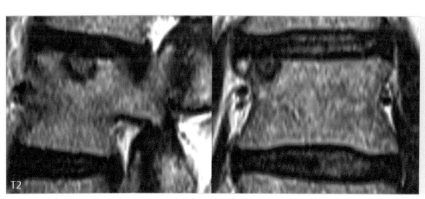

Fig. 3.97 Schmorl node. Sagittal and coronal images reveal a small lesion, immediately adjacent to the disk space, involving the endplate of a lumbar vertebral body. There is low signal intensity surrounding the lesion at its interface with the vertebra, reflecting bony sclerosis. These findings are consistent with a Schmorl node, which represents herniation of disk material vertically through a weakened vertebral body endplate, chronic in this instance (without adjacent vertebral body edema).

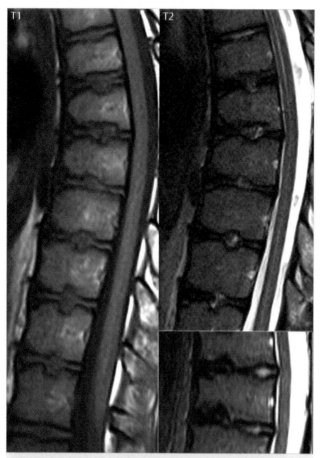

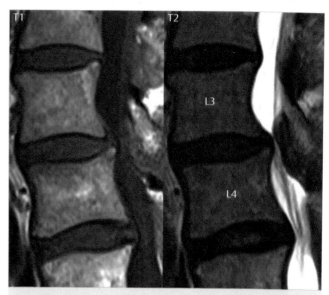

Fig. 3.99 Degenerative spondylolisthesis, grade 1. Anterior slippage of a vertebral body relative to that immediately below will result in some degree of canal compromise if there is not an accompanying spondylolysis. In this instance, there is severe central spinal canal stenosis at L3–4, despite the anterolisthesis being only grade 1. This was due to accompanying facet osteoarthritis and prominence of the ligamentum flavum (best evaluated on axial imaging, not presented).

Fig. 3.98 Scheuermann disease. Sagittal images in this adolescent patient demonstrate an exaggerated kyphosis, anterior wedging of vertebral bodies (together with elongation in the AP dimension), Schmorl nodes, endplate irregularity, and disk space narrowing. There is involvement of multiple, contiguous (≥ 3) vertebral bodies. The small insert in the right lower quadrant is from a second patient, demonstrating slightly more prominent findings, in particular the endplate irregularity and accentuation of disease anteriorly.

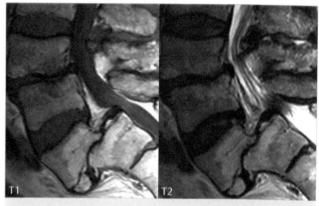

Fig. 3.100 Grade 3 spondylolisthesis. In this instance there is a grade 3 anterolisthesis (greater than 50% displacement) of L5 on S1. There were accompanying bilateral pars interarticularis defects—a finding better visualized on CT and present bilaterally in nearly all patients with grade 2 or 3 listheses. Note that despite the bilateral pars defects, due to the degree of slippage, there is severe spinal canal compromise. In chronic disease such as this, there will be accompanying loss of the intervertebral disk substance, and endplate degenerative changes, in this instance type 2 endplate disease (fatty change).

Diagnosis is also relatively easy (but less so in comparison to CT) on sagittal MR images, with reader experience important for recognition of imaging signs. An important clue to the presence of a chronic bilateral spondylolysis on MR is the presence of slippage (an anterolisthesis) without spinal canal compromise (▶ Fig. 3.102). Neural foraminal narrowing is common, and distinctive in appearance, occurring predominantly in the craniocaudal dimension (▶ Fig. 3.103). Prior to the advent of sagittal reformatted images on CT, spondylolysis was much more difficult to recognize, and the continuous facet sign was described, as follows. On axial images, from the level of the facet joints above to the level below, "facets" are seen on each image, with the intervening images between the two levels depicting the chronic fracture of the pars interarticularis.

Retrolisthesis

A retrolisthesis is a posterior subluxation of a vertebral body relative to the adjacent more distal vertebral body (the opposite of spondylolisthesis/anterolisthesis). It is most commonly caused by disk degeneration. A retrolisthesis can also occur

following surgery, with the resultant neural foraminal narrowing and nerve root impingement one cause of the failed back surgery syndrome. Retrolistheses are most common in the lumbar and cervical regions. In the lumbar region, L3–4 and L4–5 are most often involved. Retrolistheses are frequently accompanied by disk bulges and osteophytes. Spinal canal stenosis is uncommon. Neural foraminal narrowing is common. Retrolistheses are less often graded, relative to the degree of displacement, when compared to an anterolisthesis (in which the

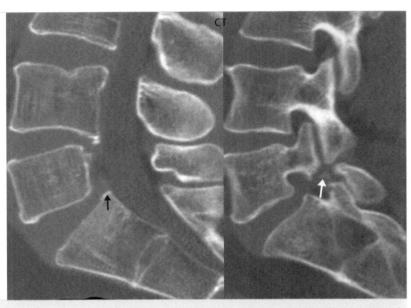

Fig. 3.101 Spondylolisthesis with spondylolysis, plain film radiography and CT. On the lateral plain film X-ray **(part 1)**, there are findings—absence of visualization of the pars interarticularis— consistent with a bilateral L5 pars defect (*black arrow*). CT **(part 2)** is however the best way to evaluate the bony spine per se, with the defect (*white arrow*) on one side illustrated and very well delineated on this sagittal reformatted image. Note that there is also a grade 1 anterolisthesis (*small black arrow*) at L5–S1. The typical accompanying broad based disk bulge is poorly visualized. A mild retrolisthesis of L4 on L5 is also present, and can be seen as well on the plain film.

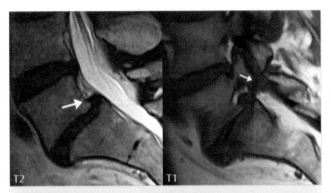

Fig. 3.102 Spondylolisthesis with spondylolysis, MR. There is a grade 1 anterolisthesis (*large white arrow*) of L5 on S1, best seen on the midline sagittal image. Note the accompanying broad-based disk bulge. Off to one side, a discontinuity of the pars (a pars defect) is noted to involve L5 (*small white arrow*), the definition of spondylolysis. There is compromise of the L5–S1 neural foramen both due to the anterolisthesis (slippage) and the disk bulge. When a mild anterolisthesis is due to a bilateral lysis, the spinal canal dimensions will be preserved, as in this case. The lack of spinal canal stenosis should clue the film reader into the need to examine the pars closely bilaterally.

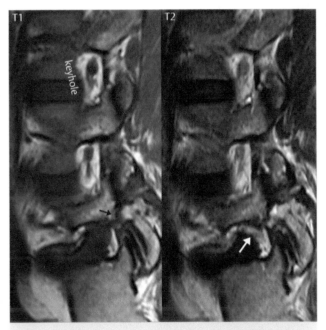

Fig. 3.103 Neural foraminal narrowing due to spondylolysis (with spondylolisthesis). On the sagittal T1-weighted scan a discontinuity (*small black arrow*) of the L5 pars is well seen, indicating spondylolysis. Normal, keyhole in shape, neural foramina are noted at L3–4 and L4–5. Although there is fat (best seen on the T1-weighted scan) both anterior and posterior to the L5 nerve in the L5–S1 foramen, the nerve (*white arrow*) is markedly compressed in the superoinferior dimension. Axial scans (not illustrated) in this instance are often misleading, showing fat anterior and posterior to the nerve, with the compression not evident due to the dimension in which it occurs. Compression both superiorly and inferiorly in the neural foramen is very common in spondylolisthesis with spondylolysis.

degree of displacement is always described), although a similar grading system can be used.

3.4.4 Surgery

Surgery for cervical spondylosis is performed to prevent further progression of myelopathic changes. For one or two level involvement, a common procedure is an anterior diskectomy, with placement either of a bone graft or a disk replacement device, with an accompanying anterior plate and screw vertebral body fusion. In the case where a bone graft is placed, the desired end result is bony fusion at the level of surgery, often without evidence of either the original bone graft or the native disk on imaging. This appearance can be differentiated from congenital nonsegmentation by the presence in the latter of narrowing in the AP dimension of the vertebrae at the level of the nonsegmentation, together with the presence on MR of a small vestigial native disk. By limiting motion at the site of surgical fusion, the patient is more predisposed to development of degenerative changes, and disk herniations, at the levels above and below the fusion, with attention thus mandatory to these levels in scan review (▶ Fig. 3.104).

A posterior cervical laminectomy is reserved for congenital narrowing or extensive, multilevel, contiguous disease. Postoperatively, on T2-weighted scans, abnormal high signal intensity within the cord at the level of surgery can represent gliosis, which could have been present preoperatively, or represent a postoperative complication including, specifically, cord contusion.

In the setting of a disk herniation with compression of the adjacent nerve, surgery may be undertaken to decompress the affected nerve. In the lumbar spine, the spectrum of surgery extends from percutaneous diskectomy to laminectomy with diskectomy, with removal of as little bone as possible preferred. Absence of the ligamentum flavum unilaterally, at the level of interest, is an important key to recognizing prior surgery.

Orthopedic spine surgery for pain generally involves stabilization of the spine. Anterior plate and screw fusion of a single level is common, with placement either of a bone graft at the disk space level to promote fusion, or of a disk replacement device. Posterior fusions can involve single or multiple levels. In the past these were often done with bone grafts only, although placement of orthopedic hardware is more common today. On MR and *CT,* iliac bone donor sites are commonly identified. Hardware complications seen in spine fusion include infection (visualized on CT as lucency surrounding a screw), fracture of a screw (▶ Fig. 3.105), migration of a disk replacement device, and misplacement of a screw (extending through the cortex of the vertebral body either superiorly, inferiorly, or anteriorly). Fatty atrophy of posterior paraspinal muscles can be seen following surgery, but also without surgery in the elderly.

Multilevel posterior decompression (laminectomy) is performed much less frequently today, due to the potential for destabilization of the spine (▶ Fig. 3.106). Removal of the

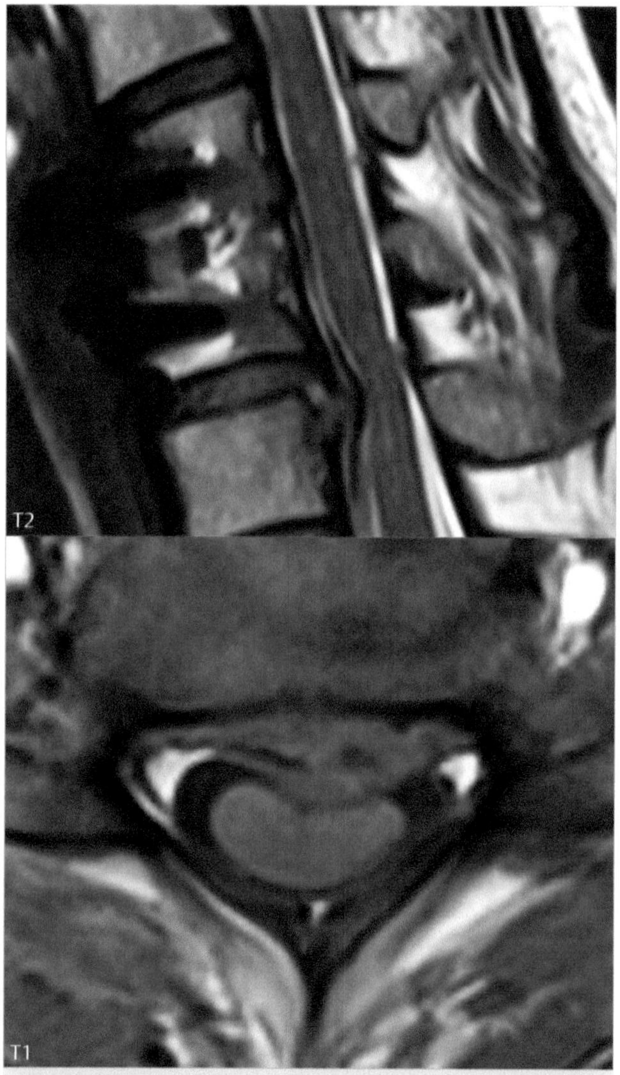

Fig. 3.104 Disk herniation following cervical fusion. Surgical fusion of a level will accentuate normal motion (in flexion and extension) at both the level above and below. This increases the incidence of disk herniation at these levels, together with degenerative disease. In the case presented, there is an anterior plate and screw fusion of a midcervical level. A central and left paracentral disk extrusion is seen on sagittal and axial images at the level below, causing moderate deformity (flattening) of the adjacent cord.

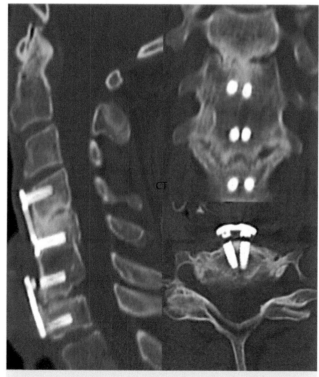

Fig. 3.105 Complications of cervical fusion. Sagittal, coronal, and axial CT scans depict an anterior plate and screw fusion of C4–5 and C6–7. There is bony fusion at C4–5 and C5–6, the latter without instrumentation. C6–7 is not fused, with sclerotic, irregular endplate margins and a slight retrolisthesis of C6 on C7. Note that both screws placed inferiorly in C6 are fractured.

posterior elements even at a single level, without other fusion or fixation, permits motion in the AP dimension that can result in either an anterolisthesis or a retrolisthesis.

In the setting of recurrent pain following lumbar diskectomy (the failed back surgery syndrome), two primary imaging diagnoses are important on MR (postoperative scar and recurrent/residual disk herniation), with intravenous contrast administration providing differentiation. Postoperative scar demonstrates homogeneous enhancement (due to intrinsic vascularity) following contrast administration on MR (▶ Fig. 3.107), although this is not consistently seen until more than 3 months following surgery.

Scar is often not masslike, but can appear as a mass lesion and thus mimic a disk herniation on unenhanced scans. Scar is one cause of persistent pain following lumbar disk surgery, with further surgery generally contraindicated. Residual or recurrent disk herniation will, however, not display enhancement on MR scans obtained within 20 minutes following contrast administration, and thus can be differentiated from scar. Thin section imaging (≤3 mm) is mandated in order to avoid partial volume effects. One important caveat is that scar is commonly present circumferential to a disk herniation, in cases both after surgery and without surgery, and is visualized as a thin rim of enhancement encompassing ("wrapping") the nonenhancing herniated disk (▶ Fig. 3.108). Scans should not be obtained post-contrast in a delayed fashion because there can be diffusion with time of contrast into the disk itself from adjacent vascular tissue (such as scar). Contrast enhancement can also be seen in a nerve that is compressed, as well as following decompression, although the latter is described as resolving by 6 months.

A pseudomeningocele is an abnormal collection of CSF within soft tissue that has formed due to a tear in the dura (in a meningocele, CSF is confined by the dura). Although strictly a brachial plexus avulsion injury is a pseudomeningocele, most of the lesions that are seen on imaging in the spine are large on presentation and a complication of surgery. Surgery involving the occiput, perhaps due to the difficulty of surgery in this area, and that involving the lumbar region, perhaps due to how common such surgery is, lead to the majority of cases.

3.4.5 Spondyloarthropathies

Diffuse Idiopathic Skeletal Hyperostosis

The criteria for the diagnosis of diffuse idiopathic skeletal hyperostosis (DISH) include flowing ossification, anteriorly, and anterolaterally (predominantly right-sided), along four or more contiguous vertebrae, with preserved vertebral height and

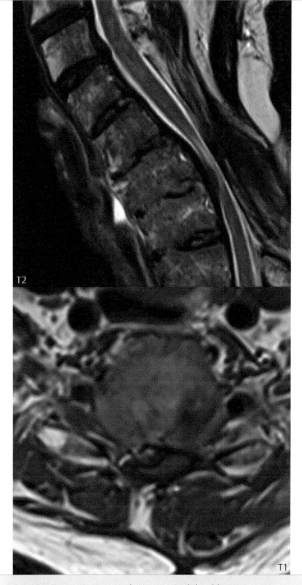

Fig. 3.106 Postoperative canal stenosis. Multilevel laminectomies, often performed in the past, can result long-term in destabilization of the spine, specifically relative to vertebral body alignment. The posterior elements in this patient are missing at four contiguous levels. Complications include canal compromise, with cord compression, atrophy, and gliosis as illustrated. A broad irregular osteophyte (posteriorly) accentuates the compression in this instance.

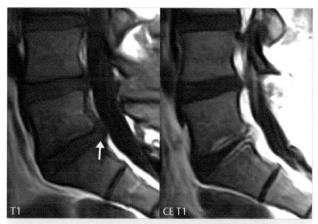

Fig. 3.107 Postoperative scar, in a patient with recurrent pain following lumbar diskectomy. On sagittal (part 1) and axial (part 2) images, prior to administration of intravenous contrast abnormal soft tissue, masslike in appearance, is seen posterior to the L5–S1 disk space level, in a right paracentral position (white arrows). This could represent either a recurrent/residual disk herniation in this postoperative patient, or scar tissue. Following contrast injection, there is enhancement of this tissue, consistent with postoperative scar. The right S1 nerve is seen on the post-contrast axial image to be encompassed by scar, lying centrally within the abnormal soft tissue identified pre-contrast.

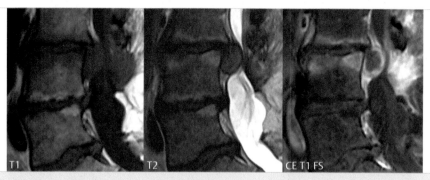

Fig. 3.108 Recurrent (postoperative) disk herniation. A large soft tissue mass is noted immediately posterior and inferior to the L3–4 disk space level. There has been prior surgery, reflected by the abnormal soft tissue posterior to the thecal sac at this level, and the extensive fat also posteriorly. On the T2-weighted scan the mass is better defined, and its appearance favors disk material. However only on the post-contrast scan is the mass definitely identified as disk material (due to the lack of contract enhancement), wrapped by enhancing scar tissue, and with some dilated enhancing epidural venous plexus both cranial and caudal to the disk. Due to the inferior extent of this disk material relative to the disk space it also likely represents a sequestered disk (free disk fragment). Note in addition the enhancement in the soft tissues posterior to the thecal sac at this level, reflecting postoperative scar.

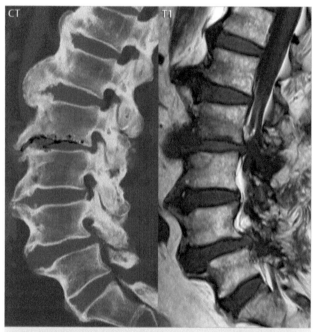

Fig. 3.109 Diffuse idiopathic skeletal hyperostosis (DISH). In the sagittal reformatted, thick section MIP from a CT exam, exuberant anterior longitudinal ligament ossification ("flowing" calcification) is noted from T12 to L5 (satisfying the requirement of involvement of four or more levels). Disk space height is generally preserved, other than at L2–3. Although there are some facet degenerative changes, these are much less prominent than the disease involving the anterior spine. On the sagittal MR exam, obtained with a slightly different obliquity, the "flowing" anterior vertebral ossification is again evident, although substantially better depicted on CT. This simply reflects once again that MR is better for visualization of soft tissue as compared with calcification or ossification, the latter being the strength of CT.

without involvement of the facet joints (▶ Fig. 3.109). It is a disease of the elderly, and is seen most commonly in the thoracic spine. Myelopathy can occur due to associated ossification of the posterior longitudinal ligament or vertebral complications (fracture or subluxation).

Ankylosing Spondylitis

This seronegative spondyloarthropathy is the most common inflammatory disease of the adult spine. Seronegative spondyloarthropathies include a variety of diseases (ankylosing spondylitis, reactive arthritis, enteropathic spondylitis associated with inflammatory bowel diseases, psoriatic arthritis, and undifferentiated spondyloarthropathies) and are all characterized by inflammation that frequently progresses to bony ankylosis.

While radiographs have traditionally played an important role in diagnosing ankylosing spondylitis, MR has today become essential both for diagnosis and monitoring ankylosing, the latter in particular with the introduction of effective but expensive drugs (e.g., the anti-tumor necrosis factor (TNF) monoclonal antibodies). MR is very sensitive for detection of inflammatory changes in the axial skeleton, and has been incorporated into the new diagnostic criteria for ankylosing spondylitis (Assessment of SpondyloArthritis, or ASAS, criteria). A MR protocol for evaluation of the axial skeleton should consist of STIR and T1-weighted sequences in order to assess both structural changes of the skeleton as well as inflammatory activity. In addition to the spine, the chest wall (including the sternum, sternoclavicular joints, and costosternal joints) is also often involved in inflammation and should be included in the imaging protocol. While contrast-enhanced T1-weighted fat-saturated images nicely depict active disease in ankylosing spondylitis, this technique has been shown to be unnecessary, as no additional information compared to STIR sequences is gained.

In ankylosing spondylitis, the sacroiliac joints are involved early in the disease course. Erosion of cortical margins, typically first on the iliac side of the joint, is seen early in the disease process (▶ Fig. 3.110). Proliferative changes subsequently dominate, with subchondral sclerosis (▶ Fig. 3.111) progressing to ankylosis (fusion) of the joint (▶ Fig. 3.112). When fusion is complete, the sclerosis resolves. Disease involvement is typically symmetric, although changes may be asymmetric on MR early in the disease process. Changes seen on MR include edema and/or fluid along the sacroiliac joints, abnormal contrast enhancement, fatty bone marrow changes adjacent to the joints,

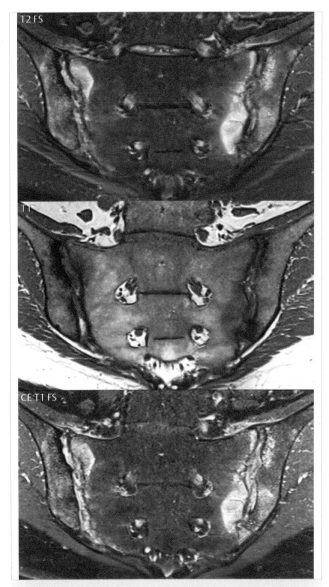

Fig. 3.110 Ankylosing spondylitis, sacroiliac joint, active disease. On the coronal T2-weighted scan, there is edema (with abnormal high signal intensity) adjacent to portions of both SI joints. Widening of the joint space is evident on the precontrast T1-weighted scan, together with subchondral sclerosis (with low signal intensity) and irregularity involving the margins of the sacrum and iliac bones bordering the joints bilaterally. On the fat suppressed post-contrast scan, enhancement is seen both within bone bordering the joint space and within the SI joints themselves, the latter reflecting inflammatory tissue.

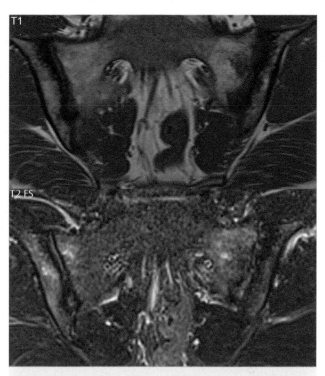

Fig. 3.111 Ankylosing spondylitis, chronic disease (prior to joint fusion). There is marked irregularity and sclerosis of the sacroiliac joints bilaterally (the latter marked by low SI on the T1-weighted scan). Mild fatty changes are noted as well, in the sacrum, bordering the joint. There is little edema within the bone adjacent to the sacroiliac joints. All are findings consistent with long standing disease.

(▶ Fig. 3.113). Syndesmophytes are slender, vertical ligamentous calcifications that extend from the corner of one vertebral body to the next, and are the hallmark of ankylosing spondylitis on radiographs, but may be difficult to visualize on MR.

MR in the active stage of the disease will show inflammatory changes involving the entheses as well as the apophyseal (facet) joints, but inflammatory changes may also be seen centrally in the vertebral bodies, unrelated to the entheses. In advanced disease, fatty changes at the entheses and ankylosed facet joints are often seen together with the appearance of a "bamboo spine," featuring multilevel syndesmophytes in addition to relative "squaring" of the vertebral bodies (▶ Fig. 3.114). Complications include fracture following minor trauma, which in the cervical spine can lead to quadriplegia.

Rheumatoid Arthritis

Findings in the cervical spine are common in rheumatoid arthritis, a chronic multisystem disease of unknown etiology featuring an erosive synovitis. The articulation of the atlas (C1) and the dens is most often involved. Characteristic imaging findings include erosion of the dens by surrounding inflammatory pannus and involvement of the transverse atlantal ligament, with the latter resulting in a retrodental soft tissue mass and increased distance between the anterior arch of C1 and the dens (due to ligamentous laxity). These changes can result in cord compression (▶ Fig. 3.115).

and bony sclerosis (the latter with low signal intensity on all pulse sequences).

Involvement of the spine is usually subsequent to that of the sacroiliac joints, and is described as occurring first in the thoracolumbar and lumbosacral regions, and then progressing cranially. In the spine, inflammation occurs often at the junction of the annulus fibrosus and the vertebral body (the enthesis, which is the connective tissue between the ligament and bone). The outer annular fibers become replaced by bone, syndesmophytes, which eventually bridge the adjacent vertebral bodies

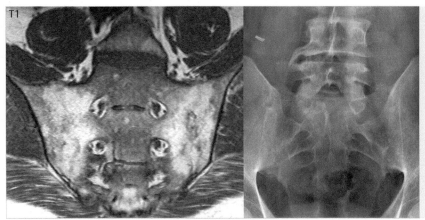

Fig. 3.112 Ankylosing spondylitis, sacroiliac joint, chronic disease. On the coronal T1-weighted scan, the sacroiliac joints are fused bilaterally (there is little evidence of the former joint spaces), with fatty marrow replacement. The AP plain film confirms bony fusion of the SI joints.

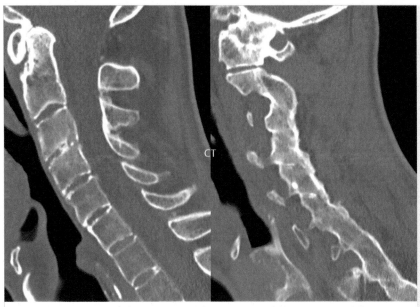

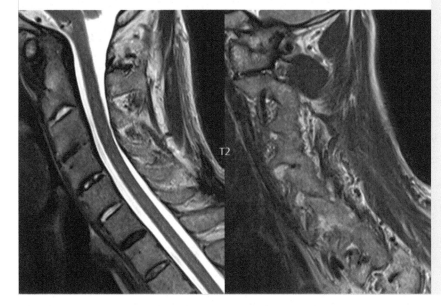

Fig. 3.113 Ankylosing spondylitis, cervical spine. Sagittal reformatted CT (**part 1**) demonstrates bony ankylosis of the facet joints from C2–3 through C7–T1, with generalized osteopenia. On both CT and MR (**part 2**), relative squaring of the vertebral bodies is evident. The bony ankylosis of the posterior elements is also evident on MR. Note that the abnormal high signal intensity of the intervertebral disks does not represent infection (there are no signal intensity abnormalities in the adjacent vertebral endplates), but rather a manifestation of the fusion in this disease process.

3.5 Arteriovascular Disease and Ischemia

3.5.1 Spinal Dural Arteriovenous Fistulas

The type I spinal dural arteriovenous (AV) fistula is the most common vascular malformation of the spine, presenting mostly in older men in the thoracolumbar region. It is a direct shunt between the arterial and venous system (between a radiculomeningeal artery and a radicular vein), with drainage retrograde into perimedullary vessels (those surrounding the cord), leading to venous congestion of the cord. The arterial stasis and venous congestion cause chronic hypoxia and (typically) slowly progressive myelopathy from venous hypertension (Foix Alajouanine syndrome). Without therapy, the result can be irreversible paraplegia.

On MR, cord edema (with hyperintensity on T2-weighted scans, predominantly centrally in the gray matter—and thus H-shaped on axial images) and dilated perimedullary vessels are seen (▶ Fig. 3.116). The latter can be seen as numerous flow voids within the CSF adjacent to the cord on T2-weighted scans, and with enhancement post-contrast. Contrast enhancement of the cord itself may also be present. Contrast-enhanced MR angiography (MRA) can be used to directly visualize the tortuous, abnormally coiled, dilated perimedullary veins within the subarachnoid space (▶ Fig. 3.117).

3.5.2 Spinal Cord Arteriovenous Malformations

About 20% of vascular malformations of the spine are arteriovenous malformations (AVMs), and these present early, in the second decade of life. Spinal cord AVMs can cause intramedullary and/or subarachnoid hemorrhage. There are both glomerular (nidal) and juvenile types. The glomerular type is more common, is usually intramedullary in location, and resembles a cerebral AVM in terms of having a vascular nidus. The rare juvenile AVM is metameric, involving cord, bone, and skin, and has a poor overall prognosis.

On MR, dilated perimedullary and intramedullary vessels are seen. Venous congestion and edema within the cord lead to cord swelling and hyperintensity on T2-weighted images.

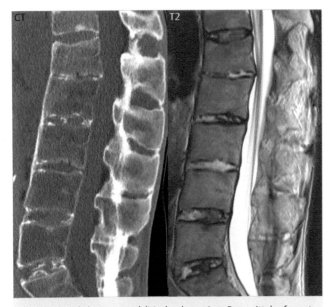

Fig. 3.114 Ankylosing spondylitis, lumbar spine. On sagittal reformatted CT, there is bony ankylosis both of the vertebral bodies and the posterior elements. Note the diffuse osteopenia and relative squaring of the vertebral bodies. There is ossification of the anterior longitudinal ligament together with the ligamentum flavum posteriorly. These findings are less evident on MR. There is abnormal hyperintensity within many of the intervertebral disks which, although nonspecific, can be seen in ankylosis.

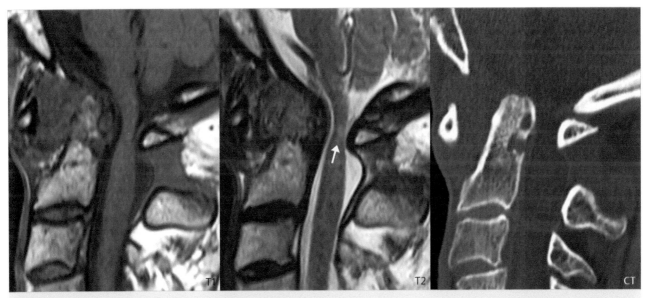

Fig. 3.115 Rheumatoid arthritis. On the sagittal images presented, increased distance between the anterior arch of C1 and the dens, erosion of the dens, and marked inflammatory pannus (surrounding the dens) are all noted. The soft tissue component of the disease, together with the compression of the cord (and gliosis therein, *white arrow*), are visualized directly only on MR.

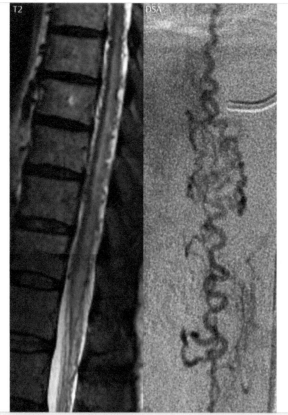

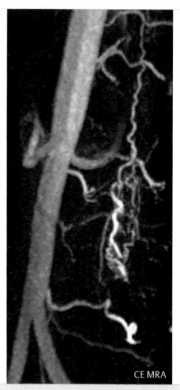

Fig. 3.116 Thoracic arteriovenous fistula (AVF). Dural AVFs lead to edema within the cord, which is typically extensive and spans the thoracic cord to the conus. This is seen on the T2-weighted scan as abnormal hyperintensity of the cord. More specific, in terms of imaging findings and diagnosis on MR, is visualization of the myriad of small flow voids along the surface of the cord and within the adjacent CSF, corresponding to enlarged veins. An AP projection from the DSA study in this patient is also presented for comparison, depicting directly the tortuous dilated perimedullary veins.

Fig. 3.117 Arteriovenous fistula, contrast-enhanced MRA. An oblique sagittal MIP from a high-resolution contrast-enhanced MR angiogram depicts the arteriovenous shunting, together with multiple dilated perimedullary veins.

3.5.3 Spinal Cord Arterial Ischemia

Arterial ischemia can be due to occlusion of intercostal/lumbar arteries or intrinsic arteries of the cord. The majority of cases involve the lower thoracic cord and conus (▶ Fig. 3.118). There is a myriad of etiologies, including specifically aortic dissection, very different from cerebral infarction where atherosclerosis is a primary cause. It should be noted that the arterial supply to the cord is highly variable and the anastomotic networks are extensive. The acute presentation is that of pain and neurologic deficit.

The specific deficits depend on the level and extent of ischemia. Symmetric involvement of the anterior two-thirds of the spinal cord is characteristic, and is well-delineated on axial T2-weighted MR images. Moderate focal cord enlargement is seen acutely, evolving to atrophy with time. Contrast enhancement of the infarct is seen in the subacute time frame. With occlusion of a segmental artery, concurrent abnormalities in the adjacent vertebral bodies (vertebral body infarctions) can be seen.

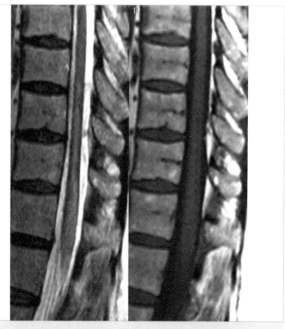

Fig. 3.118 Cord ischemia. Edema is seen within the lower thoracic cord and conus, with abnormal high signal intensity on the T2-weighted scan. There is minimal cord enlargement, best visualized on the T1-weighted scan.

3.5.4 Cavernous Malformation

A cavernous malformation (cavernous angioma) is an angiographically occult lesion, whether present in the brain or in the spinal cord, and typically silent clinically. They occur both sporadically and in a familial pattern. As in the brain, the lesions are best seen on MR. Cavernous malformations are usually small, smoothly marginated, with a border (rim) that is mildly hypointense on T1- and markedly hypointense on T2-weighted scans (a feature that is further emphasized on T2*-weighted scans) (▶ Fig. 3.119). The low signal intensity rim corresponds to a combination of hemosiderin and ferritin in macrophages that have phagocytosed blood. Centrally, these lesions have a mixture of high and low signal intensity on T2-weighted images, corresponding to a honeycomb of vascular spaces separated by fibrous strands. Mild associated cord expansion is common.

3.6 Infection and Inflammation

3.6.1 Disk Space Infection

Disk space infection can be hematogenous in origin, or a complication of spine surgery. In the latter, the clinical presentation is usually several weeks following surgery, with delays in diagnosis common. Focal pain is a prominent clinical feature, but may be absent. In hematogenous seeding, it is stated that the disk serves as the initial site of infection in children, as it is richly vascularized, whereas in adults the initial site of infection is the subchondral bone or adjacent soft tissue. On CT, only late changes are noted, including disk space narrowing, cortical endplate destruction and irregularity, and an accompanying paraspinal soft tissue mass. On MR, the most common presentation of a disk space infection is that of a narrowed irregular disk (▶ Fig. 3.120), with focal high signal intensity on the T2-weighted scan (infected fluid pockets), enhancement of the disk space (other than the fluid), and a horizontal band of edema within the vertebral body both above and below (osteomyelitis), paralleling the infected disk space. The edema within the adjacent vertebral bodies will display enhancement on post-contrast scans obtained with fat saturation (▶ Fig. 3.121).

In early disease, the extent of edema within the adjacent vertebral bodies may be mild (or absent with discitis only), and in severe disease both the vertebral body above and below can be involved in their entirety. Although often less evident than on CT, the vertebral endplates will appear indistinct on MR in a

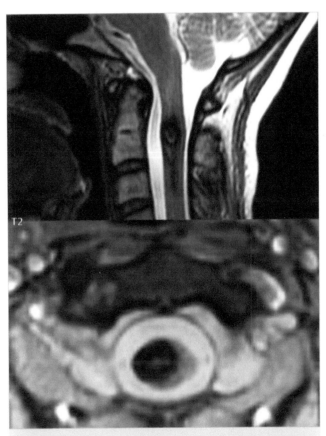

Fig. 3.119 Cavernous malformation. On the midline sagittal FSE T2-weighted scan, a focal intramedullary lesion is demonstrated, with a low signal intensity hemosiderin rim and mild cord expansion. The hemosiderin rim is emphasized due to susceptibility effects on the axial gradient echo T2-weighted scan, and is demonstrated to be complete/circumferential.

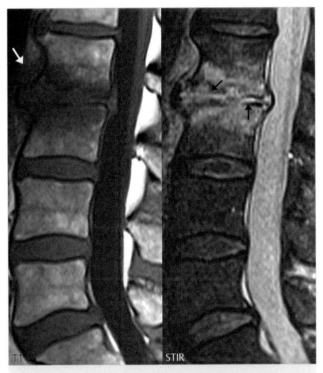

Fig. 3.120 Disk space infection with osteomyelitis, lumbar spine. On a sagittal T1-weighted midline image, abnormal low signal intensity is seen involving the vertebral endplates at the L2–3 level, with irregularity of the inferior L2 endplate, and poor visualization of portions of the superior L3 endplate. Abnormal prevertebral soft tissue is also present at this level (*white arrow*). On the corresponding sagittal STIR image, the disk space is noted to be narrowed, irregular, and with abnormal high signal intensity (*small black arrows*), the latter reflecting fluid within the disk space. The findings involving the disk space itself are consistent with infection, which is accompanied by abnormal signal intensity in the adjacent vertebral endplates (low on T1, high on STIR), consistent with osteomyelitis.

disk space infection with accompanying osteomyelitis. A paraspinal soft tissue mass is also commonly present, of varying size, with enhancement post-contrast (▶ Fig. 3.122).

Often CT-guided biopsy is performed in order to have material for bacterial culture, prior to starting antibiotic treatment. Once treatment with intravenous antibiotics is initiated, the changes on MR (reflecting recovery) lag behind that of the clinical course. Other causes of paraspinal infection, without accompanying discitis and osteomyelitis, include hematogenous seeding (e.g., with a psoas abscess) and following surgery, with infection in the operative bed posteriorly.

3.6.2 Tuberculous Spondylitis

Tuberculous spondylitis follows a more indolent clinical course than pyogenic infection. In the United States this disease is seen primarily in immigrants (from Southeast Asia and South America) and in immunocompromised patients. The disease is primarily one of adults, and occurs due to hematogenous seeding. Differentiating features on imaging from pyogenic infection include inoculum in the anterior vertebral bodies, relative sparing of the disk space due to absence of proteolytic enzymes (early in the disease process) (▶ Fig. 3.123), involvement of multiple contiguous vertebral bodies (three or more levels in half of patients),

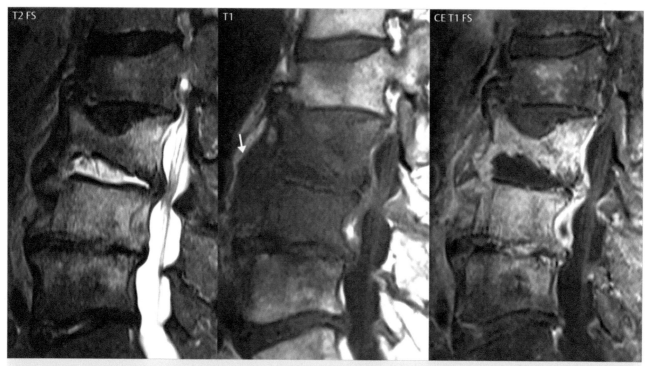

Fig. 3.121 Disk space infection with accompanying osteomyelitis (spondylodiscitis), extensive disease involvement. On sagittal images, there is fluid in the L3–4 disk space, seen as high signal intensity on the T2-weighted scan and by the lack of enhancement post-contrast. There is extensive edema (with accompanying abnormal contrast enhancement) throughout L3 and L4. These are characteristic findings in an advanced case of disk space infection, with the abnormality in the marrow indicative of osteomyelitis. There is pre-/paravertebral abnormal soft tissue (*arrow*), representing further disease extent, and loss of height of L3. There is also extension to L5 (thus involvement of 3 vertebral bodies, which is unusual), with abnormal marrow signal intensity and enhancement superiorly in L5 and involvement of the disk at L4–5 (with abnormal enhancement). The etiology in this instance was methicillin-resistant *Staphylococcus aureus* (MRSA), accounting for the unusual extent of disease.

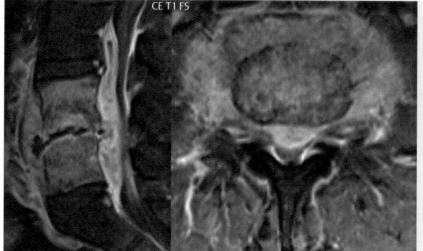

Fig. 3.122 Disk space infection, with extensive spread of infection into the adjacent soft tissues and epidural space. Abnormal enhancement, consistent with osteomyelitis, is seen throughout the L4 and L5 vertebral bodies. The L4–5 disk space is irregular and does not enhance, consistent with an infected fluid collection. There is extensive abnormal, enhancing prevertebral and paravertebral soft tissue, with extension to the epidural space and canal compromise on that basis.

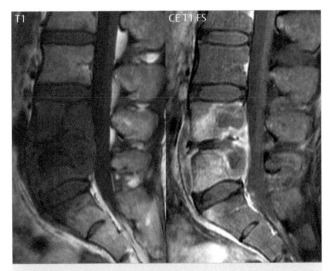

Fig. 3.123 Spinal tuberculosis. Illustrated on sagittal images is a major distinguishing feature of tuberculous spondylitis, relative sparing of the disk space, despite involvement of the adjacent vertebral bodies. Note the prominent involvement of L4 and L5, with extension of disease to the superior/anterior portion of S1, all well visualized pre-contrast with abnormal low signal intensity, and post-contrast with abnormal enhancement. Although there is loss of disk space height, anteriorly the L4–5 disk is spared, which would not be seen in pyogenic disk space infection (the primary differential in this instance).

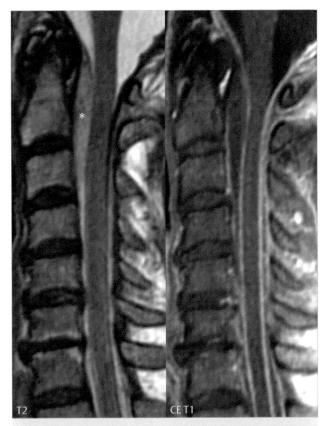

Fig. 3.124 Epidural abscess, cervical spine. An extensive infected epidural fluid collection is present, largest in bulk anteriorly in the high cervical region (asterisk), but present both anterior and posterior to the cord, effacing the thecal sac. On the sagittal T2-weighted scan, this collection is slightly lower in signal intensity in comparison to CSF, and on the sagittal T1-weighted scan slightly hyperintense. The prominent peripheral enhancement (in part representing the displaced dura) is characteristic.

and a large associated paraspinal mass. Although skip lesions are reported, these are uncommon (<5%). Spread of disease occurs under the anterior longitudinal ligament. In long standing disease there will be extensive bone destruction.

3.6.3 Epidural Abscess

In recent years, epidural abscesses in the spine have become more frequent, with a subdural abscess, though, very uncommon. Infection can occur by hematogenous spread, direct extension (e.g., anteriorly from a disk space infection with osteomyelitis), or penetrating trauma. There may be associated meningitis and myelitis. MR is the modality of choice for detection and delineation, with CT of little value. Thickened inflamed (enhancing) soft tissue (phlegmon) is seen initially, progressing to a frank abscess (with fluid centrally). Contrast enhancement on MR can thus be homogeneous, or rimlike with central low signal intensity (pus). There can be canal compromise and cord compression, due to inflammation, granulation tissue, and any associated fluid collection (▶ Fig. 3.124). Lesions usually extend over several levels, and are often very extensive (▶ Fig. 3.125).

Both sagittal and axial imaging are important, the former for definition of extent of disease, and the latter for improved assessment of the thecal sac and cord compression. Diffusion weighted scans (an abscess will demonstrate restricted diffusion), relatively recently available with reasonable image quality for spine MR imaging, are an important complementary imaging sequence (▶ Fig. 3.126).

3.6.4 Meningitis and Myelitis

In meningitis, nerve roots become congested, with exudates along their surfaces. As the disease progresses, the nerve roots

can adhere to one another. CT does not play a role in imaging of this disease. MR demonstrates characteristic findings in moderate and severe inflammation, although there is some overlap with leptomeningeal metastatic disease. A negative MR however does not exclude meningitis, with the diagnosis dependent on clinical symptoms and CSF studies.

Of all scan sequences, post-contrast images on MR are the most valuable in acute bacterial meningitis, depicting diffuse enhancement of nerve roots, together with a thin line of enhancement along the cord surface. Myelitis accompanying meningitis has been reported, with cord enlargement and increased signal intensity on T2-weighted scans as would be anticipated. Clumped nerve roots are a somewhat later finding. Adhesions and focal/diffuse obliteration or loculation of the subarachnoid space can be seen chronically.

In AIDS and immunocompromised patients, the spectrum of organisms involved is different (including, for example, cryptococcus and cytomegalovirus), and the appearance on imaging can be likewise. Abnormal enhancement is often less evident in immunocompromised patients.

3.6.5 Arachnoiditis

Arachnoiditis can be the result of infection, surgery, intrathecal drug administration, or hemorrhage within the thecal sac. In mild disease, a few nerve roots may simply be thickened and/or

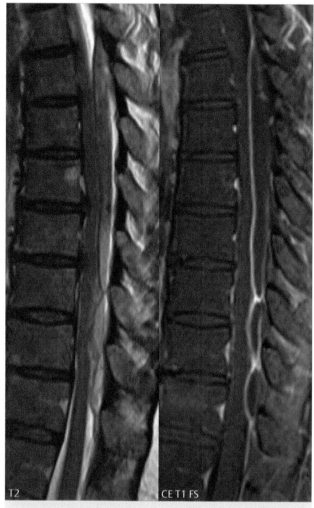

Fig. 3.125 Epidural abscess, thoracic spine. On the sagittal T2-weighted FSE scan, a posterior epidural mass with mixed signal intensity is noted to compress the cord anteriorly. The lesion is well delineated post-contrast with fat saturation, consisting of an extensive (infected) fluid collection outlined by a prominent enhancing inflammatory tissue margin.

clumped (▸ Fig. 3.127). In more severe cases, the nerve roots may be adherent to the periphery of the thecal sac (an "empty" sac), or clumped centrally to form a nodularlike mass. In severe cases, particularly postoperatively, there can be adhesions, loculation, and irregularity of the thecal sac. In acute disease, particularly infection, there will be abnormal enhancement of the nerves diffusely within the thecal sac. Note that in spinal stenosis the nerve roots will always appear clumped and redundant, in particular as they approach a focal area of stenosis, and that this should not be misinterpreted as arachnoiditis.

3.6.6 Guillain-Barré

The clinical presentation of Guillain-Barré is that of progressive motor paralysis of more than one limb (often bilateral and symmetric), with little sensory change. The etiology is felt to be immune mediated, subsequent to viral or bacterial infection, or vaccination. MR is the imaging modality of choice for diagnosis, and strongly recommended when Guillain-Barré is suspected. On MR there will be smooth mild thickening of the nerve roots of the cauda equina, with abnormal contrast enhancement (with preferential enhancement of the ventral, motor, roots in most patients) (▸ Fig. 3.128).

3.6.7 Chronic Inflammatory Demyelinating Polyneuropathy

Chronic inflammatory demyelinating polyneuropathy (CIPD) is an uncommon demyelinating disease in which thickened (hypertrophied) peripheral nerves or nerve roots can be seen. Hypertrophy (with increased signal intensity on T2-weighted scans) and abnormal enhancement of the cauda equina and lumbar nerve roots have been frequently described in the literature (▸ Fig. 3.129). Involvement in other areas appears to be less common.

3.6.8 Sarcoidosis

Sarcoidosis is a noncaseating granulomatous disease of unknown etiology, treated with corticosteroids. Symptomatic central nervous system (CNS) disease is uncommon. With

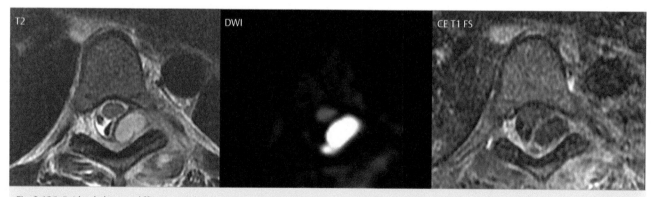

Fig. 3.126 Epidural abscess, diffusion weighted imaging. An epidural fluid collection is identified, immediately posterior and to the left of the thecal sac in the thoracic region. There is marked compression of the thecal sac and mild cord deformity. The hyperintensity of the fluid collection on DWI is consistent with an abscess, which was proven pathologically. Restricted diffusion was confirmed on the ADC map (not presented). Post-contrast there is peripheral enhancement.

spinal cord involvement, fusiform cord enlargement (with abnormal high signal intensity on T2-weighted images) together with patchy enhancement has been described.

3.6.9 Multiple Sclerosis

Cord lesions are common in multiple sclerosis (MS), although many patients demonstrate predominantly brain lesions. Our assessment of this disease, however, may be biased simply due to the development of MR, with imaging of the brain by this modality inherently markedly superior to imaging of the cord, due to differences in available coils and anatomy. Spinal cord plaques, like lesions in the brain, demonstrate abnormal high signal intensity on T2-weighted scans (▶ Fig. 3.130). An important caveat is, however, that the scan utilized should be optimized for visualization of MS plaques (with a fast spin echo STIR scan one such approach) (▶ Fig. 3.131). Standard fast spin echo T2-weighted scans are not particularly sensitive for detection of MS plaques, especially if additional radiofrequency (RF) pulses are applied at the end of the echo train (a common practice, termed driven-equilibrium Fourier transformation) to provide high signal intensity CSF with a shorter repetition time (TR). Focal cord enlargement may be present, albeit typically

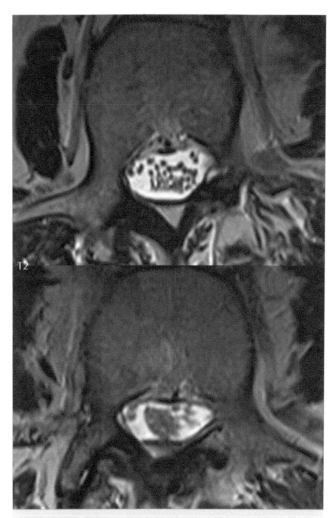

Fig. 3.127 Arachnoiditis. Two axial images at different levels are presented from the same patient. Note that the nerve roots do not layer posteriorly, and in the lower image are also clumped. Both are findings seen in arachnoiditis (acutely, as well as chronically).

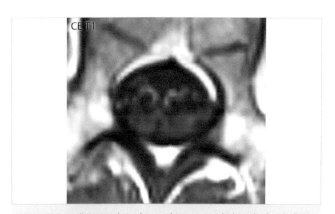

Fig. 3.128 Guillain-Barré. In this axial image just below the level of the conus, the ventral nerve roots are seen to enhance (note the higher SI of the ventral as opposed to the dorsal roots), a characteristic finding in Guillain-Barré.

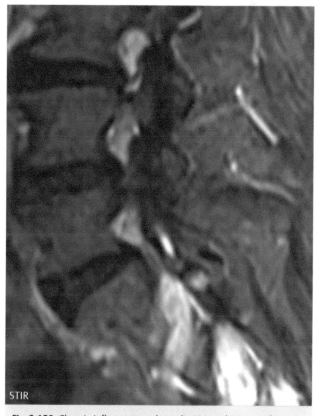

Fig. 3.129 Chronic inflammatory demyelinating polyneuropathy (CIDP). This entity presents with enlargement and hyperintensity on T2-weighted scans of nerve roots, ganglia, and peripheral nerves, as illustrated on an off-midline sagittal image. The nerves exiting in and extending beyond the neural foramina are all enlarged, and hyperintense.

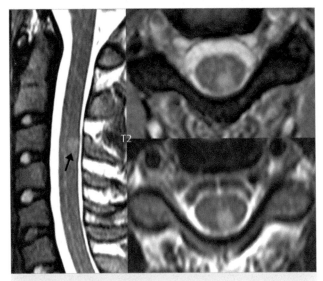

Fig. 3.130 Multiple sclerosis, imaging technique. T2-weighted techniques are most commonly used to visualize MS plaques in the cord, with a moderate size lesion at the C3 level posteriorly on the left (*black arrow*) visualized with abnormal high signal intensity on sagittal fast spin echo and axial gradient echo (GRE, upper image) and fast spin echo (FSE, lower image) scans. The low signal intensity of marrow easily identifies the axial GRE scan, with the CSF flow voids characteristic for the axial FSE scan (seen in this instance anterior to the cord). Note that this lesion, as with most MS cord lesions, does not respect gray–white matter boundaries.

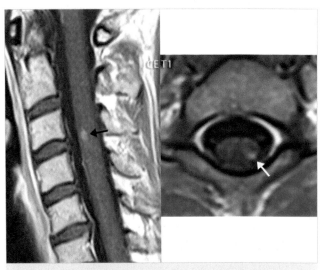

Fig. 3.132 Multiple sclerosis, two small active (enhancing) cervical plaques. Small lesions within the cord demand exacting technique, whether for detection with or without contrast enhancement. Thin sections, with high in-plane spatial resolution can depict MS plaques well in both the sagittal (*black arrow*) and axial (*white arrow*) planes, provided that motion is not a problem, there is sufficient sensitivity of the utilized scan sequence, and the slice is centered on the lesion. Slice position is a common reason for poor visualization of a small plaque in one plane, with good visualization in the other.

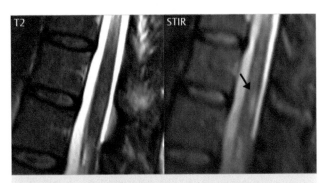

Fig. 3.131 Multiple sclerosis, optimization of MR technique for lesion visualization. Attention to imaging technique is crucial for detection of cord lesions in MS, with many pitfalls. Most variants of T2-weighted FSE technique, which display excellent cord/CSF contrast, have poor intrinsic cord/lesion contrast. This is particularly true when using scan techniques optimized to increase CSF signal intensity (e.g., RESTORE, FR-FSE, or DRIVE) or three-dimensional FSE techniques such as SPACE. Thus, the MS lesion in the conus in this patient is poorly visualized on the FSE sagittal T2-weighted scan (left image). Use of a STIR sequence (or other dedicated approaches to cord imaging), as illustrated on the right, leads to a marked improvement in lesion contrast (relative to normal cord), with excellent delineation of this small MS plaque (*arrow*) located posteriorly in the conus. Note the inherent apparent blurring on the STIR sequence, due simply to the lower spatial resolution (with STIR having inherently lower SNR compared to FSE T2-weighted scans, and thus needing to be acquired with lower spatial resolution).

MS lesions (plaques) are haphazard in distribution in the cord, both in cross-section and longitudinally, disregarding anatomic boundaries (▶ Fig. 3.133). In particular, lesions are not restricted to white matter. Plaques tend to be elliptical in shape, with greatest dimension along the craniocaudal axis (▶ Fig. 3.134). Histologically, multifocal sharply marginated areas of demyelination are seen. Focal cord atrophy, often subtle, can be seen with chronic lesions (▶ Fig. 3.135). The imaging approach to MS includes MR evaluation of the brain, cervical cord, and thoracic cord (including the conus). Only with a negative exam in these three anatomic areas can the diagnosis be excluded with any confidence. Symptoms common with cord involvement include paraparesis, and bowel and bladder dysfunction.

3.6.10 Neuromyelitis Optica

Neuromyelitis optica, also known as Devic disease, is characterized by optic neuritis (unilateral or bilateral) and myelitis, with lesions in both the optic nerve and the spinal cord visualized by MR. Lesions will have abnormal high signal intensity on T2-weighted scans, and may display abnormal contrast enhancement. The cord lesion in neuromyelitis optica is indistinguishable from that of acute transverse myelitis. Brain lesions are reported to be relatively common in patients with otherwise typical neuromyelitis optica. Whether this disease is truly distinct from multiple sclerosis is debatable.

3.6.11 Acute Transverse Myelitis

From descriptions in the literature about this disease both in terms of pathophysiology and imaging appearance, it is clear that acute transverse myelitis is poorly understood, and may

minimal, indicative of acute disease. Edema can be present, but need not be, adjacent to active lesions. In a small number of active lesions, edema is seen to extend in a flamelike manner above and below the lesion itself. Contrast enhancement is present in, and is used to define, active lesions (▶ Fig. 3.132).

represent the overlap of several entities. Acute transverse myelitis may occur as an isolated idiopathic entity (with possible viral or autoimmune etiology) or in association with systemic diseases such as lupus or sarcoidosis. The clinical presentation is one of acute or subacute motor, sensory, and autonomic dysfunction related to a focal cord lesion. The imaging appearance is generally stated to be that of abnormal cord high signal intensity on T2-weighted scans (involving the majority of the cord in cross-section), extending over multiple segments, with fusiform enlargement of the cord and in some cases abnormal contrast enhancement. An important differential diagnosis is multiple sclerosis, with multiplicity of cord lesions combined with characteristic brain lesions consistent with the latter.

3.6.12 Vitamin B$_{12}$ Deficiency

This vitamin deficiency leads to accumulation of methylmalonic acid which is myelinotoxic and results in a somewhat distinctive appearance of the spinal cord on MR. Characteristic is the focal increased signal intensity on T2-weighted images in the

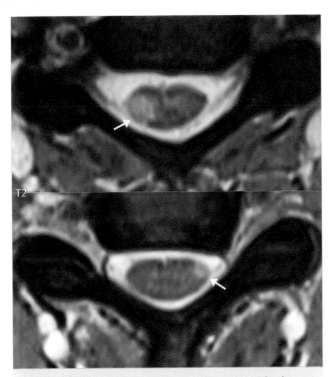

Fig. 3.133 Multiple sclerosis, lesion size. Axial GRE T2-weighted scans from one patient illustrate two different MS plaques (*arrows*) in the cervical cord, one large and one small. Note that the larger lesion involves both gray and white matter. Lesions occur of all sizes, with the larger lesions typically active and often causing focal mass effect (cord enlargement). These may also exhibit marked adjacent vasogenic edema, extending a level above and below the lesion not uncommonly.

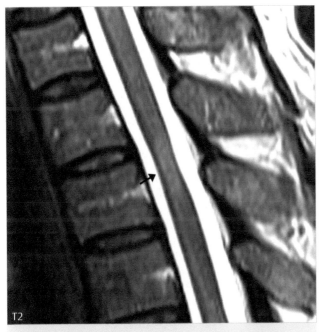

Fig. 3.135 Multiple sclerosis, chronic plaque, lower cervical spine. There is focal abnormal high signal intensity within the cord (*arrow*) on this sagittal image, indicative of an MS plaque. Note the related focal cord atrophy, best recognized due to mild indentation of the posterior cord margin, a not uncommon finding in larger, chronic MS lesions.

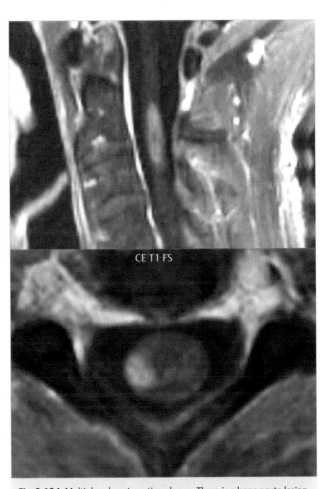

Fig. 3.134 Multiple sclerosis, active plaque. There is a large acute lesion, defined by abnormal contrast enhancement, seen on both sagittal and axial scans. Larger lesions in the cord are often elliptical in shape, with their longest dimension in the craniocaudal direction. Although the enhancement is prominent in this instance, as with most lesions that affect the blood-brain (or in this instance, blood-spinal cord) barrier, there is a spectrum of enhancement from faint to marked.

dorsal and, occasionally, lateral columns, extending over several vertebral body segments (▶ Fig. 3.136). There may be modest expansion of the cord. This entity is also known by the term subacute combined degeneration. Causes include malabsorption (most common), inadequate vitamin B_{12} intake (rare), and

nitrous oxide toxicity (inactivates B_{12}). The vitamin deficiency leads to demyelination, with early diagnosis and treatment by intramuscular injection of B_{12} important. The potential for reversal of clinical symptoms is inversely proportional to their duration and severity.

3.6.13 Paget Disease

This chronic disorder of bone remodeling is seen in older adults, with spine involvement (a single or multiple vertebrae) in perhaps half of cases. The classic chronic appearance on imaging of the spine in this entity is that of a single or multiple enlarged vertebrae (bone expansion), with accentuated, coarse trabeculae and thickened endplates/cortices ("picture frame vertebra") (▶ Fig. 3.137). The etiology is unknown, with viral, genetic, and environmental causes postulated.

3.7 Neoplasms

3.7.1 Nerve Sheath Tumors (Neurofibroma, Schwannoma)

These two tumors together represent the most common primary neoplasm of the spine, as well as the most common

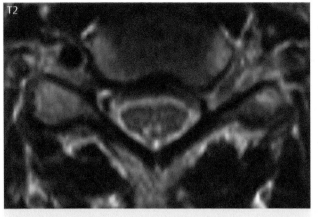

Fig. 3.136 Subacute combined degeneration of the spinal cord (vitamin B_{12} deficiency). There is abnormal high signal intensity of the dorsal columns posteriorly, forming the appearance of an inverted V. This abnormal signal intensity extended in a long continuous segment along the dorsal cord.

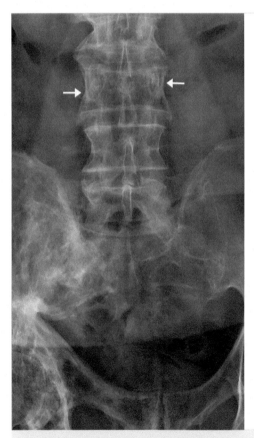
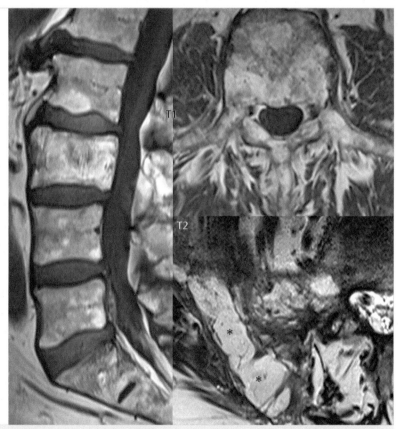

Fig. 3.137 Paget disease. On plain film (**part 1**), the L3 vertebral body is slightly expanded in left to right dimension, with its pedicles enlarged and sclerotic bilaterally (*arrows*). There is extensive disease in the right hemipelvis, with sclerosis and accentuated, coarse trabeculae. On MR (**part 2**), midline sagittal and axial T1-weighted images are presented, the latter through the L3 vertebral body, together with an axial T2-weighted image at the S1 level cropped to depict the right iliac wing and sacral ala. The L3 vertebral body is expanded, with a "picture frame" appearance seen on the sagittal image. There is associated expansion of the posterior elements, seen on the axial image at the L3 level. On the image depicting a portion of the right hemipelvis, in the axial plane, bony expansion (*asterisk*) and high signal intensity from the fatty bone marrow are demonstrated, in this late mixed active phase patient.

intradural-extramedullary neoplasm (slightly more common than a meningioma). The peak incidence is the fourth to fifth decades, with neurofibromas much less common than schwannomas. Both are World Health Organization (WHO) grade I

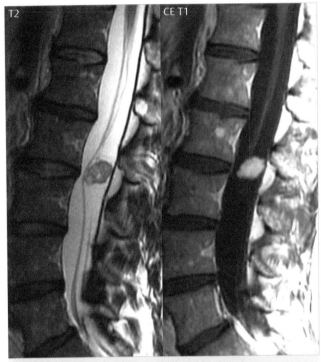

Fig. 3.138 Schwannoma. While more frequently affecting the nerve roots within the intervertebral foramina in the cervical and thoracic spine, schwannomas may also involve the roots of the cauda equina, as illustrated. Perhaps the only hints that this lesion is not a meningioma are the slightly irregular margins of the lesion and the more ovoid shape (as opposed to the typical meningioma which, with the exception of a dural interface, is very round in shape). Otherwise, this lesion is simply an intradural enhancing mass, at the L2–3 level, with the differential diagnosis being a meningioma, a small myxopapillary ependymoma, or a neurogenic tumor (schwannoma or neurofibroma).

lesions. Multiple schwannomas in a child should raise the question of NF2. The most frequent symptoms are pain and radiculopathy. Schwannomas are usually solitary. They arise from the Schwann cells of the myelin sheath. They are well encapsulated, lobulated, compressing adjacent tissue without nerve invasion. Most schwannomas are intradural (▶ Fig. 3.138), a smaller percent have both intradural and extradural components (and are dumbbell in shape), and 15% are entirely extradural (▶ Fig. 3.139). Neurofibromas are not encapsulated, contain Schwann cells, fibroblasts, and a matrix of collagen and myxoid material, enlarging the nerve itself and producing a fusiform appearance. Neurofibromas are commonly associated with NF1, particularly when multiple, but also occur sporadically. Plexiform neurofibromas in NF1 can have malignant degeneration in a small percent of cases.

CT depicts these lesions poorly, and is not the primary imaging modality (which is MR). Foraminal enlargement, erosion of the pedicles, thinning of lamina, and posterior vertebral scalloping are however well visualized. MR provides excellent delineation and localization of nerve sheath tumors (▶ Fig. 3.140). Schwannomas and neurofibromas both appear as solid well-circumscribed masses, with substantial overlap in imaging appearance. As with many lesions, both are most commonly slightly hypointense on T1- and slightly hyperintense on T2-weighted scans. Both lesions enhance post-contrast (▶ Fig. 3.141). Small cystic areas and/or a heterogeneous appearance either pre- or post-contrast favor slightly a schwannoma. Important for differential diagnostic purposes is that a lesion located within the neural foramen can be mistaken for a disk herniation, with contrast enhancement allowing differentiation.

3.7.2 Meningioma

Twenty-five percent of all intraspinal tumors are meningiomas, with this lesion second in incidence only to benign neural tumors. Meningiomas are usually solitary, with a peak age of incidence of 45 years. In terms of location, one-third are cervical (▶ Fig. 3.142) and two-thirds are thoracic (▶ Fig. 3.143). One to 3% of all meningiomas occur at the foramen magnum. Of

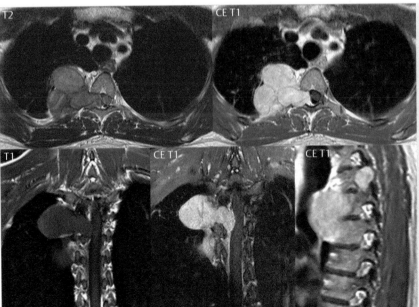

Fig. 3.139 Schwannoma (WHO grade I), thoracic. A lobulated uniformly enhancing mass lesion is noted with the bulk of the mass paraspinal in location, extending into the foramen at the T4–5 level on the right, with epidural extent and mild displacement of the cord to the left. The intervertebral foramen is enlarged. The well-circumscribed nature of the lesion, and location, favor the diagnosis of a schwannoma (with a neurofibroma also a consideration in terms of differential diagnosis). The lesion was resected via a laminectomy.

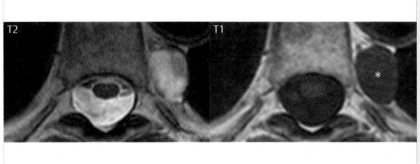

Fig. 3.140 Benign neoplasm of neural origin. A small round soft tissue mass is noted, left paraspinal in location, hyperintense on T2- and hypointense (*asterisk*) on T1-weighted images. There was uniform enhancement post-contrast (not shown). On imaging, a solitary neurofibroma cannot be distinguished from a schwannoma, and the lesion in this instance could be either pathology. Of note, most schwannomas are intradural extramedullary in location, with only 15% completely extradural. Adjacent bone remodeling is common with both entities, although not present in this instance.

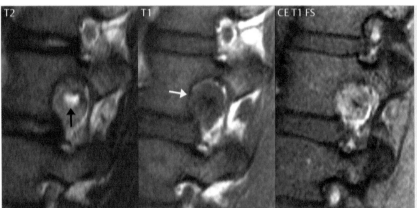

Fig. 3.141 Neurofibroma. A soft tissue mass (*white arrow*) is identified in this NF1 patient on sagittal images, scalloping the posterior margin of L2 and widening the L2–3 neural foramen. On the basis of imaging alone, this lesion could represent either a schwannoma or a neurofibroma. There is moderate enhancement of the lesion post-contrast. Although cystic degeneration is seen on the T2-weighted image as an area of central high signal intensity (*small black arrow*), a more characteristic appearance for a neurofibroma is that of a targetlike configuration with a bright rim surrounding a center of low SI.

enhancing extra-axial lesions in this specific location, three-fourths are meningiomas and one-fourth neurofibromas.

There is a 3:1 female:male incidence. An intradural location is most common, although meningiomas can be extradural. Meningiomas are benign tumors, histologically, slow growing, and cause symptoms due to cord and nerve root compression. Complete resection is achieved surgically in 95% of cases and, despite complete removal, 5% recur. On MR, pre-contrast, meningiomas are usually isointense to the cord on T1-weighted scans. Capping inferiorly and superiorly by CSF confirms the lesion to be intradural, extramedullary (by far the most common location) (▶ Fig. 3.144). Intense enhancement is seen post-contrast on MR. An enhancing dural tail is less common than intracranially. Dense calcification is often observed on CT in meningiomas, with the correlate on MR being a focal low signal intensity region within the lesion on both T1- and T2-weighted scans (which does not display contrast enhancement).

3.7.3 Ependymoma

Ependymomas are the most common spinal cord tumor of adults, with a mean age at presentation of 40 years. It is a neuroepithelial tumor arising from the ependymal cells of the central canal. An important histologic variant is a myxopapillary ependymoma, which accounts for less than 20% of all ependymomas, but which is by far the dominant type at the conus and filum terminale (and in this location is extramedullary)—and which is also the most common tumor at this location (▶ Fig. 3.145). Ependymomas are usually low grade (WHO grade

I and II). They are slow growing, well-circumscribed tumors with a tendency to compress adjacent neural tissue. On imaging, a small nodular, enhancing intramedullary lesion limited to two to three vertebral levels, with an accompanying cyst, favors the diagnosis of an ependymoma (as opposed to an astrocytoma). Hemorrhage does occur, and may produce superficial hemosiderosis involving the brainstem and lower cranial nerves, another differentiating feature. Complete surgical resection is possible. There is a very high incidence of ependymomas in NF2 patients. Ependymomas are usually well-delineated, and (disregarding the myxopapillary variant) are most common in the cervical region. On imaging, these are seen centrally within the cord, often with prominent enhancement (▶ Fig. 3.146). Reactive (nontumoral) cysts are common. Myxopapillary ependymomas may occasionally present as large lesions (scalloping the vertebral bodies), also typically display marked enhancement, and often have associated cystic components.

3.7.4 Astrocytoma

In children, spinal cord astrocytomas are more common than ependymomas, with ependymomas more common in adults. Cord astrocytomas are more likely to be low grade (WHO grade I and II) than higher grade. Clinical course parallels histologic grade. These infiltrative tumors are not amenable to surgical resection, unlike ependymomas. On imaging (MR), astrocytomas are characterized by a long segment of involvement (multiple vertebral segments), with near complete involvement of the width of the cord, poorly defined margins, and cord expansion

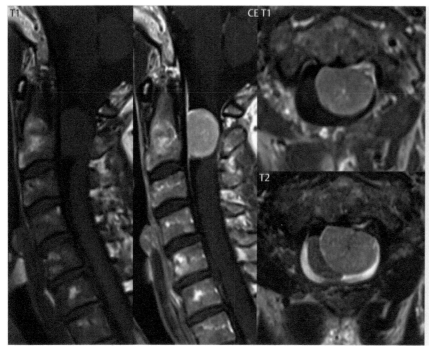

Fig. 3.142 Meningioma (WHO grade I, meningotheliomatous in type), cervical spine. A large, well-delineated, homogeneously enhancing, intradural extramedullary mass lesion is noted anteriorly within the thecal sac at the C2 level. There is prominent deformity and compression of the cord, long standing in nature, without evidence of edema or gliosis. The lesion demonstrates characteristic slight hyperintensity to the cord on the T2-weighted scan, and avid, homogeneous enhancement post-contrast. Note also the flat margin of the lesion along the dura (a broad dural base).

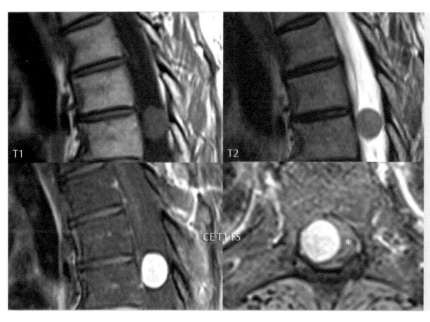

Fig. 3.143 Meningioma (thoracic). Sagittal images slightly off midline demonstrate a round intradural extramedullary, homogeneously enhancing soft tissue mass. Note the marked compression and deformity of the cord (which is displaced to the left, *asterisk*) on the axial scan. Clinical symptoms are often minimal, consistent with a very slow growing benign neoplasm.

(▶ Fig. 3.147). As with most tumors, the lesion will be of lower signal intensity than normal cord on T1-weighted scans, and of higher on T2-weighted scans. Contrast enhancement can be homogeneous, heterogeneous, seen only with delayed scans, or not present, and does not differentiate between tumor grades.

3.7.5 Hemangioblastoma

This tumor is the third most common intramedullary neoplasm of the spine, after ependymoma and astrocytoma. Hemangioblastomas can be solitary or multiple, the latter specifically with von Hippel-Lindau disease. These are slow growing lesions, generally diagnosed in adults. Hemangioblastomas are well-circumscribed, highly vascular (and thus with prominent enhancement on MR), small nodular lesions (▶ Fig. 3.148). On MR, there may be associated cord edema. In a minority of cases in the spine, a hemangioblastoma will lie along the wall of a large cyst. Prominent associated vessels are common, and can be visualized by contrast-enhanced MRA. Hemangioblastomas occur anywhere along the spinal cord, and in patients with von Hippel-Lindau disease small nodular lesions can be seen along nerve roots as well (▶ Fig. 3.149).

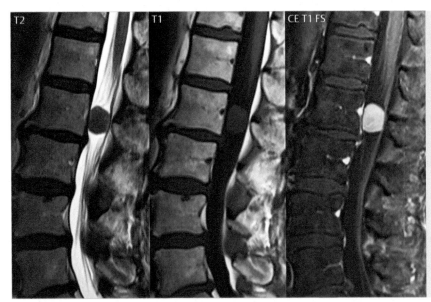

Fig. 3.144 Meningioma (lumbar). Sagittal images demonstrate a meningioma that lies just below the conus, which despite its size is easily identified as intradural in location. Note on the T2-weighed scan the arc of CSF both superior and inferior to the lesion, marking it as intradural, as opposed to an extradural lesion, which would displace and compress the thecal sac. There is also characteristic, prominent homogeneous contrast enhancement.

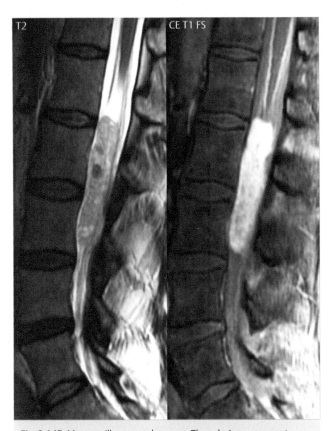

Fig. 3.145 Myxopapillary ependymoma. These lesions represent < 20% of all spinal ependymomas, but > 80% of those involving the conus or filum terminale. They are extramedullary, slow growing, and low grade, as with all ependymomas. As illustrated, myxopapillary ependymomas often span multiple vertebral body segments, and may fill the spinal canal. They are slightly hyperintense on T2-weighted scans, due to the presence of mucin, with intense enhancement post-contrast. The enhancement adjacent to the conus, in the case illustrated, represents leptomeningeal tumor spread, which was confirmed at surgery.

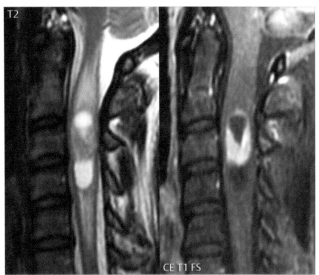

Fig. 3.146 Ependymoma (cervical). An intramedullary mass lesion causing focal cord expansion is demonstrated, with its epicenter at C3. There are both solid (enhancing) and cystic components. The lesion itself is relatively short in length, extending only two vertebral body segments. Edema is seen within the cord, extending both cranial and caudal to the lesion, with abnormal high signal intensity on the T2-weighted scan.

3.7.6 Leptomeningeal and Spinal Cord Metastases

Contrast-enhanced MR is the most sensitive imaging modality for the detection of leptomeningeal metastases. CT myelography can demonstrate leptomeningeal seeding (as nodular filling defects), but is less sensitive and rarely employed. Although contrast enhancement on MR markedly improves detectability, abnormal enhancement is not seen in all instances. In areas of the spinal axis where the cord is present, the imaging appearance includes focal irregularity of the cord surface (tumor adherent to or encasing the cord) (▶ Fig. 3.150), a thin coating of the cord by tumor (▶ Fig. 3.151), and small focal nodules within the subarachnoid space. In the lumbar region, distal to the conus, the imaging appearance of leptomeningeal disease includes large and small nodules, and coating of nerve roots (which may appear "beaded" in appearance) (▶ Fig. 3.152). The entire spinal axis (cervical, thoracic, and lumbar regions) should be studied to rule out leptomeningeal involvement, with attention to the lumbar region. Due to the effect of gravity, if the patient is ambulatory, the disease as depicted by imaging may be restricted to the distal thecal sac (▶ Fig. 3.153).

Leptomeningeal metastases are seen with many different primary tumors, but in particular with (amongst CNS primary tumors) ependymoma and medulloblastoma and (of non-CNS tumors) lung carcinoma and breast carcinoma. The clinical presentation is varied, but includes pain, nerve deficits, and gait disturbance. The prognosis is poor. CSF cytology is the gold standard for diagnosis, but can require multiple samples and large volumes of CSF.

Spinal cord metastases are rare. Their appearance is nonspecific, that of a small focal mass lesion within the spinal cord, with associated vasogenic edema, that demonstrates contrast enhancement and causes mild focal cord expansion. Bronchogenic carcinoma is the most common primary.

3.7.7 Vertebral Body Hemangioma

A hemangioma is a common, benign incidental finding on spine MR. In autopsy series, they have been found in about 10% of patients, and on the basis of MR imaging are likely to be even

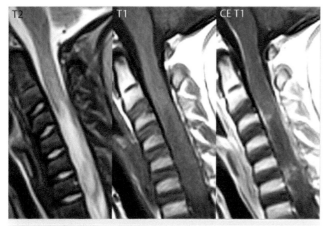

Fig. 3.147 Astrocytoma. On sagittal images of the cervical spine, there is a long segment, spanning in this instance more than four vertebral bodies, of marked, diffuse cord expansion, with abnormal high signal intensity on the T2-weighted scan and heterogeneous enhancement. Low grade (WHO grade I and II) astrocytomas of the spinal cord, the most common type, show variable enhancement, which may be homogeneous, heterogeneous, or lacking.

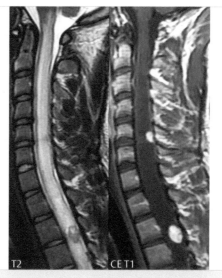

Fig. 3.148 Spinal cord hemangioblastomas. A midline sagittal T2-weighted scan reveals extensive cord edema. Post-contrast, two enhancing focal intramedullary cord lesions are noted, at the C5 and T2–3 levels. In this patient with von Hippel-Lindau syndrome, both hemangioblastomas are located in the more posterior aspect of the cord, with lesions rarely present anteriorly. Multiple cord lesions of varying size are common in von Hippel-Lindau syndrome; however, the extensive cord edema noted in this instance is unusual.

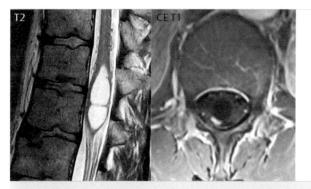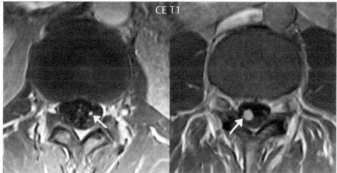

Fig. 3.149 Hemangioblastoma. A characteristic imaging appearance for a spinal cord hemangioblastoma is that of an intensely enhancing lesion with an associated cyst and serpentine flow voids, the latter due to lesion vascularity. These features are all illustrated (part 1), with the enhancing component small in this instance relative to the size of the cyst, also a characteristic finding. About a third of all hemangioblastomas are seen in patients with von Hippel-Lindau syndrome. In such cases, as with this patient, there may be multiple small hemangioblastomas—with a small pinpoint lesion (arrow) involving a nerve root, and a larger nodular lesion (arrow) in the lumbar region illustrated (part 2) on axial scans.

more common. They can be solitary or multiple, and vary in size from small to involving the entire vertebral body and posterior elements. Very rarely these lesions may be aggressive (extending posteriorly and causing cord compression). Histologically, hemangiomas contain thin-walled capillary and cavernous sinuses (angiomatous tissue) interspersed between sparse, coarse osseous trabecule and fatty stroma. On imaging, thick vertical striations/trabeculation will be evident. Lesions are focal and well-circumscribed, and on CT hypodense other than the accentuated vertical trabeculae. On MR, hemangiomas are hyperintense on both T1- and T2-weighted images, with the thickened trabeculae visualized as thin vertical low signal intensity lines (▶ Fig. 3.154).

Hemangiomas show prominent enhancement on postcontrast MR scans obtained with fat saturation. Unfortunately, atypical hemangiomas (in terms of imaging characteristics) are common. The primary differential diagnosis is focal fat (within vertebral bodies), another common benign entity. Focal fat follows the signal intensity of fat on all MR pulse sequences, and does not display abnormal contrast enhancement (▶ Fig. 3.155).

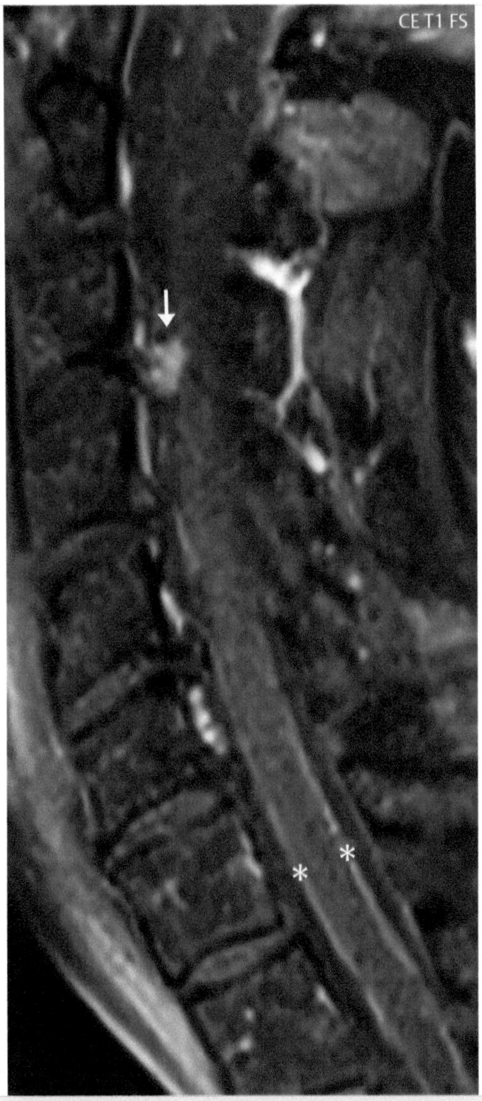

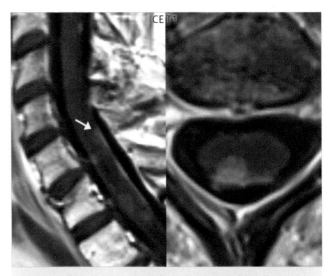

Fig. 3.151 Leptomeningeal metastatic disease (cervical). A small enhancing intramedullary lesion is seen on both sagittal (*arrow*) and axial T1-weighted scans. The lesion could represent either a metastasis to the cord, or extension to involve the cord from metastatic disease to the pia-arachnoid. Additional, mild enhancement along the surface of the cord is indicative of more extensive involvement of the pia-arachnoid.

Fig. 3.150 Leptomeningeal metastatic disease (cervical), the utility of fat saturation post-contrast. In certain instances, as demonstrated in this patient, fat saturation can be useful for improved detection of disease (on the basis of abnormal contrast enhancement), even for lesions within the thecal sac. The absence of high signal intensity from fat (and fatty marrow) in this scan improves detection of both a nodular focus of leptomeningeal disease within the subarachnoid space (*white arrow*), as well as the coating (also termed "icing") of cord surface (*asterisk*).

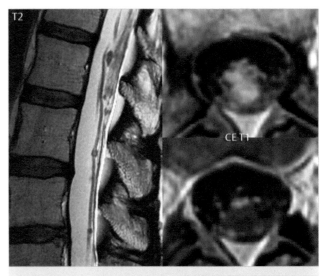

Fig. 3.152 Leptomeningeal metastases (lumbar). If very high-resolution images are acquired, small nodular leptomeningeal metastases may be well visualized on a T2-weighted scan, as illustrated with a midline sagittal image. However, contrast enhancement offers the most sensitive approach, with axial post-contrast scans illustrating a large, irregular, enhancing nodular metastasis involving the conus and innumerable small enhancing foci adherent to nerve roots in the cauda equina.

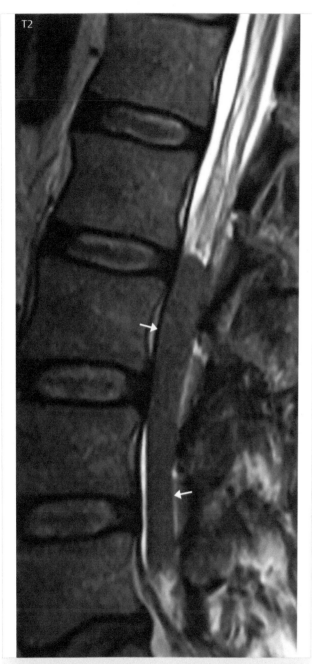

Fig. 3.153 Leptomeningeal metastases (lumbar, confluent mass). In ambulatory patients, gravity may result in involvement primarily of the caudal thecal sac, mandating careful inspection of the low lumbar and sacral regions. In advanced disease, as illustrated, leptomeningeal metastatic disease can present as a confluent mass in the lumbar region. Such lesions are easily visualized on a T2-weighted scan, with the soft tissue mass (*arrows*) being of intermediate SI in distinction to the very high SI CSF.

3.7.8 Aneurysmal Bone Cyst

This entity is seen mainly under the age of 20 and, although benign, is generally considered within the category of neoplastic disease and often requires treatment. An aneurysmal bone cyst on CT and MR is classically lytic, multiloculated, expansile, lobular, and highly vascular. About 20% arise in the spine, with the majority of these in the posterior elements (▶ Fig. 3.156).

Aneurysmal bone cysts have both cystic and solid components, with the latter enhancing. The cystic components often contain blood degradation products, with fluid-fluid levels present.

3.7.9 Osteoid Osteoma

An osteoid osteoma is a common benign bone tumor composed of vascular fibrous connective tissue. An osteoid osteoma is small by definition (<2 cm in diameter, with a lesion above this size defined as an osteoblastoma) and sharply demarcated from surrounding bone, with variable surrounding sclerosis. This lesion occurs primarily in pediatric patients and young adults, presenting with pain (relieved by aspirin) and sometimes scoliosis. Ten percent of osteoid osteomas occur in the spine, most commonly in the posterior elements of the lumbar spine. On CT the lesion will be lytic, with surrounding sclerosis commonly present, with calcification of the central nidus seen in more than half of cases (▶ Fig. 3.157). On MR, both the nidus and accompanying edema (often prominent) can be visualized in most cases. Attention to imaging technique, specifically avoiding partial volume effects due to large voxel size, is important. Enhancement of the nidus is consistently seen (and best visualized) on subtracted or fat-suppressed images, specifically in the early phase of dynamic contrast enhancement on MR (▶ Fig. 3.158).

3.7.10 Osteochondroma

An osteochondroma is simply an osteocartilaginous exostosis: a bony excrescence covered by cartilage with the cortex and medullary cavity contiguous to parent bone. It is the most common benign bone tumor, although it is rare in the spine. Osteochondromas are usually asymptomatic and an incidental finding (malignant transformation is known, and more common with hereditary multiple exostoses, but still rare). In the spine, the most common location is a spinous or transverse process.

3.7.11 Giant Cell Tumor

Giant cell tumors are rare in the spine, with the most common location being the sacrum. This tumor is lytic, vascular (thus enhancing), expansile, and low grade but locally aggressive. Giant cell tumors present with back pain at night or following pathologic fracture. On CT the margins of the lesion are usually not sclerotic. The signal intensity characteristics on MR are nonspecific, intermediate to low on T1-, and intermediate to high on T2-weighted scans, with heterogeneous enhancement. Giant cell tumors of the spine have a better prognosis than when located elsewhere in the body, with a low rate of recurrence following resection.

3.7.12 Chordoma

Chordomas are usually large at presentation. Fifty percent occur in the sacrum/coccyx, 35% skull base/clivus, and 15% vertebral body. They are midline, locally invasive, destructive, lytic, lobular, slow growing malignant lesions. In the spine, they can involve two or more vertebral segments and extend into the disk. Intratumoral calcifications may be present.

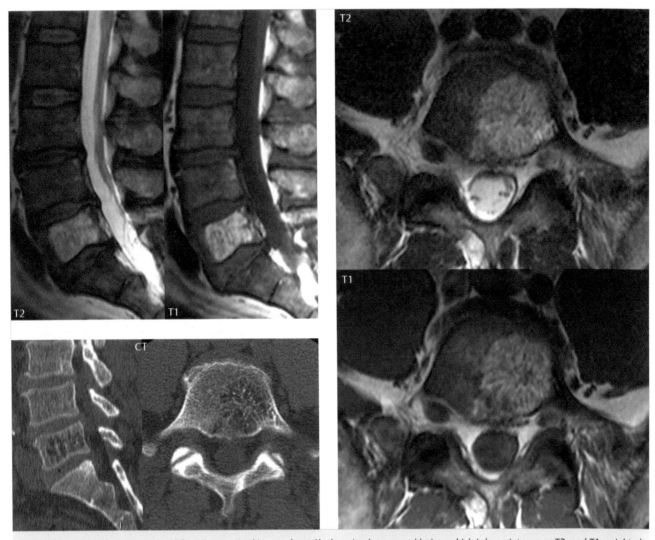

Fig. 3.154 Vertebral hemangioma. Within L5, on sagittal images (**part 1**), there is a large round lesion, which is hyperintense on T2- and T1-weighted images (consistent with fat), with characteristic accentuated vertical trabeculae. On axial MR images (**part 2**), this classic hemangioma exhibits almost a radial appearance to the accentuated trabeculae. On CT (**part 3**), sparse thickened vertical trabeculae are seen on the sagittal reformatted image, with a spotted appearance on the axial image. (Courtesy of Lee Nakamura, MD.)

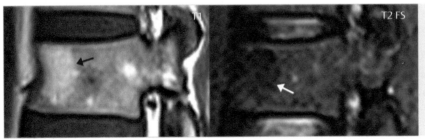

Fig. 3.155 Focal fat (with in a vertebral body). Focal collections of fat within a vertebral body are common, particularly in the elderly patient population. These are felt to be of no clinical significance. Focal fat will appear as a focal lesion with higher SI (*black arrow*) than the adjacent hematopoietic marrow on a T1-weighted scan. Suppression of the high SI (*white arrow*) will be seen on a T2-weighted FSE scan with fat saturation.

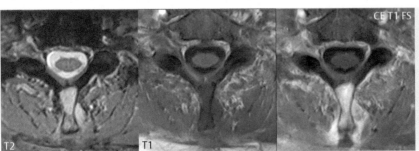

Fig. 3.156 Aneurysmal bone cyst. There is an expansile mass of the spinous process (of this cervical vertebra), with abnormal high signal intensity on the T2-weighted scan and prominent enhancement. There is mild involvement of the adjacent para-spinal soft tissue. This expansile benign neoplasm consists of blood-filled spaces, with enhancement present in solid portions of the lesion.

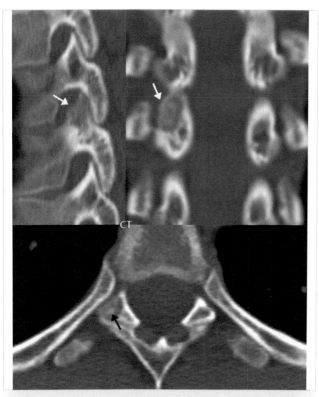

Fig. 3.157 Osteoid osteoma (CT). Sagittal, coronal, and axial images depict a small lucent lesion (*white arrows*), with adjacent sclerosis, and a small intranidal calcification (*black arrow*). As depicted, this small benign bone tumor, when it occurs in the spine, is most common in the posterior elements. In this instance, the lesion lies near the junction of the superior articular process, pedicle and transverse process.

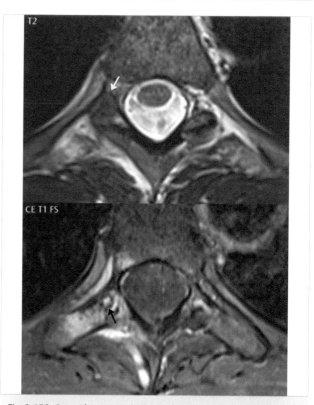

Fig. 3.158 Osteoid osteoma (MR). Axial images, at two slightly different slice locations, depict the same small lesion (*white arrow*) as presented in the prior case. The nidus enhances (*black arrow*), together with the extensive associated edema, here seen within the marrow of the transverse process.

3.7.13 Sacrococcygeal Teratoma

A sacrococcygeal teratoma is a rare congenital tumor, and is the most common presacral mass in a child. There is a four to one female preponderance. These lesions are usually lobulated and sharply demarcated, with both cystic and solid components (▶ Fig. 3.159).

3.7.14 Focal Vertebral Body Metastatic Disease

Vertebral metastases are a major cause of morbidity in cancer patients (▶ Fig. 3.160). The vertebrae are involved in up to 40% of patients dying of metastatic disease. Vertebral metastases may cause bone expansion, cord compression, and pathologic fractures. Lung carcinoma is the most common cause of metastatic disease to the vertebral column. Other common etiologies include breast, prostate, and renal cell carcinoma. Lung carcinoma also has the highest incidence of epidural disease. Cord compression due to epidural metastatic disease presents typically with pain at the level of involvement and neurologic deficits. Motor impairment is seen early, due to anterior cord compression. Compression, when present, is usually only at a single level (▶ Fig. 3.161). Upper cervical metastatic lesions have high morbidity, with extensive sensory and motor deficits

(▶ Fig. 3.162). Spread to the skull base can cause cranial neuropathies. Squamous cell carcinoma of neck spreads by local invasion, and with extensive disease can also involve the cervical spine and skull base.

Plain radiographs are insensitive for detection of vertebral metastases. Nuclear medicine bone scans have moderate to high sensitivity (lower than MR), and low specificity. CT is relatively insensitive, with poor evaluation of soft tissue extension and (often, due to radiation dose concerns) limited anatomic coverage (▶ Fig. 3.163). MR has high sensitivity and specificity, excellent anatomic coverage, and excellent evaluation of soft tissue. Sagittal images provide an initial screen for metastatic involvement, with axial images important for assessment of epidural extent and canal compromise (▶ Fig. 3.164).

Lytic metastatic lesions have, on MR, low signal intensity on T1-weighted scans, focally replacing the normal high signal intensity fatty marrow. Pre-contrast T1-weighted imaging is the primary scan used for detection of bony metastatic disease, both for MR and for imaging in general (▶ Fig. 3.165). T2-weighted scans without fat saturation are very insensitive for detection of bony metastatic disease (▶ Fig. 3.166). With fat saturation, however, many but not all metastatic lesions will be visualized, with abnormal high signal intensity, on T2-weighted scans. Blastic metastases are sclerotic on CT (▶ Fig. 3.167) and appear with very low signal intensity on T1-weighted scans, and low signal intensity on T2-weighted scans (▶ Fig. 3.168). Blastic metastases are common in prostate carcinoma.

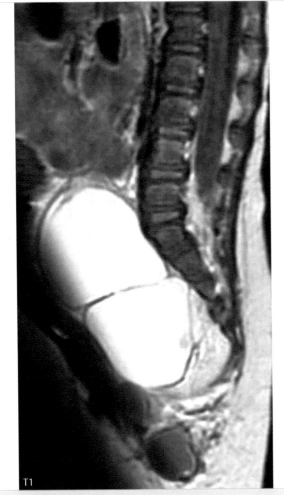

Fig. 3.159 Sacrococcygeal teratoma. A midline sagittal T1-weighted scan of the lower lumbar spine and pelvis is presented in a 6 month old. A large hyperintense presacral mass is present. Although relatively homogeneous in this example, a more typical appearance would be that of a heterogeneous mass, with cystic and solid components, containing fat, soft tissue, and fluid.

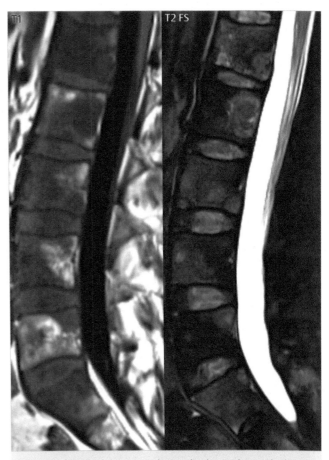

Fig. 3.160 Vertebral metastatic disease, lumbar, widespread. There is near complete replacement of the normal fatty marrow by low signal intensity metastases on the T1-weighted scan. L5 and S2 are partially spared. The T2-weighted scan in this instance is performed with fat saturation, thus differentiation of the metastases from normal marrow is improved in comparison to a FSE T2-weighted scan without fat saturation, although still with lower sensitivity to focal lesions in comparison with the T1-weighted scan.

Lung and breast carcinoma metastases are usually lytic, but may be osteoblastic when treated. Following intravenous contrast administration, lytic bony metastases enhance to near isointensity with normal marrow on T1-weighted scans without fat suppression. Such scans poorly visualize metastatic disease. However, with fat saturation, in certain instances (and in particular for very small lesions) post-contrast scans can be the most sensitive sequence for detection of metastatic disease (▶ Fig. 3.169 and ▶ Fig. 3.170). Contrast administration can also be useful for improving definition of both paraspinal soft tissue and epidural extension of metastatic disease (▶ Fig. 3.171). Careful evaluation of the prevertebral soft tissues is important for tumors that spread via lymphatics—for example, prostate carcinoma.

Radiation therapy changes are often recognizable due to their nonanatomic distribution, being restricted to the treatment area ("port"). Uniform fatty replacement of bone marrow occurs as early as 2 weeks following initiation of therapy, with temporal progression, and is well depicted on noncontrast T1-weighted scans (▶ Fig. 3.172).

3.7.15 Pathologic Compression Fracture

When the entirety of the vertebral body is involved, differentiation between a benign acute vertebral and a pathologic compression fracture can be difficult. Both entities will demonstrate diffuse low signal intensity on T1- and high signal intensity on fat suppressed (or STIR) T2-weighted scans. Low ADC (restricted diffusion), presence of a paraspinal mass, involvement of the pedicle or posterior elements, and the presence of an epidural mass all favor a pathologic compression fracture. Coexisting healed benign compression fractures and focal retropulsion (superiorly or inferiorly) favor a benign compression fracture. Regardless of etiology, MR and CT offer valuable information regarding canal compromise.

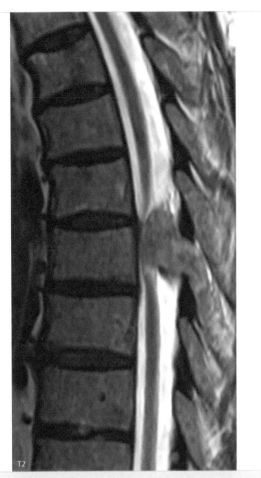

Fig. 3.161 Vertebral metastatic disease, posterior compromise. Involvement by metastatic disease has led to the expansion of the posterior elements of T7, with resultant compression of the cord. On this FSE T2-weighted sagittal scan, there is however little differentiation on the basis of signal intensity between normal vertebral bodies and those involved with metastatic disease, a pitfall of this choice of imaging technique.

3.7.16 Langerhans Cell Histiocytosis

Langerhans cell histiocytosis is a benign disease with its pathogenesis a matter of debate (in terms of a reactive versus a neoplastic process), usually affecting children. The manifestations of this disease range from isolated bone lesions to multisystem involvement, with the classic appearance of Langerhans cell histiocytosis in the spine being vertebra plana (a single collapsed vertebral body) (▶ Fig. 3.173). Treatment for this entity is typically conservative.

3.7.17 Diffuse Marrow Disease

Diffuse marrow low signal intensity on T1-weighted scans can have many origins. Marrow replacement disorders cause this appearance, and include leukemia, lymphoma, and multiple myeloma (▶ Fig. 3.174). Diffuse metastatic disease (e.g., from breast or prostatic carcinoma) is typically somewhat heterogeneous, and thus differentiable on this basis. Marrow reconversion (myeloid hyperplasia) is an additional cause, and occurs with severe chronic anemia (specifically sickle cell disease and thalassemia) as well as treatment with granulocyte macrophage colony stimulating factor during chemotherapy. Myelofibrosis, in which there is replacement of marrow by fibrotic tissue, can also have diffuse low signal intensity on a T1-weighted scan.

3.7.18 Lymphoma

Paravertebral, vertebral, and epidural (▶ Fig. 3.175) lesions all occur with lymphoma, and simultaneous involvement of two or three regions is not uncommon. The most frequent area of involvement is paravertebral, due to local spread from retroperitoneal nodes. Epidural disease can result in cord compression. Isolated epidural lesions do occur, presumably from either

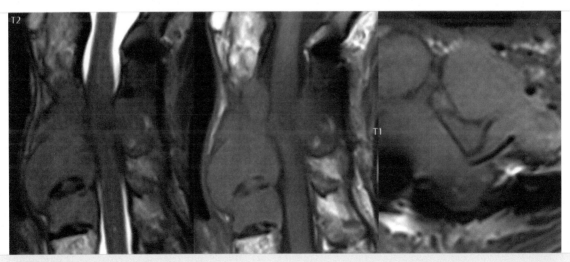

Fig. 3.162 Spinal canal compromise by vertebral metastatic disease (cervical). The most urgent complication, requiring rapid intervention, from vertebral body metastases is compromise of the spinal canal and resulting cord compression. The hyperintensity of CSF on a FSE T2-weighted scans allows excellent delineation of the subarachnoid space, with this sequence typically preferred for demonstration of cord compression, as illustrated. T1-weighted scans may not visualize as well the canal compromise. Although the two sagittal scans presented appear to well delineate the involved region, axial imaging (as illustrated) is also mandatory. The axial scan, in this instance, provides the best assessment of canal and cord compromise, with severe cord compression and deformity due to circumferential bony metastatic involvement.

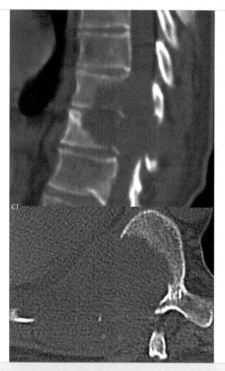

Fig. 3.163 Vertebral metastatic disease, CT. A large lytic lesion consistent with metastatic disease is noted involving T9 and T10. On the axial reformatted section (at the T10 level), there is destruction of a portion of the vertebral body, the right pedicle, lamina, transverse process, and proximal portion of the right rib. There is an accompanying large soft tissue mass, paraspinal in location but somewhat poorly defined, extending both anteriorly and into the posterior paraspinal musculature. The mass extends into the spinal canal; however, the degree of canal compromise and cord compression cannot be evaluated. This is one of the pitfalls of CT, and a reason it is not used for evaluation of vertebral metastatic disease, since compromise of the spinal canal cannot be well evaluated.

hematogenous spread or epidural lymphatics. Contrast enhancement on MR is typically homogeneous, regardless of location. Lymphoma, leukemia, and myeloma may all present with diffuse marrow infiltration, and thus uniform abnormal low signal intensity marrow on T1-weighted scans (isointense to the intervertebral disk) (▶ Fig. 3.176).

3.7.19 Leukemia

In leukemia, bone involvement is most often diffuse, but can be focal. It is critical in review of spine MR images to always assess the relative signal intensity of the vertebral body and the intervertebral disk on T1-weighted scans. Loss of the normal higher signal intensity of the (fatty) vertebral marrow, when diffuse, can be easily overlooked. Although the differential is broad for diffuse marrow involvement as demonstrated by MR, it encompasses many important disease categories including specifically hematologic neoplasms and hemoglobinopathies.

3.7.20 Multiple Myeloma

As with the other hematologic malignancies, MR is the imaging modality of choice for the spine, with CT less sensitive to disease involvement. However, within this category of disease (and, as emphasized multiple times in this section), the findings are nonspecific to any one entity (▶ Fig. 3.177). Common findings on CT include multiple lytic lesions and vertebral destruction/fracture. Marrow involvement in multiple myeloma as depicted by MR can be focal, diffuse (▶ Fig. 3.178), display an inhomogeneous pattern of tiny lesions, or be *normal*.

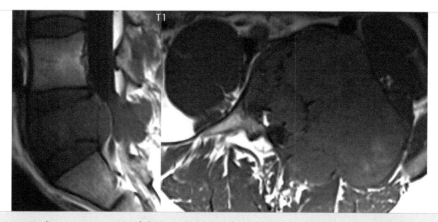

Fig. 3.164 Vertebral metastatic disease, compression of the lower lumbar and sacral spinal canal. MR is the modality of choice both for detection of metastatic disease involving the spinal axis and for visualization of the extent of this disease, and its impact on adjacent critical structures. In this instance, visualized on sagittal and axial unenhanced T1-weighted scans, there is near complete replacement of L5 by metastatic disease. Concomitant involvement of the anterior body and posterior vertebral elements is noted. The sagittal image reveals loss in height of the L5 vertebral body compared to L4, and diffuse hypointensity within the former, consistent with replacement of normal vertebral body fatty marrow. While compression of the thecal sac and posterior extent of this mass are clearly evident on this image, improved delineation of the tumor's extent and resulting canal compromise is possible on the axial image. Evident here is obliteration of the left L5 lamina, pedicle, and transverse process. The compressed spinal canal itself is hypointense to this large mass and displaced posterolaterally to the right, posterior to the remaining hyperintense epidural fat. Contiguous spread of this metastatic lesion is seen posteriorly to involve the paraspinal musculature on the left and laterally to displace the nearby left psoas muscle anterolaterally. There is involvement of multiple lumbar and sacral nerves. This extensive metastatic lesion was found to be secondary to a ganglioneuroblastoma primary.

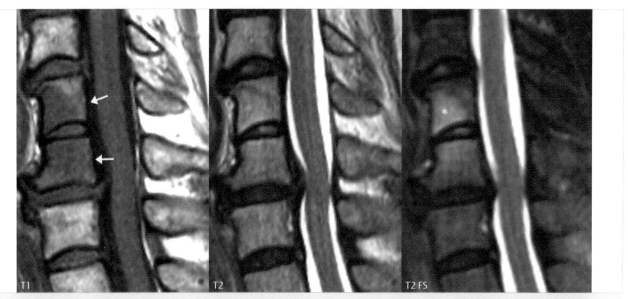

Fig. 3.165 Vertebral metastatic disease (cervical). In patients with abundant fatty marrow, metastatic disease to the bony spine is well visualized on T1-weighted scans, as foci of abnormal low signal intensity. Metastases to two midcervical vertebral bodies (*arrows*) are illustrated, with degenerative disk disease both above and below the involved levels. Fast spin echo (FSE) T2-weighted scans do not typically display vertebral metastatic disease well, an important pitfall, due to the relatively high signal intensity of normal marrow. Fat saturation is critical for visualization of bony metastatic disease on such scans, with lesions then demonstrating abnormal high signal intensity (*asterisk*) relative to normal adjacent marrow.

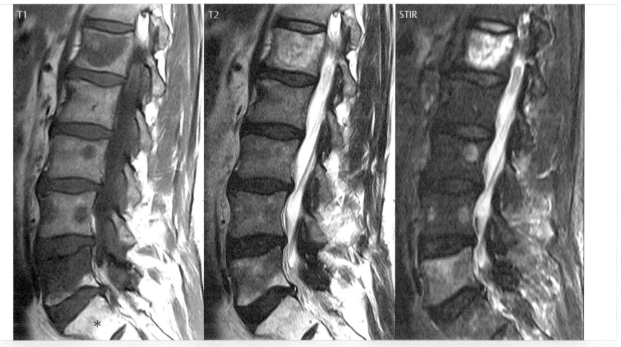

Fig. 3.166 Vertebral metastatic disease, imaging technique (T2). Multiple metastatic vertebral body lesions are noted on the unenhanced T1-weighted sagittal image, with abnormal low signal intensity contrasting with the normal higher signal intensity of fatty marrow. These involve L1, L3, L4, and nearly the entirety of L5. S1 on the T1-weighted scan has abnormal homogeneous high signal intensity (*asterisk*), consistent with fatty replacement in this patient with prostate carcinoma, who previously received radiation therapy to the prostate and surrounding region. The fast spin echo (FSE) T2-weighted scan is relatively insensitive to bony metastatic disease, in this instance revealing only the L1 lesion, with marrow fat signal not suppressed and thus many metastatic lesions isointense to the normal adjacent marrow. STIR, as illustrated in this instance, or fat suppressed FSE T2-weighted scans, should be employed for imaging with T2 contrast in patients with suspected vertebral body pathology, and reveal well both edema and focal abnormal tissue within the marrow space. STIR suffers from low SNR when compared to FSE T2-weighted scans, and thus is typically acquired with lower in-plane spatial resolution, but is more robust in terms of magnetic field homogeneity (fat-suppressed FSE scans can be more inhomogeneous with old magnet designs, and in the presence of metal). STIR is also favored by many radiologists for evaluation of elderly patients with possible acute compression fractures, likely due to slightly improved depiction of marrow edema when compared to fat suppressed FSE T2-weighted scans.

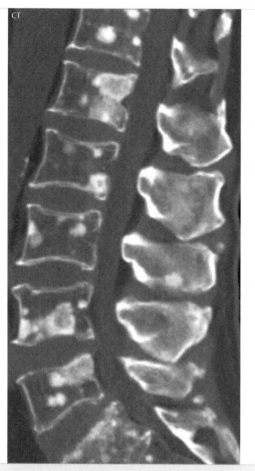

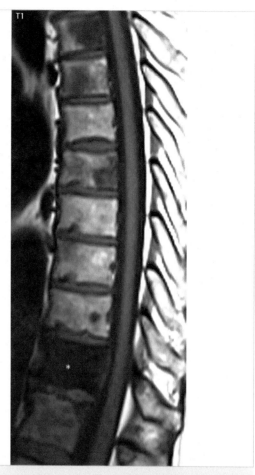

Fig. 3.167 Vertebral metastatic disease, CT, blastic metastases. CT is relatively insensitive to metastatic disease involving the spine when compared to MR. However, in the case of osteoblastic metastases, these are well seen, as illustrated. This elderly patient presents with widely metastatic adenocarcinoma of the prostate, with the relative osteopenia of the spine improving further the visualization of blastic (sclerotic) metastases, which are seen in every vertebral body. However, lytic lesions may also be present in such patients, and are poorly visualized by CT.

Fig. 3.168 Lytic and blastic metastases. A blastic metastasis (*asterisk*), which is more commonly seen with prostate and breast cancer, can be recognized by its substantially lower signal intensity on T1-weighted scans, when compared to the more common lytic metastases. In this instance, there are multiple lytic metastases in the upper thoracic spine.

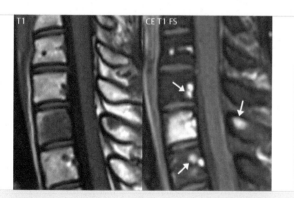

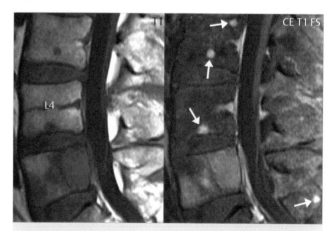

Fig. 3.169 Vertebral metastatic disease (cervical), the utility of contrast enhancement. A further improvement in sensitivity to metastatic disease can be achieved in some patients by the use of fat-suppressed, post-contrast T1-weighted scans. As illustrated, multiple small vertebral body and spinous process metastases are seen with abnormal low signal intensity on the T1-weighted scan pre-contrast. Post-contrast, with fat saturation, there is improved visualization of these lesions, which markedly enhance (*arrows*) in comparison to the adjacent, now suppressed, normal fatty marrow.

Fig. 3.170 Vertebral metastatic disease, imaging technique (contrast enhancement). Although pre-contrast T1-weighted scans are the mainstay in terms of detection of vertebral metastases, post-contrast scans with fat saturation can improve in certain instances lesion sensitivity/visualization. In this patient, there is near complete replacement of the L5 vertebral body by metastatic disease. However, note the excellent visualization, post-contrast, of four small enhancing lesions (*white arrows*), with the lesion superiorly in L3 and that in the spinous process of S1 best seen post-contrast.

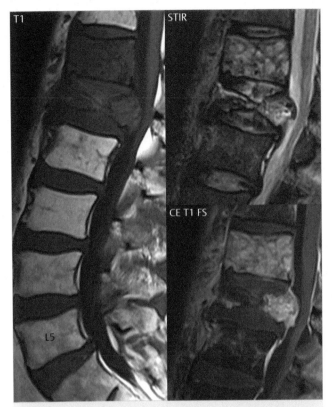

Fig. 3.171 Vertebral metastatic disease, compression of the thecal sac. There is replacement of marrow, loss of vertebral body height, and retropulsion involving L1, all consistent with metastatic disease. Note also the extension of metastatic disease into the prevertebral soft tissue. The canal compromise is below the level of the conus, thus bowel and bladder function were preserved. The case is complex, however, because of prior therapeutic radiation. Note the very high signal intensity of the L2 and L3 vertebral bodies on the T1-weighted scan that were included in a prior radiation port, due to fatty marrow replacement. The ill-defined, mild enhancement within L2 is of unknown etiology, although radiation necrosis is a consideration. There is complete replacement of T12 by metastatic disease, with little loss in vertebral body height.

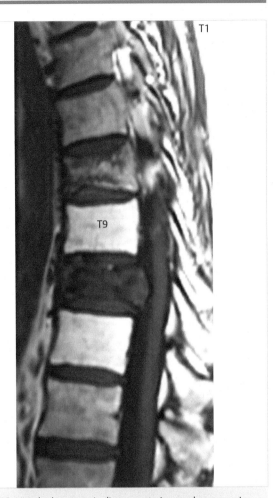

Fig. 3.172 Vertebral metastatic disease, anterior canal compromise, and the effects of therapeutic radiation. The signal intensity of the T9 and T11 vertebral bodies is markedly higher than that of the normal T6, T7, and T12 vertebral bodies. T8–T11 were irradiated to treat the metastatic tumor within T10. Long-term following radiation therapy, there is compensatory hypertrophy of the fatty elements of the marrow, leading to an increase in signal intensity (as seen) on T1-weighted imaging. Unfortunately radiation therapy in this case was not curative, and recurrence of metastatic disease within the T10 vertebral is seen. Abnormal soft tissue (tumor) also extends posteriorly at this level, producing mild canal compromise and cord compression. Loss of T8 vertebral body height is consistent with an additional compression fracture. Acute fractures due to either osteoporosis or tumor are difficult to distinguish on MR since similar abnormal signal intensity is present in both. In this instance, an irregular low signal intensity band within the inferior half of T8 suggests a distinct fracture and thus osteoporosis, without a definite metastatic focus identified.

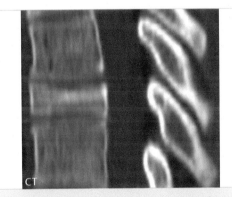

Fig. 3.173 Vertebra plana. In this young male patient, there is near complete loss of height of a single thoracic vertebral body (T8) on a sagittal reformatted midline CT section. The adjacent disks and posterior elements are uninvolved. In the spine, this is a very characteristic presentation for Langerhans cell histiocytosis, as was confirmed in this patient.

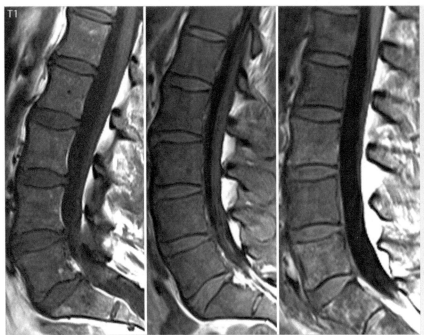

Fig. 3.174 Diffuse marrow replacement—myeloma, lymphoma, and acute lymphocytic leukemia (from left to right). It is essential to evaluate the relative signal intensity of the vertebral bodies and the intervertebral disks on T1-weighted scans on every acquired spine exam. Diffuse loss of the normal higher marrow signal intensity (when compared to the disk space) is indicative of either a generalized marrow disorder or a very active marrow. Myeloma, lymphoma, and leukemia can all present in this fashion, with the appearance nonspecific in terms of etiology.

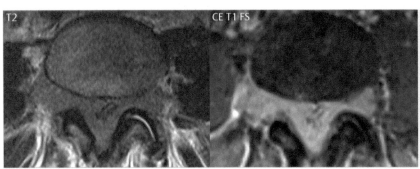

Fig. 3.175 Lymphoma (epidural). The epidural/extradural space may also be involved in metastatic disease. In this case of lymphoma metastatic to the epidural space, there is marked compression of the thecal sac by abnormal soft tissue, which also extends into the neural foramina bilaterally. There is moderate to prominent diffuse enhancement, typical for lymphoma.

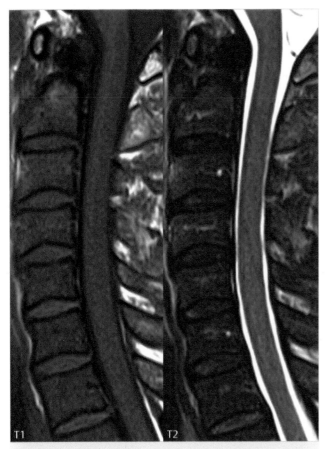

Fig. 3.176 Hodgkin lymphoma. There is a diffuse marrow abnormality, with the vertebral bodies on the T1-weighted scan isointense to the intervertebral disks (replacing the slight hyperintensity normally seen due to a combination of *red* and *yellow* marrow). The abnormality is more difficult to recognize on the T2-weighted scan. This appearance is not specific for any one etiology, but rather reflects diffuse marrow replacement, and can also be seen with a very active marrow.

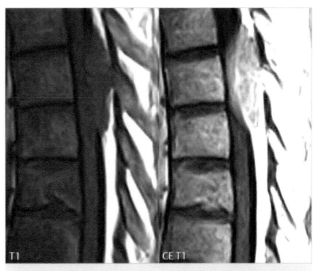

Fig. 3.177 Epidural mass, myeloma. A soft tissue mass lesion, arising from the epidural space (note that its epicenter is in the epidural fat), causes prominent mass effect upon the cord. The marrow is also diffusely abnormal, with isointensity to the intervertebral disks pre-contrast, and prominent diffuse enhancement—when pre- and post-contrast scans are compared using the same pulse sequence and imaging parameters. In this instance, there is diffuse marrow infiltration by myeloma, with an additional, focal, extradural soft tissue tumor mass.

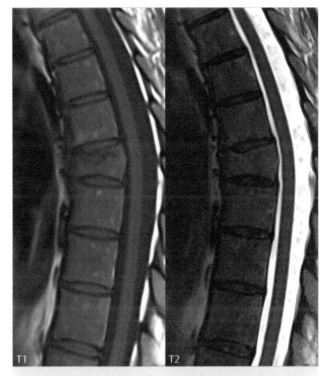

Fig. 3.178 Multiple myeloma. There is a diffuse marrow abnormality. This is best recognized on the pre-contrast T1-weighted scan, where the vertebral bodies demonstrate homogeneous abnormal low signal intensity, isointense to the intervertebral disks. There is an anterior wedge compression fracture of a midthoracic vertebral body, in this instance likely not due to osteoporosis or major trauma, but rather to neoplastic involvement compromising the structural integrity of the vertebral body.

Index

Note: Page numbers set **bold** or *italic* indicate headings or figures, respectively.